HUMAN
CEREBRAL
ASYMMETRY

THE CENTURY PSYCHOLOGY SERIES

James J. Jenkins
Walter Mischel
Willard W. Hartup

Editors

JOHN L. BRADSHAW
Monash University

NORMAN C. NETTLETON
Monash University

HUMAN CEREBRAL ASYMMETRY

PRENTICE-HALL, INC.   *Englewood Cliffs, New Jersey 07632*

Library of Congress Cataloging in Publication Data

Bradshaw, John L.   (date)
  Human cerebral asymmetry.

  (Century psychology series)
  Bibliography: p.
  Includes index.
  1. Cerebral dominance. 2. Left and right (Psychology)
3. Brain—Localization of functions. I. Nettleton,
Norman C.   (date). II. Title. III. Series: Century
psychology series (Prentice-Hall, Inc.) [DNLM: 1. Brain—
Anatomy and histology. 2. Brain—Physiology. 3. Later-
ality. WL 335 B812h]
QP376.B693 1983   612'.825   82-10159
ISBN 0-13-444646-1

Editorial production/supervision by Marion Osterberg
Manufacturing buyer: Ron Chapman

Printed in the United States of America

10 9 8 7 6 5 4 3 2 1

ISBN 0-13-444646-1

Prentice-Hall International, Inc., *London*
Prentice-Hall of Australia Pty. Limited, *Sydney*
Editora Prentice-Hall do Brazil, LTDA, *Rio de Janeiro*
Prentice-Hall Canada Inc., *Toronto*
Prentice-Hall of India Private Limited, *New Delhi*
Prentice-Hall of Japan, Inc., *Tokyo*
Prentice-Hall of Southeast Asia Pte. Ltd., *Singapore*
Whitehall Books Limited, *Wellington, New Zealand*

Contents

CHAPTER TEN

Handedness: Behavioral and Genetic Accounts   189

CHAPTER ELEVEN

Sex Differences in Cognition and Lateralization   214

CHAPTER TWELVE

Developmental Aspects of Lateralization   228

CHAPTER THIRTEEN

Developmental Dyslexia, Schizophrenia, and Left Hemisphere Dysfunction   242

Preface

The topic of human cerebral asymmetry is almost a microcosm of the whole network of empirical psychology in its major forms—perceptual, cognitive, physiological, neuropsychological, clinical, developmental, and comparative. The recent enormous increase in interest in the topic owes much to the dramatic demonstrations of divided cognitive function after the commissurotomy operations of the 1960s. However, there has been a long tradition, dating back at least to the nineteenth century, of assigning functions to specific brain areas, and studies of hemispheric asymmetries of function are very much part of that tradition. Nevertheless, the topic is not uncontroversial, partly because of the profound philosophical implications which arise from the idea (itself going well back into the nineteenth century) of the brain's duplex structure, and partly because findings have not always been consistent and verifiable.

Of the three major approaches to human cerebral asymmetry, we have been engaged most deeply in studying its manifestations in normal subjects. However, we also have had some experience in the other two approaches, wherein the effects are documented of lateralized lesions and commissural section upon perception, thought, and action. Moreover, we have successfully employed in our empirical studies all three major sensory modalities.

Strangely, given the long history of this topic, no single treatment had appeared when we started this book, though a number addressed more or less specialist or circumscribed aspects, and there were several co-authored and edited compilations which again tended to address a number of idiosyncratically chosen issues. The initial opportunity to start this book came when we were each able to take a sabbatical year away from teaching and administrative commitments. Nettleton spent 1979 working full time on our research at Monash University. Bradshaw spent the latter part of 1980 at Cambridge University, and at the University of Victoria, Canada, and the first half of 1981 back in our own laboratory at Monash, with access to the collection of several thousand relevant reprints which we have built up over the years.

The book attempts to survey and review the entire field of human cerebral asymmetry. After an initial brief account of the question of left and right in biology, evolution, medicine, mythology, and anthropology, it reviews the evidence for left/right asymmetries at the structural and anatomical levels (both central and peripheral), as well as the behavioral, in species other than man. After surveying the recent evidence for morphological asymmetries in the human brain, it deals with the three lines of evidence for cerebral asymmetry in man—the clinical and the commissurotomy studies, and the evidence from experimental work with normal subjects. Thereafter a number of logically related topics are sequentially considered —the effect of load, novelty, and arousal on behavioral asymmetry, the extent of language mediation by the nondominant (right, minor) hemisphere, the question whether the verbal/nonverbal distinction is the basic dichotomy with respect to cerebral asymmetry or whether there are more fundamental modes of specialization, human handedness and its relation to cerebral asymmetry, sex differences in these respects, developmental issues, and clinical syndromes such as developmental dyslexia and schizophrenia insofar as they might relate to cerebral asymmetry. The book concludes with a chapter on educational and clinical implications.

Although the book is an attempt at a neutral and eclectic survey, its issues spread into a number of enormously interesting related areas—art, aesthetics, mythology, anthropology, and evolution. Multidisciplinary issues tend to exert a fascination and a potential for interactive fertility out of all proportion to the mere algebraic sum of the contributing disciplines. We have tried to be dispassionate judges of the empirical evidence, but feel that the intrinsic interest of the subject matter permits us to slacken slightly the reins of speculation in two places—in the first introductory chapter, and in Chapter Nine where we discuss possible scenarios for the evolution of language and tool use, and their joint lateralization. As Neisser observes in his own Preface to his seminal book *Cognitive Psychology* published in this selfsame series, rationalization and discovery can never be entirely separated, and even *reading* a book is a constructive process.

Although we do not claim to have reviewed the literature exhaustively, we hope to have been comprehensive. No doubt our selection has at times been idiosyncratic, and we therefore apologize to those whose work we have either left out or misunderstood. The material is presented in such a way as, we hope, to be useful at a number of levels—advanced undergraduate, graduate, scholar, teacher, researcher, neurologist, clinician, psychologist, and educationalist, whether or not they have a formal background in the topic with which the book deals. The provision of an extensive Summary and Conclusions section at the end of each chapter should provide the reader both with a general overview and a balanced judgment

Acknowledgments

The writer of a book is indebted to many people. We would like to thank all those research workers whose work we have described and whose ideas we have borrowed and embroidered. We trust that we have not unduly misrepresented them. The fact that the book has been produced at all is entirely due to the support and assistance of our families, who inevitably found themselves shouldering more than their fair share of domestic management. We thank the Council of Monash University for providing us with Sabbatical leave and the opportunity to undertake the project, and the Biomedical Library of Monash University for their unparalleled resources and resourcefulness in obtaining primary sources. We are extremely grateful to Professor Ross Day (Chairman, Department of Psychology, Monash University) for the support and encouragement he has given us both over many years. We also thank Professors Oliver Zangwill (Cambridge University) and Otfrid Spreen and Lou Costa (University of Victoria, Canada) for providing one of us (JLB) with a place to read, think, and write. We thank Judy Sack and Vladimir Kohout, respectively, for their drafting and photographic skills, Karen Spehr and Diane Nettleton for helping with proofreading, and Pam Ward and Dessi Green for handling all the multitudinous secretarial matters so efficiently. Above all, we are grateful to Kay Kinnane, who so expeditiously typed the manuscript from our handwritten drafts, and to Judy Bradshaw who spent an enormous period of time checking all the references, preparing the References and Author Index, and assisting with proofreading. Without their willing and friendly help this book may have never been finished. We also wish to acknowledge, with gratitude, all the help and encouragement which we have received from our Senior Editor, Ted Jursek, and Production Editor, Marion Osterberg, at the various stages in the planning and production of this book. We thank our numerous colleagues and students, undergraduate and postgraduate, without whose intellectual interaction our own research work would have been the poorer. This research, much of which is described in the book, has been consistently supported by the Australian Research Grants Committee for thirteen years, and we are duly grateful.

CHAPTER ONE

Biological
and Mythological Aspects
of Human Cerebral Asymmetry

The naked, unadorned human body, and the bodies of most vertebrates for that matter, display an almost perfect left–right symmetry. This symmetry, however, like beauty (and indeed in many cultures the two have been at times almost synonymous) is only skin deep. Beneath the surface are a number of unpaired organs (heart, liver, spleen, alimentary system, and so on) that are either highly asymmetrical, laterally displaced, or both. When a person extends a hand in greeting or threat, one hand, the right, is more likely to be employed.

Faces and Profiles:
Left and Right Sides and Mirror Reversal

We are of course mostly right-handed (or, as a minority, left-handed). We show other minor superficial departures from perfect symmetry: The distribution of our head, body, and even pubic hair is not perfectly even, the sizes of the two female breasts are usually not quite identical, and Greek sculptors over two thousand years ago "knew" that the two male testicles are asymmetrical in size and level. (We now know that the right testicle is both higher and larger; however, the ever-rational Greeks got the height but not the weight right: They thought that the lower left testicle was naturally the heavier; see, e.g., McManus, 1976.)

Even the two sides of the face are not quite identical. The classical demonstration for this is photographically to recreate two composite faces, one from two left halves of a face (reversing one of the halves and abutting the two midlines), one

1

from the two right halves (see Figure 1-1). It is claimed that the composite made from the two (real-life) left halves not only looks *different* from its fellow—the one made from the two right halves, (see, e.g., Gilbert & Bakan, 1973)—but typically is judged as indicating the subject's current emotional state more clearly and strongly (Sackeim, Gur, and Saucy, 1978). This has the slightly paradoxical consequence that in a face-to-face situation the side of the face (the left) that is more likely to portray emotional expression with greater intensity is the one more likely to be projected to the viewer's left, or verbal, hemisphere, which is relatively inferior in face recognition and the processing of emotional information (see Chapter Seven). It is possible that the greater expressiveness of the left side of the face has evolved to compensate for the relative inferiority of our left hemisphere in such nonverbal functions as the recognition of faces and emotions.

FIGURE 1-1 A normal photograph of a human face with left-left and right-right composites of the same face, each made from one half alone.

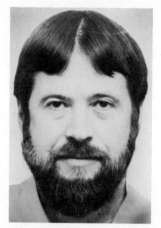

NORMAL

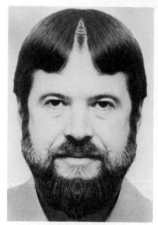

RIGHT-RIGHT

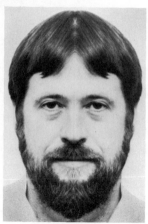

LEFT-LEFT

We can easily demonstrate the asymmetry of our own face with a double reversing mirror or that of someone very well known to us with a single reversing mirror. With a double reversing mirror we can see ourselves "live" exactly as others see us, with our familiar mirror image reversed. It is intuitively probable that we gradually habituate to any small departures from our preconceived stereotype of facial symmetry through long experience with our own reflections, ceasing to notice any small characteristic discrepancies. As we look at our own face in a double-reversing mirror system or as we look at the mirror image of the face of an *extremely* close acquaintance (spouse, parent, child or sibling), the unfamiliar left–right transposition will briefly augment rather than reduce the numerous small asymmetries to which we have gradually habituated. Such a symmetry-constancy phenomenon, if it can be so labeled, appears as yet not to have been formally investigated.

One aspect of the two sides of the human face that has received some recent attention is the question of whether there is a preferential direction for profiles in portraiture. McManus and Humphrey (1973) and Humphrey and McManus (1973) reopened the issue when they reported that portrait painters tend to show more of the left than the right cheek. They considered a number of possible explanations, such as its being easier for right-handed painters to draw a convex-out profile to the left of the canvas (just as it is easier for right-handers to write from left to right); another possibility considered was that there are systematic biases in the positioning of artist, sitter, easel, and palette that lead to such an outcome, or systematic biases in social interaction or in head turning, and so on. Others have either disputed the generality of the above findings (e.g., Freimuth & Wapner, 1979) or have invoked conventions (whether innate or acquired) of bottom-left to top-right scanning of pictures (Coles, 1974; Freimuth & Wapner, 1979), which possibly interact with perceived light sources illuminating the sitter's face. The question is intriguing and is not yet fully resolved, nor is the related issue of whether people prefer art in its original rather than its left–right mirror-reversed orientation (Coles, 1974; Blount, Holmes, Rodger, Coltheart, & McManus, 1975; Freimuth & Wapner, 1979).

To turn to the looking-glass world of fiction, Alice's preoccupation with the question of mirror reversals may itself stem from the apparently quite marked asymmetry of her creator. Lewis Carroll, the Reverend Charles Dodgson, Oxford mathematician and favorite raconteur and companion for a generation of little girls (incidentally, he also stammered and mirror-wrote, traits sometimes associated with left-handedness), is described by Martin Gardner, in his Introduction to *The Annotated Alice,* as follows:

> In appearance, Carroll was handsome and asymmetric . . . one shoulder was higher than the other, his smile was slightly askew and the level of his blue eyes was not quite the same.[1]

[1] From the Introduction of Martin Gardner to *The Annotated Alice* (New York: Bramhall House), p. 10. Copyright © 1960 by Martin Gardner. Used by permission of Clarkson N. Potter, Inc.

As an extremely competent portrait photographer in the early days of the art, Carroll might first have become aware of his own asymmetry through his medium, seeing himself as others saw him and not as the looking glass showed.

Left and Right in the Natural World

We can imagine the consequences of entering, like Alice, a mirror-reversed world, without actually experiencing such reversal. As Corballis and Beale (1971) point out, we would never notice the difference were it not for *man-made, unidirectional* objects or constructs such as writing, roads (where one drives on one side), cork-screws, water taps, and such, which would all appear to function the wrong way around. We can easily simulate such a world by looking at back-to-front reversed slides. We are only able to notice the reversal of these asymmetrical man-made objects because we ourselves are not perfectly left–right symmetrical. Were we perfectly symmetrical, we would never notice their reversal (nor would we be able differentially to cope with *d* and *b*, *p* and *q*, to drive on one side of the road and not the other, and so on) since entry to a mirror-reversed Alice world is *logically* equivalent to the world being unreversed and our own bodies instead being subjected to reversal; such a reversal, were we *perfectly* left–right symmetrical, would be completely trivial and without consequence.

It is perhaps a consequence of our high degree of symmetry that we *do* often have difficulty in telling left from right. Pooh Bear was well aware of this problem:

> Pooh looked at his two paws. He knew that one of them was the right, and he knew that when you had decided which one of them was the right, then the other one was the left, but he never could remember how to begin.[2]

Children are notoriously prone to confuse *d* and *b*, *p* and *q*, and occasionally to write or read words in the wrong direction, for example, reading *saw* for *was*. The letters *N, S,* and *Z* are often written, even by untutored adults, as И, Ƨ, and Ƨ, but curiously letters such as *E, F, K,* and *L* rarely seem to be reversed. It is even said that army recruits in nineteenth-century Europe learned to drill, turning left and right on command, with a bundle of straw tied to one leg to introduce a helpful asymmetry. Pavlov attempted, unsuccessfully, to condition a dog to salivate differentially to a tickle on one side but not the other (a conditioned salivatory response to other types of stimuli than those involving mirror discriminations is normally well within the animal's repertoire). Pigeons *may* learn differentially to peck or not to peck at obliquely slanting lines, / and \, but if successful they appear to employ an ingenious strategy: They tilt their heads to one side, converting the two above obliques respectively into − and |, which are no longer confusing. This strategy,

[2]From A. A. Milne, *The House at Pooh Corner* (London: Methuen, 1928), p. 116. Courtesy of the publishers—Methuen London Ltd., Curtis Brown Ltd., E. P. Dutton & Co., Inc., and McClelland & Stewart.

however, only works if they "remember" always to tilt their heads in the *same* direction. Consequently, they must be able to capitalize on some *preexisting* asymmetry in solving this discrimination (see Corballis & Beale, 1970a, 1971, 1976, for further discussion on this and related issues.)

Why is it that members of at least the phylum Chordata are so very nearly left–right symmetrical? An explanation that has enjoyed long currency considers the evolutionary environment of developing organisms in terms of optimal surface-to-volume packaging and the imposition of externally and internally generated forces. An organism floating *within* a supporting medium, unexposed to unidirectional forces such as gravity (i.e., not against any substrate) or light (not floating on or near the surface) will optimally adopt a spherical shape as the most economical. Many simple free-floating organisms like *Radiolaria* are spherically symmetrical. On their sinking to the bottom or floating to the surface, an upper and a lower region is likely to differentiate. Radial symmetry is pronounced in such animals as the jellyfish. Upon their acquiring directional locomotion, a leading and a trailing edge will differentiate, probably with a propulsive system at the rear end and sensors at the front. Further topological distortions can be superimposed on this laterally symmetrical ground plan—for example, the coiling of the gastropods, the migration of the eye and other structures across the upper surface in flatfish (see Chapter Two), and morphological and biochemical asymmetries in the brains of a number of vertebrate species, including ourselves (see Chapter Three). However, we shall return later to evolutionary issues, to alternative accounts of cerebral asymmetry in the evolution of humans, and to the question of whether lateral symmetry or mild asymmetry is likely to be the more fundamental condition in vertebrates (see Chapter Nine).

Left and Right in Disease and Health

Our own most manifest asymmetry, as we pointed out earlier, is our handedness: Most of us are dextral (right-handed). However, most of our other paired organs, limbs, and other bones and structures, including skinfold thickness, are now known to often exhibit very small but highly consistent asymmetries, though neither normal nor anomalous developmental asymmetries favor one particular side over the other *overall* (McManus, 1979; Whitaker & Ojemann, 1977). Moreover, quite apart from instances where particular mechanical factors might predispose toward one side rather than another, a large number of disease states and other syndromes (listed by McManus, 1979) tend consistently to strike one side of the body in preference to the other, for reasons as yet unknown but in a manner curiously reminiscent of the systematized tradition of the ancient Greeks, to which we shall shortly turn. (Indeed, Robin and Shortridge, 1979, record a massive predominance in humans of left-sided tumor incidence in bilateral organs such as breast, kidney, testis, adrenals, ovary, nasal cavity, and paranasal sinuses.) In the meantime it should be noted that our dextrality antedates the Greco-Roman civilization, the

Hebrews of the Bible, and the ancient Egyptian and Mesopotamian civilizations (see, e.g., Coren & Porac, 1977; Hardyck & Petrinovich, 1977; Hicks & Kinsbourne, 1976a). Tomb and cave paintings (e.g., the leftward-facing profiles typically drawn by right-handers, though this is disputed by Perelló, 1970) and the hand stencils of primitive and ancient peoples (Hicks & Kinsbourne, 1976a, 1978, see Figure 1-2) all attest to our primeval dextrality. Ornaments, weapons, and especially tools from the paleolithic seem largely to have been constructed by and even *for* the right hand, to judge by the distribution of concavities that fit the thumb, finger tips, and palm of the right hand. The paleoanthropologist Dart (1949) even claims that *Australopithecus* (our evolutionary cousin, though not our ancestor, of some three million years ago) was right-handed, from forensic examinations of the locus of penetrating head wounds in kills associated with his remains. This being so, it is of interest to note the suggestion that modern primitive peoples may possibly be somewhat less lateralized in terms of brain function (see the following section) than their civilized literate counterparts (Paredes & Hepburn, 1976; Scott, Hynd, Hunt, & Weed, 1979). With respect to handedness, however, intercultural differences probably reflect differential permissiveness (Dawson, 1977).

As Corballis (1980a) notes, the left–right distinction has long evoked, throughout almost all the world's cultures, a fascination that seems out of all proportion to its practical importance. Yet, curiously, it is only in the last fifteen or twenty years that human experimental psychology has taken more than a passing interest in left–right differences. What originally was studied in the context of differences in skill between the two hands (which were themselves often seen merely as useful tools in

FIGURE 1-2 Examples of stencils made by Australian aborigines in caves in Western Queensland by pressing the hand or other object against a surface and spattering pigment (ochre) from the mouth around it.

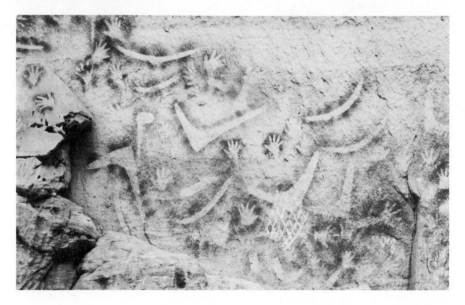

studying the effects of practice and transfer between otherwise equivalent motor systems) has recently burgeoned into an important area in its own right. One possible reason for this is the way that human cerebral asymmetry has come to be seen by many as a sort of microcosm of psychology and as a point of intersection for a number of important areas (clinical and neuropsychology, psycholinguistics, cognitive and perceptual psychology, behavior genetics, and so on). Indeed, its variously grounded biological foundations on the one side and its strong associations with anthropology, mythology, symbolism, and mysticism on the other, together with its potential relevance to a number of clinical and applied areas, have strongly attracted interdisciplinary researchers. Unfortunately, as we shall see, this has also led at times to loose experimental and frankly speculative and dubious work on cognitive style, hemispheric activation, conjugate eye movements as an index of personality, psychopathology, and emotionality, hand posture in writing, and so on.

Left and Right in Mythology and Etymology

Humans and the cosmos of which they are a part are almost universally seen as subject to two opposing influences, possibly as a consequence of a simplistic tendency in peoples, ancient and modern, philosopher and scientist, to dichotomize reality and to see it in terms of polar opposites rather than as a whole range of shades of gray (Newell, 1973). Thus we have the pre-Confucian concepts of *yin* and *yang* and the Hindu ideals of *Buddhi* and *manas* (Ornstein, 1977). Almost equally universally, the left-handed are seen as a suspect minority. They are *sinistral* (with all the etymological connotations associated with this word), *gauche* (from an old French verb meaning "to bend," a meaning that persists in the associated derivative *gawky*), *cackhanded* (*kak* is an ancient Indo-European root meaning "feces," cf., Latin *cacare*) as opposed to *dextral, adroit, right* (i.e., correct) handed. Indeed, the concept of ill omen runs through at least two putative Indo-European roots associated with *left*: the common origin of the words *laevus* (Latin), λαιϝος (Greek), *lubberly,* and *left,* on the one side and on the other the words *scaevus* (Latin), σκαιϝος (Greek) and *skew* (old English). We can contrast *dexter,* δεξιος, *digit, (in)dicate,* all from the root **dek,* which seems to imply hand, handing, or receipt. Likewise in German *link* (left) is also equivalent to *clumsy,* and *mancino* (Italian: *left* or *deceitful*) and *nalevo* (Russian: *left* or *surreptitious,* as opposed to *pravo, right* or *true*) carry on this tradition. Only the ancient Greeks, with a euphemistic attempt at averting ill fortune, labeled the left hand ἡ ἀριστερα (the better(er) hand). For at least seventy years, anthropologists have been aware of almost exactly parallel beliefs in cultures and civilizations ranging from the Maori of New Zealand (Hertz, 1909) to ancient Israel. To the Maoris, the right was the sacred side, the side of the gods, strength, and life, while the left was associated with profanity, demons, and death. In the Bible, the blessed sit at the right hand of God.

    Closer to our times and culture, Michelangelo appears as a good, right, male chauvinist, like most of his contemporary artists, when we view the ceiling of the

Sistine Chapel. God creates Adam with his right hand, and Adam raises his *left* (or weak) hand to receive the charge of life. Eve is created via the right hand of God from Adam's *left* side. When tempted, Eve turns to a *female* serpent, which hands the fruit with its *left* hand to Eve's *left*. In disgust, God sends an angel to expel them from the Garden, and the angel is *left*-handed. No wonder we continue to sin!

The link between handedness and the sexes is made manifest in the Pythagorean Table of Opposites, a mixture of numerology, number magic, mysticism, and prehistoric mythology, cited by Aristotle (*Metaphysics,* A5, 985b23). Left is linked with female, cold, dark, bad, crooked, and other pejoratives, and right with the opposites. These ideas may be a reaction against the half-forgotten mysticism of the old neolithic and chalcolithic cultures of Central (Danubian and Aegean) Europe (Gimbutas, 1974). These cultures were pre-Indo-European, sedentary, matrilinear, and with a religion, as the numerous artifacts attest, dominated by a steatopygous Earth Mother or Great Goddess (i.e., female) who was symbolized by the Moon, as regulator of growth, fertility, seasonal variation, and the female cycle. Life force was possibly represented by the left side, the locus of the heart and where the baby is nursed by its mother. (In other matriarchal societies there may be a reversal of traditional values and a corresponding preference for the left. As Corballis (1980a) notes, in the Isis cult of ancient Egypt, honor was given to Isis over Osiris, to mother over son, to night over day, and the Isis procession was led by a priest carrying an image of the left hand.) The Danubian and Aegean cultures, largely destroyed in Europe during the aggressive Indo-European invasions three to four thousand years ago, left lingering elements in the form of nature cults, mysticism, and witchcraft, which were largely suppressed in classical times as suspect, evil, dark, or Chthonic. The Great Goddess herself survived as at best a minor deity, Hecate-Cybele-Artemis of the moon cycle, associated with death, childbirth, and the nighttime. Some might even claim that the Virgin Mary is a modern surviving epiphany.

The ruling Indo-European warrior elite spread into Northern Europe, the Mediterranean, Persia, and India and gave rise to the epic traditions celebrated by the skalds, bards, and poets of the Norse, Teutonic, Celtic, and Homeric cycles. As a patriarchal society, a male sky or sun god was worshipped, the daytime (bright) father (Dyaus Pitar of Indian Sanskrit, Jupiter and Ζευς Πατηρ of the Romans and Greeks, and Tiw or Ziu of the Teutons). There was a corresponding emphasis on warlike qualities, the sword, and the right hand. Parenthetically, the following modern parallelism may therefore not be entirely fortuitous: *blue* (sky color) for *boys* and the political *right* wing and to ward off *evil,* and *pink* (blood, earth, or ochre color) for *girls* and the political *left* wing.

The Pythagorean Table of Opposites as we saw linked the right side with maleness, the left with femaleness. Parmenides, the Greek philosopher of the sixth century B.C., thought that the embryo's sex was determined by the side of the womb in which it lay (male embryos on the right, female on the left). Anaxagoras (his contemporary) conversely believed intuitively, and as we now know correctly, that the *father* was responsible for an offspring's sex. However, he held that semen from the right testis develops into males, and that from the left into females (see, e.g., Lloyd, 1966, for further thoughts on left and right as viewed by the pre-Socratic philosophers). Despite empirical evidence to the contrary from such philosophers as Aristotle, these beliefs persisted via the Greco-Roman physician Galen and the Arab Avicenna into the Middle Ages. Potential fathers even tied one testicle in order to "determine" their offspring's sex, and pregnant mothers with an enlarged left breast were believed to be carrying a daughter (Mittwoch, 1977). Parenthetically, Harlap (1979) reports that infants conceived just before or just after ovulation (defined in terms of the period of maximum temperature rise) are more likely to be male, and those conceived *on* the day of ovulation are slightly more likely to be female. This is almost the exact opposite of the schema offered by the Greek philosopher and physiologist Empedocles ("male embryos result if the semen falls into the womb when it is hotter, females when it is colder"). The contemporary explanation is based on possible acidity changes in the cervix occurring around ovulation, and/or aging of the male sperm, differentially affecting the X or Y chromosomes carried by the sperm.

Left and Right in Biological Hermaphroditism

According to Mittwoch (1977), there may indeed be some truth in the old superstitions linking sex and left and right. Sex is determined by whether one of our twenty-three pairs of chromosomes is an XX (as in females) or an XY (males). Only the father can contribute a Y, so he therefore determines the offspring's sex. The Y chromosome imposes masculinity on the developing embryo and turns undifferentiated gonads into ovaries or testes. Sometimes, however, things may go wrong. The first such possibility is for one of the sex chromosomes to be damaged around the time of fertilization. If the remaining undamaged chromosome is an X, the egg may survive—XO, or Turner's Syndrome, resulting in a viable if abnormal and infertile individual. The converse (YO) condition is apparently nonviable, leading to the pleasing (for the feminists) consequence that human embryos may be regarded as basically female. Eve was indeed the first to enter the Garden of Eden! However, the feminists' joy must be short-lived with respect to a second chromosomal abnormality whereby, in addition to the normal Y, the egg contains two or even three Xs. The result is always male, suggesting that if the Y chromosome is the junior of the two, it can still triumph over several of its rivals. A third chromosomal fault, perhaps the most interesting in the context of sidedness, relates to hermaphroditism. While many hermaphrodites may merely have composite ovotestes, some possess a differentiated testis and an ovary. When this occurs, the single testis is preferentially found on the right side and the ovary on the left, a situation that must surely not have gone unnoticed by the prurient Greeks and Romans, who were ever fascinated by hermaphroditism. Moreover, in *normal* humans the right gonad generally exceeds the left in weight, protein, DNA content, and number of cells, with a greater relative left–right difference for the (smaller) ovaries than for the testes.

Mittwoch (1977) consequently concludes that when things go wrong, undifferentiated gonads on the right side must have a greater potential of developing into testes and those on the left into ovaries—a situation reminiscent of the first two entries in the Pythagorean Table of Opposites. Curiously, this XX (female) and XY (male) relationship in mammals is reversed in birds, where the left gonad is the larger and the basic blueprint appears to be for maleness: A hen turns into a cock if supplies of female hormones dry up.

Summary and Conclusions

Vertebrates display a superficial and often only skin-deep left–right symmetry. Since natural forces tend to operate along a body's vertical axis, lateral symmetry could be expected; unidirectional horizontal movement would make leading and trailing edges asymmetrical and leave the two sides of the body laterally symmetrical since they are unlikely to be exposed to systematically asymmetrical forces on the left and right. However, many paired organs are slightly and consistently asymmetrical, and many disease states tend to strike one side of the body more than the other. Even in hermaphroditism there seems to be a systematic left–right disposition of male and female gonads.

The two sides of the face are usually slightly asymmetrical, though long exposure to our own face (via the mirror) and our friends' faces may blind us to any such asymmetries unless special procedures are taken to highlight them. As a possibly related phenomenon, portrait painters tend to show more of the left than the right cheek, though the reasons for this are still debated.

If we were not slightly asymmetrical ourselves, we would not notice the presence of left–right asymmetries, nor would we be able to correctly use asymmetrical man-made objects. However, the degree of brain and body asymmetry is indeed slight, as indicated by the difficulty that adults as well as small children and lower vertebrates have in discriminating between left–right mirror-image stimuli or in making discriminative responses with a left or a right limb.

Human dextrality probably antedates paleolithic times. It has long fascinated scientists, anthropologists, myth makers, and myth researchers as well as common people down the ages. Many cultures seem quite independently to link the right with the good, warm, bright, and male and to contrast it pejoratively with the left, cold, dark, and female. Reasons for this may be found deep within the cultural and religious organization of pretechnological societies.

FURTHER READING

CORBALLIS, M. C. Laterality and myth. *American Psychologist,* 1980, *35,* 284–295.

CORBALLIS, M. C., & BEALE, I. L. Bilateral symmetry and behavior. *Psychological Review,* 1970, *77,* 451–464.

CORBALLIS, M. C., & BEALE, I. L. *The psychology of left and right.* Hillsdale: Lawrence Erlbaum, 1976.

COREN, S., & PORAC, C. Fifty centuries of right handedness: The historical record. *Science,* 1977, *198,* 631–632.

HARDYCK, C., & PETRINOVICH, L. F. Left handedness. *Psychological Bulletin,* 1977, *84,* 385–404.

HARRIS, L. J. Left handedness: Early theories, facts and fancies. In J. Herron (Ed.), *Neuropsychology of left-handedness.* New York: Academic Press, 1980.

LLOYD, G. E. R. *Polarity and analogy: Two types of argumentation in early Greek thought.* Cambridge: Cambridge University Press, 1966.

MITTWOCH, U. To be right is to be born male. *New Scientist,* 1977, *73,* 74–77.

NEEDHAM, R. *Right and left: Essays on dual symbolic classification.* Chicago: University of Chicago Press, 1973.

CHAPTER TWO
Asymmetries in Species Other Than Man

In the first chapter we saw that humans exhibit various bodily asymmetries, of which a prevailing tendency toward dextrality is but one manifestation. While such a *population* lateralization is almost unique to humans (although gastropod species also tend to be highly consistent in the direction of shell coiling), at an *individual* level many other species of animal exhibit left–right asymmetries, though their direction may not be consistent between individuals.

Asymmetries in the Animal Kingdom

Detailed reviews of the many variations from strict lateral symmetry in the animal kingdom are provided by Chapple (1977), Corballis and Morgan (1978), Dimond (1977), M. Morgan (1977), Neville (1976), Nottebohm (1979), and Walker (1980). In certain crab species, for example, the left claw (chela) is consistently the larger, while in others it is the right. The mandibles of certain species of termite are asymmetrical, as are the lungs of some species of snake and the antlers of certain deer. Genital asymmetries are common in insects, cephalopods, certain fish and reptiles, and possibly even in marsupials and ungulates. With flatfish, the left side has become the bottom and the right the top in some species, while with others the reverse is true. Amid the odontocete suborder of the cetaceans, the narwhal has a better-developed right side of the skull, from which the single tusk usually grows. In the brain, as we shall see shortly, the habenular nucleus is frequently considerably larger on one side for various species of lower vertebrates (lamprey, fish, and amphibians), though again *between* species the direction is not systematic. This lack of systematicity *across* species, and the presence of aberrant individuals *within* species, argue against the proposition of Corballis and Morgan (1978) that there is a general tendency within the animal kingdom for a leftward growth gradient (see Chapter Ten). There are anecdotal accounts of locomotor asymmetries in the baleen whale, the African elephant, and the horse, although studies have generally not yet been systematic (but see Meij & Meij, 1980, on the horse).

Pawedness, Clawedness, and Handedness
in Animals Other Than Man

Many species of animal inhabit ecological niches where they must manipulate food or other objects in order to survive. While manipulative dexterity has reached an evolutionary peak in humans, such skills in varying levels are certainly not confined to our species, nor even to carnivores or fruit eaters. They are well developed in rodents, racoons, cats, bears, monkeys, and the apes. Only rats, mice, cats, and primates have been extensively studied. All of these animals and the brush-tailed possum of Australia (*Trichosurus vulpecula*) (though possibly not the apes and monkeys), may show strong, stable, and consistent paw or hand preferences at the *individual* subject level for food reaching, playing, and such. These preferences, certainly among the rodents, are unsystematic *between* subjects (which divide about equally into left- and right-handers) and often *within* subjects for different tasks (see Walker, 1980, for a detailed review). The preferences appear not to be acquired during testing as a result of experience but seem to be innate, being relatively resistant to attempts to change them and to the effects both of fatigue and of imposed disuse. Selective breeding does not alter the fifty-fifty distribution of right- and left-pawed mice in later generations (Collins, 1977a); the *degree* of lateralization may possibly be subject to genetic variability but apparently not its *direction*. Such idiosyncratic left–right preferences may depend upon idiosyncratic and equally slight asymmetries in the availability of catecholamines in the nigrostriatal (i.e., *extrapyramidal*) motor pathway; these latter asymmetries may be enhanced by the administration of amphetamine and lead to turning biases (Glick, Jerussi, & Zimmerberg, 1977). In humans (see Chapter Five) the *pyramidal* motor system is probably the more important for hand control.

　　With monkeys (see, e.g., Lehman, 1980), hand preferences, while again consistent *within* tasks and nonsystematic like those of the rodents, are often initially weak and task specific, fail to predict later performance, and are strongly affected by experience and practice (J. M. Warren, 1977, 1980). As a result of such practice, monkeys may subsequently develop strong idiosyncratic preferences. Even the appearance of handedness in monkeys may be an artifact produced by the methods used in repeated experiments. Although monkeys seem to learn to prefer one hand for a particular sort of manipulation, such spontaneous hand preferences can be quickly and permanently reversed by contingent reinforcement of the nonpreferred hand, which suggests that handedness in monkeys is not homologous to that in humans. Anecdotal and somewhat cursory observation of the apes has also suggested unsystematic preferences, except for one report (Schaller, 1963) of a right-hand preference in chest-beating behavior in mountain gorillas. Curiously, however, there are recent reports (e.g., Rogers, 1980) that many species of parrot are predominantly *left-footed* for food manipulation, suggesting the possibility of *analogous* (though not *homologous*) functioning with humans. Such observations are particularly interesting as we shall shortly discuss another great similarity between humans and certain species of bird—the left-brain control of song (in birds) and speech (in humans). Notwithstanding, parrots are *not* among those avian species that exhibit this left-dominance for calling and song.

Brain Asymmetries in Vertebrates

If the brain ultimately controls the various manifestations of behavior, it is to the brain that we should perhaps look for an explanation of such phenomena as hand or paw preference. In vertebrates the brain is a paired organ; its left side largely mediates the initial perception of stimuli impinging on the right side of the body, and vice versa. We shall return later (Chapter Nine) to discuss possible reasons for this contralateral (crossed-over) relationship, and how it manifests itself in vision among lateral- and frontal-eyed species. At this stage we should note that a largely contralateral arrangement also exists at the motor level. The left half brain (the left *hemisphere,* or forebrain, with its heavy mantle of cortex in the higher vertebrates) generally controls responses made by muscles on the right side of the body and vice versa. Consequently, if an individual (rat or human) "prefers" to use the right hand, it would seem appropriate to seek corresponding left–right asymmetries in brain anatomy or biochemistry, perhaps initially in those areas of the brain known to be involved in such functions. We should remember that a *structural asymmetry* does not necessarily imply a *functional asymmetry,* nor does *structural symmetry* rule out a *functional* or *biochemical asymmetry.*

The habenular nuclei. As mentioned earlier, within the diencephalon of lower vertebrates the habenular nuclei (which are thought to be involved in olfaction and the mediation of emotional responses) are often of unequal size, though *between* species the direction is unsystematic. What functional significance this has for the individual animal is unclear, but in humans, as we shall see in Chapter Seven, emotional reactivity appears to be partly lateralized to one side of the brain and the same (right) side may also be involved in responses to novel cognitive tasks (Goldberg & Costa, 1981); in rats, as we shall see in the next section, the right hemisphere has been implicated in the mediation of arousal, territoriality, aggression, and responses to novelty (Denenberg, 1981). In rats and humans, of course, these effects may be primarily telencephalic and cortical, rather than diencephalic, but diencephalic signals may possibly also initiate the corresponding and appropriate behaviors in rats and humans.

Studies with rats. Denenberg, Garbanati, Sherman, Yutzey, and Kaplan (1978) reported a complicated series of experiments that demonstrated that handling and environmental enrichment experiences in very young rats affected the right hemisphere more than the left, as measured by activity levels after brain lesions in one of the hemispheres. Enriched environments and handling both increased open field activity. Handling was crucial in determining the response to brain damage: Unhandled rats increased activity when either the left or right hemisphere was damaged. Handled rats were made either very active or virtually immobile by right hemisphere damage, depending on whether they were reared in groups or in isolation; they were unaffected by left hemisphere damage.

In a subsequent study Sherman, Garbanati, Rosen, Yutzey, and Denenberg (1980) found no difference in mouse-killing behavior between unhandled rats with either left or right hemisphere lesions; however, handled rats with left hemisphere lesions killed mice far more rapidly than rats with right hemisphere lesions. This suggests the general involvement of the right hemisphere in aggression and emotional responses. Similarly, R. G. Robinson (1979) showed that lesions in the right frontoparietal cortex of rats led to a temporary increase in activity and a short-term decrease in noradrenalin content in several ipsilateral brain areas; damage to the left hemisphere had no such effect. Glick, Meibach, Cox, and Maayani (1979) likewise found that the frontal cortex and hippocampus of rats initially exhibit greater glucose metabolism on the left side, but that the bias shifts to the right hemisphere after amphetamine arousal. Finally, Diamond, Dowling, and Johnson (1980, cited in Denenberg, 1981) found that the cortical thickness of the right hemisphere is greater than that of the left, particularly in posterior regions, for male (but not normal female) rats and for females with ovaries removed at birth, suggesting the important role of hormones. These conclusions, implicating the importance of the right hemisphere in complex behavioral tasks, novelty, emotionality, and aggression, are discussed in more detail by Denenberg (1981).

Studies with birds. Historically, the first convincing example of functional asymmetry in a nonhuman nervous system was that of vocal control in several species of songbird, reported by Nottebohm in the early 1970s (see, e.g., Nottebohm, 1979): Sectioning of the left hypoglossus nerve of the adult male chaffinch leads to the loss of most of the song components; sectioning of the right hypoglossus has very little effect. In the former case the bird silently mouths, although a very few vocal elements are retained at the correct points in an otherwise silent sequence. With right-sided damage, only a few components of the song drop out. The song organ in birds (see Figure 2-1), the syrinx, has two parts, one in each bronchus, and each is separately innervated by a branch of the left or right hypoglossus (the tracheosyringalis nerve), which ultimately originates in a brain center

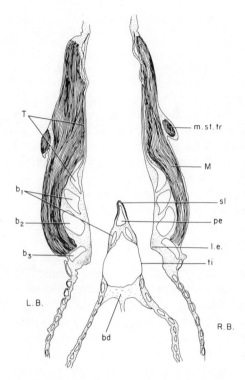

FIGURE 2-1 Longitudinal section of the syrinx of an adult male canary. Note that the muscle mass serving the left syringeal half is heavier than its right counterpart. R.B. and L.B. = right and left bronchi; M = section through the lateral mass of the intrinsic syringeal muscles; T = tympanum; b_1, b_2 and b_3 = bronchial half rings; db = bronchidesmus; pe = pessulus; sl = semilunar membrane; l.e. = labium externum; t.i. = internal tympaniform membrane; m.st.tr. = sternotrachealis muscle. (From F. Nottebohm, "Origins and Mechanisms in the Establishment of Cerebral Dominance," Figure 13, page 331, in M. S. Gazzaniga, ed., *Handbook of Behavioral Neurobiology, Vol. 2, Neuropsychology.* New York: Plenum Publishing Corporation, 1979. Courtesy of the publisher and author.)

known as the hyperstriatum ventrale, pars candalis. The control is ipsilateral, thus damage to the left hyperstriatum has the same detrimental effect on song as damage to the left hypoglossus. Loss of song is irreversible if the left-sided damage occurs in the adult male chaffinch (females do not sing, and their relevant brain centers are smaller). However, if damage occurs before song is fully developed, centers on the right can take over. This plasticity is apparently hormone-dependent. (As we shall see in Chapter Eight, this is reminiscent of the ability of the right hemisphere in humans to take over the mediation of speech from the left if the left is damaged in infancy but not if it is damaged in adulthood.) This period, therefore, can be prolonged with castration and terminated with testosterone treatment. Such effects are demonstrable with chaffinches and several species of sparrow and canaries but not, as we noted earlier, with the parrot. In canaries, the effects are not permanent beyond a year, since the bird normally develops a new song repertoire each year, and the right hemisphere can then take over.

Apart from lateralized song control in certain species of birds, there is very recent evidence of lateralization of certain other complex behaviors (discrimination learning, habituation, fear, attack and copulation, and responses to novelty; see, e.g., Rogers, 1980, for review). Learning that is known to be lateralized to the *left* forebrain includes imprinting, visual discrimination learning, auditory habituation, and attention switching. The left forebrain is more likely to activate a pecking response and also to *inhibit* it when it ceases to be rewarded. Conversely, responses to novelty seem to be activated by the right hemisphere (cf. Denenberg's 1981 findings discussed above with rats) and inhibited by the left, as are attack and copulation. Generally, the right forebrain in chicks seems to control the hypothalamic-pituitary-gonadal axis. Rogers demonstrated these effects by injecting cycloheximide (an antibiotic inhibiting ribosomal protein synthesis) into one or the other forebrain of two-day-old chicks. The observed effects depended on the injected side: If the left forebrain was injected, visual discrimination learning and auditory habituation decreased, and switching was reduced between equally available and acceptable (but differently colored) foods. Right-forebrain injections had no effects on these aspects of performance. Likewise, only with left-sided injections did attack and copulation increase, suggesting that the right forebrain activates these behaviors, being more reactive generally to novel or threatening stimuli, while the left forebrain inhibits them.

It is possible that all the above effects, including the lateralized control of song, occur because just before hatching the chick's head is turned up on its left shoulder, shielding the left eye and ear, and only the right eye and ear receive sensory inputs to transmit to the left hemisphere; therefore, only the left hemisphere is activated. According to Rogers (1980) there is some evidence that the above lateralizations may fail to appear if eggs are kept in a dark and quiet location before hatching. We shall see in Chapter Twelve that a similar argument (position *in utero*) has been developed to explain head-turning reflexes in human neonates, which some believe might underlie subsequent handedness patterns.

Studies with monkeys. After an extensive review of the literature, J. M. Warren (1980) found no evidence of *generally* inferior cognitive or problem-solving performance when the brains of monkeys were lesioned on one side or the other, the same or opposite to their preferred hands. Studies using *reversible* inactivation of one or other cerebral hemisphere (achieved by placing certain chemical substances on the cortex) did not show one hemisphere to be superior to the other in discrimination learning. Likewise, with split-brain monkeys where the commissures (which neurally connect the two forebrains at the level of the cortex) are cut, either hemisphere can learn visual discriminations with equal facility at all levels of processing (Hamilton, 1977; see also Chapter Five).

However, when Japanese macaques (Petersen, Beecher, Zoloth, Moody, & Stebbins, 1978) were tested on their ability to perform discriminations on taped versions of the calls specific to their own species, the calls being fed to one or the other ear (each projects largely to the hemisphere on the opposite side), the right ear (left hemisphere) proved superior. It would be of interest, as Walker (1980) observes, to determine whether a similar effect occurs with songbirds (i.e., whether there is lateralization at the *receptive* as well as at the *expressive* end), and whether monkeys have any left hemisphere superiority for *call production*.

There is some further, if weak, evidence for left lateralization of (nonvocal) auditory function in the macaque monkey. Dewson (1977) presented one of two auditory stimuli (a pure tone or white noise), followed by two panels lighting up simultaneously, one red and one green (randomly left or right) after a varying interval. The monkey had to press the red one if it had heard the tone, the green one if it had heard the noise, or vice versa. Dewson found that lesions to the left auditory cortex (superior temporal gyrus) led to greater deficits with longer (or possibly more variable) delays than lesions to the right, which had little effect. Walker (1980), however, reviews a number of experimental problems with this study, such as the sample size and the existence of certain other lesions, leading to some doubt as to whether the results can be accepted at face value. Were there any significant degree of functional lateralization in the monkey brain, as the Petersen et al. and the Dewson studies suggest, we might possibly expect an indication of anatomical or morphological asymmetries between corresponding left–right cortical areas. In the next section we shall see evidence for this in the great apes, and in the next chapter the even stronger evidence for it in humans. In the monkey, all evidence to date has proved negative, with the exception of one study. Falk (cited by Witelson, 1977a) found that in Old World monkeys, structures occupying areas thought to be analogues of the human language areas were larger in the *right* than in the left hemisphere. If confirmed, this will prove an interesting finding, as it is the opposite of what one would expect from the human studies, which indicate that speech-related areas are generally larger on the left.

Studies with apes.   In the next chapter we shall review the evidence for left–right anatomical asymmetries in the human brain, particularly in the region of the auditory cortex of the temporal lobe. Suffice to say that after the very recent demonstration of such effects in humans, similar if weaker effects have been found in the apes but not in the monkeys. Most studies have measured the length of the Sylvian fissure (see Chapter Three) either directly or indirectly via skull or skull endocast measurements. The Sylvian fissure is more often longer on the left, and there may be comparable left–right differences to those of humans in its point of inflexion (Witelson, 1977a). Such observations go back to the days of Cunningham (1892) who studied human, chimpanzee, orangutan, and baboon brains, but only very recently has interest revived. LeMay and Geschwind (1975) found that the point of termination of the Sylvian fissure was higher on the right side than on the left in the chimpanzee, gorilla, and orangutan, the effect being strongest in the orangutan and weakest in the gorilla. Yeni-Komshian and Benson (1976) found that the length of the Sylvian fissure was longer on the left in twenty out of twenty-five chimpanzees, just as in humans, but there was a smaller relative effect, with no significant differences, for rhesus monkeys. Finally Cain and Wada (1979) found that in baboons, as in humans, certain *frontal* lobe measurements are greater in the *right* hemisphere.

The implications of these findings for human speech will be discussed in the next chapter. Suffice to say that humans alone have the capacity to communicate by speech, though chimpanzees can apparently be taught to communicate by versions of American Sign Language (Terrace, 1980). However an extremely acrimonious debate is currently raging as to whether they are really using *language*.

The argument centers on whether or not they do in fact generate novel proposi-tions. Either way, chimpanzees probably are *not* using those areas of the brain that correspond to the human speech areas (see Chapter Four), that is, parts adjacent to the auditory association cortex in the temporal lobe (Wernicke's area), and areas adjacent to the motor cortex for the face in the frontal lobe (Broca's area). We can at most conclude that apes and possibly monkeys are perhaps *preadapted* for the evolutionary development of lateralized control systems. If we include the un-doubted lateralization of birdsong, we must conclude either that such phenomena are instances of independent, parallel evolution, with lateralization developing inde-pendently in different species when the environment favored it, or that some prior factor (e.g., Corballis and Morgan's, 1978, leftwards growth gradient) underlies all such evolutionary developments. In any case the whole question of left–right ana-tomical asymmetries in the brain is a vexed one: How do you define a functional area? Cytoarchitectonically? In terms of boundary gyri and sulci? In terms of measured performance change as a function of localized lesions (if lesions ever *can* be strictly localized)? As we shall see in the next chapter, all such criteria are open to various interpretations and often fail to correlate.

Summary and Conclusions

Many animal species display left–right bodily asymmetries, but human dextrality is almost unique in terms of lateralization at a *population* level, though some species of parrot do apparently show consistent left-foot preferences. Manipulative dex-terity in perhaps all other species is associated with strong individual or paw pref-erences, which are, however, unsystematic *between* individuals and even *within* subjects for different tasks. Such preferences seem not to be acquired by experience but to be innate, resistant to change and to selective breeding. Idiosyncratic left–right paw preferences in the rat may be subject to idiosyncratic asymmetries in the availability of catecholamines in the extrapyramidal motor system. Hand prefer-ences in the monkey may initially be the weakest and least systematic and may be strongly affected by experience and practice.

Within the brain, the habenular nuclei involved in emotional responses in the lower vertebrates are often systematically asymmetrical, though the direction is not constant at an *interspecies* level. Handling and environmental enrichment affects the right hemisphere of rats more than the left, the right seeming to be involved in arousal and possibly possessing a slightly thicker cortex. Left-brain control of song, which is apparently hormone-dependent, is evident in several species of songbird. In chicks there may also be differential lateralization of discrimination learning, habituation, fear, attack and copulation, and responses to novelty in birds, though it is also possible that some or all of these latter effects stem from the position of the chick's head before hatching.

Monkeys show no evidence of lateralization of cognitive functions, though the left hemisphere may possibly be involved in the discrimination of species-specific calls in particular and auditory functions in general. Apes alone show similar (though smaller) left–right morphological asymmetries of the brain to humans in the peri-Sylvian regions, which are speech-related in humans. It is uncertain, however, to what extent this could be related to communication, unless apes are simply preadapted for the evolutionary development of lateralized control systems.

FURTHER READING

CORBALLIS, M. C., & MORGAN, M. J. On the biological basis of human laterality. *Behavioral and Brain Sciences,* 1978, *2,* 261–336.

DENENBERG, V. H. Hemispheric laterality in animals and the effects of early experience. *Behavioral and Brain Sciences,* 1981, *4,* 1–50.

NOTTEBOHM, F. Origins and mechanisms in the establishment of cerebral dominance. In M. S. Gazzaniga (Ed.), *Handbook of behavioral neurobiology, Vol. 2: Neuropsychology.* New York: Plenum, 1979.

ROGERS, L. Lateralization in the avian brain. *Bird Behavior,* 1980, *2,* 1–12.

WALKER, S. F. Lateralization of functions in the vertebrate brain: A review. *British Journal of Psychology,* 1980, *71,* 329–367.

WARREN, J. M. Handedness and laterality in humans and other animals. *Physiological Psychology,* 1980, *8,* 351–359.

CHAPTER THREE
Morphological Asymmetries of the Human Brain

Before the end of the last century a major landmark on the surface of the human brain, the Sylvian fissure, a lateral fissure that separates the temporal and parietal lobes, was known to be usually longer on the left side (Cunningham, 1892). This asymmetry was later shown to be accompanied by asymmetries in the surface area of the parietal and posterior temporal cortex, including the region of the temporal planum, which is known to be very important in mediating the receptive and semantic aspects of speech. Von Economo and Horn (1930) showed that the temporal planum is longer on the left side. These morphological asymmetries, however, received very little attention, being thought too slight to account for general human dextrality and left-hemisphere dominance for language. (We shall see in the next chapter that for over one hundred years clinicians have been aware of asymmetry in the representation of speech in the brain.)

Only in the last dozen or so years has the often fairly extensive nature of some of these morphological asymmetries been realized. They are generally visible to the naked eye post-mortem or by radiological methods of examining the living brain, including newer noninvasive computerized tomographic techniques. The latter techniques scan the brain by means of numerous low-dose X-ray exposures taken from carefully chosen locations under computer control and build up a whole series of composite pictures. (Scans of the living brain, incidentally, seem to demonstrate the asymmetries even more strongly, since on post-mortem fixing the brain is liable to shrinkage and distortion.) Gross asymmetries in the brain may also be inferred from routine arteriographic or pneumoencephalographic studies. In arteriographic studies the position of major blood vessels, which tend to follow major cortical landmarks or boundaries, can be plotted radiographically by the injection of radio-opaque dyes. In pneumoencephalographic studies the injection of air into the ventricles shows, with X-radiography, their position and size, and by inference the extent and position of overlying structures.

Peri-Sylvian Asymmetries

Recent studies of the Sylvian fissure (Hochberg & LeMay, 1975; Rubens, 1977) show not only that it is generally longer on the left but that it continues further, horizontally, on the left before it bends upward (see Figure 3-1). Moreover, the posterior end of the Sylvian fissure (the "Sylvian point") is generally higher on the right side, a situation that is often apparent by the sixteenth week in fetal brains (LeMay & Culebras, 1972) and has been noted in the skulls of at least two species of fossil humans, Neanderthal and Peking man (LeMay, 1976).

The Temporal Planum

As mentioned earlier, the temporal planum, a most important language-related area of the temporoparietal region through which the Sylvian fissure passes, may be measured indirectly in terms of the latter landmark or more directly. It lies between Heschl's gyrus (the primary auditory cortex in the central portion of the temporal operculum) rostrally and the posterior end of the Sylvian fissure caudally, on the superior surface of the temporal lobe. Including much of Wernicke's area, (see Chapter Four), it is a part of association cortex devoted to language and has recently undergone massive evolutionary development.

Geschwind and Levitsky (1968) found that where an asymmetry *was* apparent, the temporal planum was larger on the left in 65 percent of cases, and on the right in only 11 percent (the remaining brains not being easily assignable to one or the other category). Similar findings were reported by Wada, Clarke, and Hamm (1975), Witelson and Pallie (1973), and Teszner (1972). LeMay and Culebras (1972) reported that the parietal operculum (the inferior portion of the postcentral gyrus and also part of Wernicke's area, which is concerned with the kinesthetic

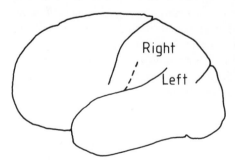

FIGURE 3-1   Left (solid line) and right (broken line) Sylvian fissures, the right shown superimposed (and mirror-reflected) on the appropriate part of the left hemisphere. Note that the Sylvian fissure is generally longer on the left, but terminates at a lower level than the right. (Figure redrawn from samples published by Rubens, 1979.)

afferentation of the articulators) is also larger on the left. Rubens (1977) questioned whether findings such as Geschwind and Levitsky's could possibly be partly an artifact of relying on inflexions in the Sylvian fissure as an indicator of a boundary of the temporal planum. However Galaburda, Sanides, and Geschwind (1978) provided the much needed cytoarchitectonic confirmation that, in terms of cell structure also, the relevant regions of the temporoparietal auditory cortex around the Sylvian fissure are generally larger on the left. Moreover, they showed that the superior portion of the superior temporal gyrus is the most markedly asymmetrical part of the temporal planum. Cytoarchitectonic methods also avoid the problem of morphological asymmetries otherwise being masked by the fact that large extents of cortex may be buried in sulci as a consequence of folding.

Asymmetries of the temporal planum are apparently observable in the fetus, as early as the thirty-first week of gestation (Chi, Dooling, & Gilles, 1977). These authors also confirmed in the fetus the observation of Campain and Minckler (1976) in the adult that immediately anterior to the temporal planum there may be additional transverse temporal gyri—additional, that is, to Heschl's gyrus—which are more common on the *right* side.

Left–right asymmetries of the temporal planum are generally larger for some brains than others, and are sometimes in the opposite direction, indicating that such differences are continuously distributed. The *relative* magnitude of these left–right asymmetries could possibly correlate with the extent of functional brain lateralization of language. (Indeed, differences are generally smaller and more likely to be reversed with known sinistrals; see, e.g., LeMay, 1977). The *absolute* magnitudes of the language-related structures, on the other hand, could possibly reflect or determine the likelihood of a subject's experiencing difficulty in developing language (e.g., developmental dysphasia or dyslexia) or even of withstanding the effects of local cerebral lesions, with language functions either surviving intact, rapidly recovering, or perhaps never recovering. However, the location, direction, magnitude, and consistency of these morphological asymmetries do support the conclusion that they are almost certainly the neurological substrate of language.

Frontal Asymmetries and Regional Connectivity

Nevertheless, a problem initially seems to arise for the above conclusion when we examine the prefrontal regions. Such regions, which include Broca's motor-speech area (see Chapter Four) appear to be *smaller* on the left side (LeMay, 1977; Wada et al., 1975). There is, however, some evidence that total folding may be greater on the left, perhaps still leading to a greater *overall* (i.e., extended) cortical surface; moreover, Broca's area, which is included *within* such prefrontal regions, is difficult to measure and has no clear boundaries. Indeed, according to Galaburda (1980, cited in Goldberg and Costa, 1981) the pars opercularis of the inferior frontal gyrus (which together with the inferior portion of the precentral gyrus is thought to constitute Broca's area) is in fact larger on the left. Goldberg and Costa (1981) go on to argue that since cortical asymmetries also occur outside the classical speech zones (Broca's and Wernicke's areas), we should not view such asymmetries purely in terms of linguistic versus nonlinguistic modes of processing. In Chapter Nine we shall argue that some other dichotomy (e.g., analytic–holistic modes of information processing) probably underlies the linguistic–nonlinguistic distinction. Goldberg and Costa incline to the related view that the right hemisphere is characterized more by *inter*regional connectivity and integration, and the left by *intra*regional organization; the right hemisphere (which, as we shall see in Chapter Seven, apart from nonverbal, visuospatial, holistic processing, also seems in both human and animal studies to be involved with novelty and emotionality) has more associative cortex for multimodal processing, and the left has greater capacity for unimodal processing and specific representation of sensory and motor functions. Whatever the truth of these speculations, there is some anatomical support for them. Gur, Packer, Hunger-buhler, Reivich, Obrist, Amarnek, and Sackeim (1980) found that the ratio of grey to white matter is higher in the left hemisphere, especially in the frontal and pre-central regions; they suggest this finding supports the hypothesis that the left hemi-sphere is organized to mediate processing *within* and the right hemisphere *between* discrete regions.

Gross Asymmetries of Length and Breadth

Overall, there appears to be more tissue in the right hemisphere (Whitaker & Oje-mann, 1977), and the right hemisphere tends to be the heavier (LeMay, 1976). The left occipital pole is wider and protrudes more posteriorly than the right ("left occipitopetalia"; the smooth indentations made by the larger lobes on the inside of the skull are known as petalia and were one of the possible indices for determining the anterior or posterior extent of the poles). Anteroparietal and posterooccipital regions are generally larger on the left. The right frontal pole and the central (pre-frontal) portion of the right hemisphere tend to be the wider, and the right frontal pole tends to extend beyond the left ("right frontopetalia") (LeMay, 1976; similar findings were reported also by Chui & Damasio, 1980). The left occipitopetalia is generally more pronounced and is evident even in fetuses and neonates. These generally greater values in terms of both width and length for right anterior and left posterior regions are sometimes described as giving the human brain a counter-clockwise torque (see Figure 3-2).

Asymmetries of the Pyramidal Tracts

Morphological asymmetries are also found below the level of the forebrain. They appear as far down as the medulla oblongata and the spinal cord, in the level and pattern of decussation, and cross-section size, of the pyramidal motor tracts. The pyramidal motor system is the more direct and important of the two routes from the motor regions of our brain and is concerned with the mediation of fine, skilled,

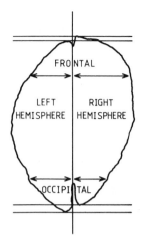

FIGURE 3-2 Asymmetries of frontal and occipital lobes. Note the wider right frontal and left occipital lobes and the more extensive left occipital and right frontal poles. (Redrawn from the computerized axial tomograms of Galaburda, LeMay, Kemper, & Geschwind, 1978, and of Chui & Damasio, 1980.)

distal movements (see Chapter Five). There is one-to-one topographic representation in the posterior strip of the frontal lobes. Most fibers decussate (unlike what happens with the extrapyramidal motor system), though some continue ipsilaterally, leading to two distinct tracts in the spinal cord. The patterns of decussation and other characteristics of the pyramidal tracts were studied in detail by Yakovlev and Rakic (1966) and Yakovlev (1972). Of 179 fetal and 130 adult specimens, 80 percent were found to have more fibers going from the left motor cortex via the contralateral pathway to the right side (e.g., right hand) and from the right motor cortex via the ipsilateral pathway to the right side, than they had fibers going via the contralateral and ipsilateral tracts to the left side. Thus, the right hand received the stronger innervation by motor fibers. Moreover, the contralateral tract from the left hemisphere usually crossed at a higher level in the medulla than did the contralateral tract from the right hemisphere (see Figure 3-3). Kertesz and Geschwind

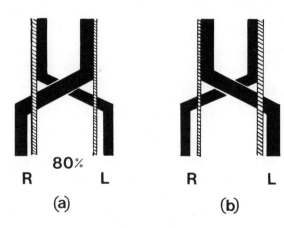

80%

R   L   R   L

(a)   (b)

FIGURE 3-3 Schematic drawing of pyramidal tracts showing various patterns of decussation and distribution of tracts. Pattern (a), which occurs in approximately 80 percent of the population, shows the higher level of the crossing of the left contralateral tract and the more numerous fibers leading to the right side (based on Yakovlev, 1972). (From S. Witelson, "Neuroanatomical Asymmetry in Left Handers," Figure 2.6, p. 96, in J. Herron, ed., *Neuropsychology of Left Handedness*. New York: Academic Press, 1980. Courtesy of the publishers and author.)

(1971) also studied pyramidal decussation in 125 dextral adults, many of whom were included in the previous study, and found that 73 percent had higher left-to-right pyramidal crossing and 17 percent the opposite. These figures are very similar to those reported for other morphological indices of hemispheric asymmetry and for behavioral asymmetries (ear and visual field differences; see Chapter Six), which lend credence to the idea that such morphological patterns are probably the substrate of the behavioral phenomena.

In summary, then, bundles of descending nerve fibers in the left medullary pyramid are larger and cross to the opposite side before descending the spinal cord at a higher level than those of the right pyramid. The right pyramidal tract is the larger overall.

Asymmetries of the Venous System

Left–right asymmetries in the venous system can also be used to index morphological asymmetries in the cortex. The predominant vein in the left hemisphere (Vein of Labbé) is situated close to language-related regions; the predominant vein in the right hemisphere (Vein of Trolard) covers the supero-parietal region (Hochberg and LeMay, 1975), which (as we shall see in Chapters Four to Six) is involved in spatio-perceptual processing. According to LeMay and Geschwind (1978) we can accurately judge difference in width of posterior parieto-occipital regions by means of the posterior end of the sagittal sinus and the transverse sinus. These venous channels can be seen during cerebral angiography (see Chapter Four) and also from the impressions they leave on the inside surface of the vault. The position of the sagittal sinus to the right and the lower transverse sinus on the left are said to predict accurately the width of the posterior portion of the brain. The posterior end of the sagittal sinus usually lies to the right, and the right transverse sinus is usually higher, all reflecting the smaller occipital brain mass in the right hemisphere. LeMay and Geschwind claim that differences in hemispheric size in the parietal region are probably responsible for the position of the sagittal sinus.

Arterial blood pressure may also be used as an indirect measure of brain asymmetry. Carmon and Gombos (1970) measured the pressure within the ophthalmic arteries in young adults by means of ophthalmodynamometry. Ophthalmic arterial pressure reflects the pressure within the ipsilateral internal carotid artery, which in turn reflects the blood flow to the ipsilateral hemisphere. They found a significant correlation between left–right differences in systolic ophthalmic pressure and the side and strength of hand preference. Dextrals showed a greater *right*-sided ophthalmic pressure. Likewise, hemispheric blood volume can be measured by the intravenous injection of radioactive material (Carmon, Harishanu, Lowinger, & Lavy, 1972). Higher irradiation (measured by radiation detectors over the head) and therefore presumably greater blood volume was more frequently found in the hemisphere *ipsilateral* to hand and ear preference—that is, in the *non-speech-dominant* hemisphere, exactly as in the Carmon and Gombos study above. One can only speculate as to why there should be greater blood volume to the minor hemisphere, especially when it may be shown that *increases* in blood flow can index engagement of left or right hemisphere function during cognitive tasks such as verbal or spatial problem solving (see Chapter Six). Presumably the latter effects are superimposed on the other preexisting base-line asymmetries.

Some Problems of Interpretation

The findings we have discussed so far all indicate that in the last ten or fifteen years a considerable number of left–right morphological asymmetries have become apparent, particularly in language-related areas of the cortex. These differences are often small, apparent only in reasonably large samples, and continuously distributed, not all or none, as in the position of the spleen or liver in the two sides of the body. They are, however, usually present at or before birth (Witelson & Pallie, 1973; Wada et al., 1975; Chi et al., 1977), and so cannot be due simply to experience or even posture. Do these facts, and the fact that the extent and sometimes the direction of such anatomical asymmetries correlate generally with hand preference, the effects often being reduced or even reversed with nondextrals (Witelson, 1980) and females (Wada et al., 1975) suggest that the asymmetrical anatomical structures are the *substrates* of language functions? As Ratcliff, Dila, Taylor, and Milner (1980) observe, the hypothesis of a correlation between cortical asymmetries and hand preference would seem to fit the data at least as well as an interpretation in terms of cerebral dominance for speech, and the possibility that morphological asymmetry has no functional significance has not been definitely excluded. These authors did, however, find further support for the interpretation in terms of cerebral speech dominance when they determined the asymmetry of the posterior Sylvian branches of the middle cerebral artery on the carotid angiograms of fifty-nine patients in whom speech laterality was known from amytal testing (see Chapter Four). The usual asymmetry of these vessels (which on leaving the posterior part of the Sylvian fissure typically slope more sharply down on the left side) was found in subjects with left-sided speech but was substantially reduced and more variable in patients with atypical cerebral speech dominance.

We shall discuss further evidence for the idea that asymmetrical anatomical structures are the substrates of language functions in later chapters. Generally, as we noted earlier, the percentage of cases showing asymmetries in a particular direction tends to correlate fairly closely with behavioral measures of ear and visual field superiority, though not, it should be noted, with clinical findings. Instead of around 70 percent of dextrals showing a left hemisphere mediation of language, as suggested by the anatomical asymmetry studies and the behavioral work with normal subjects, something of the order of 95 percent is usually reported (see Chapters Four and Eight). It used to be said that the lower figure with the behavioral studies reflected unreliability in the techniques. Criticisms can indeed be levied against the anatomical studies, but it seems likely that different aspects of language lateralization (e.g., receptive vs. expressive) are probably being tapped by the different approaches.

One problem in interpreting the gross morphological findings is the fact that the superficial topographical landmarks of gyri and sulci are highly variable, making it very difficult to delineate functional areas in this way. Of the two other alternative procedures, determination of the cytoarchitectonics or of the patterns of connectivity, the former is the easier and is the only one so far attempted (Galaburda et al., 1978). If we do continue to attempt to measure discrete anatomical areas, our findings will be subject to the limitations of fixed brains tending to shrink and distort, and radiological and other *in vivo* scans being unable to tell us too much about discrete bounded areas such as the temporal planum. Certain measures such as gross lengths and widths of the hemispheres, and of petalia, could possibly be in part due to such environmental factors as preferred side of head for sleeping on in infancy, though LeMay and Geschwind (1978) did find left occipitopetalia to be present even in fetal and newborn brains. There may, in a given area, be more fissuring, despite less *superficial* surface area, with a resultantly greater *total* cortical area (Wada et al., 1975). Surface mapping can therefore be deceptive. In any case, what does a larger neurological region indicate? Are there more cells, more dendritic growth and connectivity, larger cells, or more of the same tissue? Only sophisticated cytoarchitectonic studies can resolve this. Does more necessarily mean *better*? Certainly, there tends to be more primary and association cortex for the more important sensory and motor functions. Finally, as Walker (1980) observes, the correlations between left–right morphological and left–right functional asymmetries are not strong outside the area of language reception. Thus with respect to both fine motor control and language production, it is uncertain whether the relevant left-frontal region is the larger; indeed, with respect to visuospatial processing, the left occipital lobe is the bigger.

This chapter has been concerned with morphological asymmetries of the human brain. It has, however, dealt almost exclusively with asymmetries that relate directly or indirectly (e.g., the pyramidal asymmetries) with the neocortex, since to date there is little evidence of systematic asymmetry outside of these regions. Perhaps the only noteworthy exception is the thalamus, for which there is (as we shall see in Chapter Four) electrophysiological evidence of asymmetrical language involvement. Oke, Keller, Mefford, and Adams (1978) report higher concentrations of norepinephrine on the left in the pulvinar region, which may link the anterior and posterior speech zones, and higher concentrations on the right in somatosensory regions, which may possibly be concerned with the perception of spatial relationships. We shall repeatedly encounter this verbal–spatial dichotomy in later chapters.

Summary and Conclusions

Left–right asymmetries in the human peri-Sylvian (speech-related) cortex, especially in the region of the temporal planum, have been known for over a century but were long thought to be insufficient to account for the asymmetrical representation of language. The Sylvian fissure is generally longer on the left and continues further horizontally before bending upward. Its posterior end (the Sylvian point) is usually higher on the right, even as early as the sixteenth week of gestation and has been observed in at least two species of fossil humans.

The temporal planum, especially the superior portion of the superior temporal gyrus, an important language area through which the Sylvian fissure passes and which includes much of Wernicke's (speech comprehension) area, is generally larger on the left as early as the thirty-first week of gestation. The same holds for another part of Wernicke's area, the parietal operculum. As defined in cytoarchitectonic terms, the temporoparietal auditory cortex around the Sylvian fissure is larger on the left. Such effects are smaller and less consistent with nondextrals.

Broca's motor speech area, on the other hand, may be smaller on the left, as viewed superficially. However, it has no clear boundaries, and the total folding may in fact be greater on the left, leading to a greater overall extended cortical surface on that side.

There are repeated suggestions that the right hemisphere is characterized both anatomically and behaviorally more by *inter*regional connectivity and integration, the left by *intra*regional organization. The left has a higher ratio of grey to white matter; the right has more tissue and is heavier. The left occipital pole is wider and protrudes more posteriorly than the right, even in neonates. Anteroparietal and posterooccipital regions are generally larger on the left. The right frontal pole extends beyond the left and, together with the central (prefrontal) portion of the right hemisphere, is the wider. Overall, the brain may be said to have a counterclockwise torque.

The bundles of descending fibers in the left medullary pyramids are larger and cross to the opposite side, before descending the spinal cord, at a higher level than those of the right pyramid. Overall, the right motor pyramidal tract is the larger.

Asymmetries of the venous system may also be used to map surface asymmetries of the brain, either directly or via the impressions left on the inner surface of the vault. Asymmetries in the blood pressure of the ophthalmic arteries correlate with the side and strength of hand preference.

The question remains whether these morphological asymmetries are the neurological substrates of language, of handedness, or of both. They probably correlate more directly with language, especially at the motor or expressive level, despite the fact that the morphological asymmetries may be more apparent and obviously related to language in regions mediating speech comprehension. It is not always easy to assign landmarks and boundaries in determining cortical asymmetries. What does a larger region indicate? More cells, more connectivity, more of the same tissue? Is more necessarily *better*?

FURTHER READING

GALABURDA, A. M., LEMAY, M., KEMPER, T. L., & GESCHWIND, N. Right-left asymmetries in the brain. *Science,* 1978, *199,* 852–856.

GALABURDA, A. M., SANIDES, F., & GESCHWIND, N. Human brain: Cytoarchitectonic left–right asymmetries in the temporal speech region. *Archives of Neurology,* 1978, *35,* 812–817.

LEMAY, M. Morphological cerebral asymmetries of modern man, fossil man and nonhuman primate. *Annals of the New York Academy of Sciences,* 1976, *280,* 349–366.

RUBENS, A. B. Anatomical asymmetries of human cerebral cortex. In S. Harnad, R. W. Doty, L. Goldstein, J. Jaynes, & G. Krauthamer (Eds.), *Lateralization in the nervous system.* New York: Academic Press, 1977.

WITELSON, S. F. Anatomic asymmetry in the temporal lobes: Its documentation, phylogenesis and relationship to functional asymmetry. *Annals of the New York Academy of Sciences,* 1977, *299,* 328–354.

WITELSON, S. F. Neuroanatomical asymmetry in left handers: A review and implications for functional asymmetry. In J. Herron (Ed.), *Neuropsychology of left-handedness.* New York: Academic Press, 1980.

CHAPTER FOUR
Evidence
from Clinical Studies
of Cerebral Asymmetry
in Man

We have seen in the previous chapters that humans are not unique in the animal kingdom in exhibiting anatomical and behavioral asymmetries, though the magnitude and extent of their asymmetries are far greater than in any other species. Apart from the recent discoveries of anatomical asymmetries in the human brain, there are three major lines of behavioral evidence for asymmetrical functioning: neurological or clinical studies, split-brain (commissurotomy) studies, and investigations employing normal healthy subjects. This chapter will explore the first of these; the remaining two will be considered successively in the next two chapters.

Problems with the Neurological Approach

The neurological or clinical approach is certainly the oldest, extending back several thousand years, and the most extensively documented, though in many respects the information it provides is the least clear and unambiguous. One problem, at least in modern times, is the right and proper aversion to intervening unnecessarily in otherwise healthy human tissue. Clinicians must wait for suitable cases, usually the result of accident, disease, or war injury, all of which only rarely produce discrete well-localized lesions. When the surgeon decides to remove tissue to prevent or restrict disabling seizure activity, he or she obviously has far greater control over the extent of tissue removal, but even then mechanical trauma and interruption in blood supply, to say nothing of preexisting anomalies in brain structure or operation, will render any findings potentially nonrepresentative of the general population. Moreover, the resultant symptoms themselves are rarely clear, distinct, unitary, or unique, and cannot be attributed in any simple way to any given brain area.

Rarely does a particular cognitive function depend exclusively on either a single, unitary mental operation or on a single corresponding brain center. If a function such as reading is found to be disrupted by damage in widely different areas, it does not mean that reading is *mediated* by a multiplicity of centers, only that such centers, each of which may play a particular role in reading, contribute to the ultimately manifested capacity to read. Moreover, if *several* such centers are independently damaged, we may get not only *additive* but maybe even *multiplicative* effects on the capacity to read. Furthermore, given the nature and complexity of the excitatory and inhibitory pathways that run through and between the hemispheres, though lesions may be localized, symptoms often are not. A damaged area may not necessarily mediate the affected faculty, since deficits may result from the release of inhibition to some other area where the faculty is mediated. Thus area A may normally inhibit area B, which, were it not so inhibited by A, would in turn inhibit area C. If area A is damaged, B is freed from inhibition from A and is now free to inhibit C. If C mediates some function such as language, a deficit in that faculty (i.e., aphasia or dysphasia) will appear upon injury to A, leading to the erroneous conclusion that A (rather than in fact C) mediates language functions.

We shall see in Chapter Eight that there is evidence for the operation of such inhibitory chains at the interhemispheric level in the case of language. Moreover, we can also ask whether defective performance observed after, for example, unilateral injury results from the damaged area or hemisphere striving to achieve its maximum potential in the face of injury, or from another less specialized area (or hemisphere) doing its best in the face of an inherent lack of the requisite capacities, or even of noise transmitted from the damaged, specialized area. We shall see that in some circumstances an impaired function may even improve if a damaged area is totally removed. In any case, when the brain is left to its own devices, considerable improvement over time is far from uncommon and may itself reflect the new establishment of appropriate excitatory and inhibitory pathways.

Another problem facing the clinician is that all patients are different, not only genetically but also phenotypically, for example in their background, culture, education, intelligence, sex, and so on. All these factors almost certainly interact with brain development and function. Moreover, the clinician may know little of the preexisting history of morbidity, prior to injury or surgery. If morbidity has been long-standing or gradually incremental, or if it has occurred in a child, the effects on both brain function and performance are likely to be very different from cases where the injury is sudden, massive, or involves an older person. In the former circumstances, neural plasticity is far more likely to lead to a successful reorganization.

Finally, two potentially serious sources of statistical bias can easily affect any final attempt to gain an overview of the incidence of certain conditions. First, at least in our Western society, it is socially and economically far more disruptive and incapacitating to lose the faculty of language than, say, not to be able to produce or appreciate art or music. Many of us may never become aware of having lost a faculty we never knew we had. Only if we are painters, sculptors, architects, or musicians would we tend to become aware of the loss, sudden or gradual, of an artistic faculty. For this reason left hemisphere functions have until now tended to receive a perhaps undue emphasis, and minor hemisphere symptomatology has frequently been dismissed by patients (and occasionally by the clinician), posing a problem for balanced neuropsychological study. A second, not dissimilar problem is the fact that journals are organized to publish the rare or the unusual rather than the frequent or commonplace; as a result rare conditions may come to be over-represented, giving the reader a false idea of their relative frequencies.

Clinical Techniques

Apart from observing and reporting the consequences of accidental injury or deliberate surgery, which will be the main concern of this chapter, the clinical neuropsychologist has other techniques at his or her disposal. In principle, many of these can be employed on normal subjects, for example, recording electroencephalograms (EEGs) or auditory or visual evoked potentials (these techniques will be described in Chapter Six when we discuss normal subjects). However, some techniques are normally used only with clinical patients, either because the technique is difficult or because it is potentially somewhat hazardous and its use can be sanctioned only if it is likely to lead to an improvement in the patient's condition. A number of radiological techniques fall into this category. Arteriography or cerebral angiography, used to determine the width and position of major blood vessels in the brain, involves injecting a radio-opaque fluid directly into the blood stream. Air-(pneumo) encephalography involves introducing air into the cerebrospinal fluid to outline the ventricular system and to examine for possible atrophy or wasting of the cortex; this technique is based on differences in the opacity of air and the rest of the brain to the passage of X-rays. A more recent technique, computerized axial tomography, uses a computer to obtain information about soft tissue, information that was previously lost because of the insensitivity of earlier methods of recording radiographic images. It depicts the condition of a thin slice, or plane, through the head in a roughly horizontal position, several "cuts" being made at different levels.

In addition to radiographic techniques, electrostimulation of the surface of the exposed brain of a conscious patient, a mapping technique performed under local anaesthesia as an alternative to lesion mapping, will be discussed in detail in a later section of this chapter. Typically, the initiation, facilitation, and inhibition of language processes is observed as a function of the location and the intensity of the stimulation. There are two other major approaches, which again could in principle be applied to normal subjects, but because of their slightly hazardous and rather unpleasant nature, they are generally only employed with clinical patients. These are the Wada test and lateralized electroconvulsive therapy.

The Wada amytal test is used to determine the locus of language lateralization prior to surgery, so that critical structures can be located and, if possible, be avoided. Wada (1949) first developed the procedure now known as the Wada test: an injection of the barbiturate sodium amytal (amobarbital) into one (left or right) of the common carotid arteries that supplies its ipsilateral hemisphere. A temporary loss of function is produced on the affected side of the brain: a flattening of the EEG, along with hemiparesis, hemianaesthesia, and hemianopsia. It is in effect reversible hemispherectomy, permitting tests of higher mental functions in the other hemisphere. If the drug is injected into the dominant hemisphere, there is usually total and abrupt cessation of speech. In view of the slight but definite risk accompanying the insertion of a needle or catheter into the carotid artery, the Wada test is employed only when absolutely necessary, and consequently such patients usually have more or less severe existing abnormalities of cerebral function. More-over, since the unilateral suppression lasts only five to ten minutes and the experi-ence itself is probably disturbing to the patient, usually all that can be determined is which hemisphere is specialized for speech production. Typically, the upraised contralateral arm and leg fall to the bed with a flaccid paralysis a few seconds after the injection. If the injected hemisphere is nondominant for speech, the patient can continue to count and carry out verbal tasks during the temporary paralysis. If the injected hemisphere is dominant for speech, there is an abrupt and more or less total cessation of speech shortly after the injection; it lasts until recovery from the hemiparesis is well advanced. The patient makes characteristic dysphasic responses (perseveration, misnaming, mixing up the sequence of numbers and of days of the week, etc.) for several minutes before speech returns to normal (Wada & Rasmussen, 1960; Rasmussen & Milner, 1977). The Wada test has shown that dextrals have a clear left hemisphere language dominance in over 90 percent of the cases, and sinis-trals in 70 percent of cases.

Electroconvulsive therapy (ECT) was originally prescribed for severe depres-sion (though the exact mechanisms of its operation are not thoroughly understood, and some even doubt its long-term effectiveness). Its therapeutic effects seem to be relatively undiminished if it is presented unilaterally to the minor hemisphere, a procedure that avoids the often disturbing and distressing consequences of disrupt-ing language and verbal memory in the patient. The degree of dysphasia during the recovery period after successive unilateral ECT treatments to left or right sides of the head has been used to determine language laterality in depressed patients (War-rington & Pratt, 1973; Annett, Hudson, & Turner, 1974). The effects of unilateral ECT are very similar to those of unilaterally injected sodium amytal. Left-sided ECT in dextrals leads to much greater impairment in verbal tasks than right-sided ECT, and the results are more variable in sinistrals (Pratt, Warrington & Halliday, 1971; these authors in fact recommend it as a less hazardous and less unpleasant technique than the Wada method for determining language dominance). Kriss, Blumhardt, Halliday, and Pratt (1978) reviewed the evidence that, in the immedi-ately postictal period after ECT to the dominant hemisphere, patients have signs of dysphasia, which usually resolve within half an hour of treatment; more persistent deficits in verbal memory last for more than an hour after treatment. Nonverbal and spatial deficits after treatment to the minor hemisphere can apparently last for hours or even days; the deficits in higher neurological functioning resemble the deficits found with lateralized cerebral lesions (see below), including unilateral spatial neglect. Findings such as these raise the possibility, which no one seems yet to have commented on, that because of the much longer time period at the disposal of the investigator, unilateral ECT, unlike the Wada test, may even be useful in determining the fine-grain receptive or perceptual aspects of language lateralization (and see also Fedio & Weinberg, 1971) rather than just the expressive or productive aspects, which have always been the more obvious, dramatic, and easier to assess. The reliability of the method and its correlation with other indices of language lateralization were assessed by Geffen, Traub, and Stierman (1978), who found that the ear contralateral to the dominant hemisphere for speech, as determined by unilateral ECT, was superior in hit rate or reaction time or both in a dichotic monitoring test.

The picture described so far is of a double dissociation, with disruption to left hemisphere processes (at least in dextrals) producing deficits of an essentially verbal nature and disruption to processes in the minor hemisphere affecting non-verbal (loosely, visuospatial) forms of processing. This is the picture whatever the methodological approach—application of the Wada (amytal) test, unilateral ECT, or observation of patients with unilateral cerebral lesions. As stated earlier, the Wada test and unilateral ECT are, in effect, forms of reversible lesioning. At the perceptual level such a double dissociation from the viewpoint of unilateral cerebral lesions is nicely demonstrated by the work of Warrington and Taylor (1978) who investigated visual object recognition in patients with left- or right-sided lesions. One task maximized perceptual categorization in terms of physical identity (the ability to recognize two representations of a familiar object, with one viewed from an unfamiliar angle). The other task maximized semantic categorization in terms of functional identity: The patient had to decide whether pictures of two objects (e.g., different types of chair such as a deck chair and a wheelchair) both represented the same superordinate category (chairs). Patients with right hemisphere damage were inferior in the first task, and those with left hemisphere damage were inferior in the second. Similarly, at the memory level, B. Milner (1977) reviewed the evidence for the proposition and herself further demonstrated that left temporal lesions led to verbal memory disorders and deficits in verbal IQ; damage to corresponding areas in the right hemisphere were detrimental to learning, recall, and recognition of non-verbal visual and auditory patterns and to performance in nonverbal IQ. She concluded that this supported the proposition that two memory codes exist, a verbal and an imaginal code, and that both are needed for efficient long-term recall. We shall further discuss the idea of two such memory codes, and whether there is possibly a more fundamental underlying dichotomy or mode of hemispheric specialization, in Chapter Nine.

Finally, Jones-Gotman and Milner (1977) noted that while right frontal and frontocentral lesions led to impairment in the ability to produce rapidly a number of different abstract, meaningless designs, similar lesions in the frontal regions of the left hemisphere reduced verbal fluency in an exactly analogous manner.

Aphasia

The written history of aphasia goes back at least four and a half thousand years, to the Ebers papyrus of Egypt, where there is the record of a man who, as a result of a head injury, "lost his ability for speech without paralysis of his tongue" (Hécaen & Albert, 1978). Likewise, the Edwin Smith papyrus, of similar date, contains the earliest known anatomical, physiological, and pathological descriptions of the effects of localized brain damage on body functions (e.g., paralysis and paresis) with a hint that the contralateral nature of brain-body motor control was known (Walsh, 1978). Historically, however, this latter knowledge first appears to have become explicit with the writings of the Hippocratic group of classical Greece, between the latter part of the fifth century and the middle of the fourth century B.C., when the reader is warned against prodding blindly at a wound in the temporal area of the skull lest paralysis of the contralateral side should ensue (Walsh, 1978; Giannitrapani, 1967). According to Giannitrapani, the Hippocratic school was even aware of the connection between left-sided head wounds and right hemiplegia and aphasia. By the first century A.D. Aretaeus the Cappadocian reported on the decussation of nerves from the left to the right side of the brain "in the form of the letter X," though it is unknown whether he was referring to the optic chiasm or the decussation of the pyramidal motor system. Cassius circa A.D. 450 explicitly addressed himself to the question of contralateral paralysis, and Lancisi in 1718 was the first to determine that the corpus callosum consisted of parallel transverse fibers and thought, because of its prominent central position, that it was the seat of the soul (Giannitrapani, 1967). In the first two decades of the nineteenth century, at the height of the misplaced enthusiasm for phrenology, when every bump on the skull was thought to indicate the presence of some positively or negatively valued faculty, Gall and Spurzheim proved anatomically the decussation of the pyramidal motor system.

Broca's aphasia. Aphasia, however, as currently recognized, dates from 1861 with the French neurologist Paul Broca's public exhibition of the brain of his patient Tan, so named because after loss of his power of speech the only sounds he could utter were the monosyllables "tan tan." The brain showed a lesion in the posterior-inferior portion of the left frontal lobe. It was not, however, until 1885 that Broca published his famous dictum *"nous parlons avec l'hémisphere gauche"* (Walsh, 1978). Broca's (eponymously entitled) aphasia is now a neurologically accepted and much described condition, consequent on injury (in dextrals) to the posterior portion of the third, or inferior, frontal gyrus or convolution (the frontal operculum), just in front of the primary motor zone for muscles of the lips, tongue, jaw, palate, vocal cords, and diaphragm—that is, the speech musculature (see Figure 4-1). However, it should be emphasized that the condition does not itself depend on paralysis of this musculature (which as we noted earlier, had been observed nearly five thousand years ago). Patients with this form of aphasia are normally said to show relatively good comprehension, though comprehension deficits are less

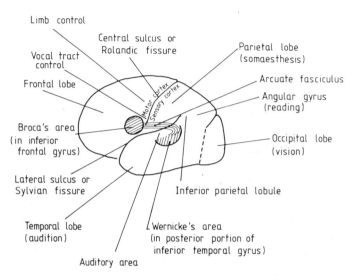

Limb control

Central sulcus or
Rolandic fissure

Vocal tract
control

Parietal lobe
(somaesthesis)

Frontal lobe

Arcuate fasciculus

Angular gyrus
(reading)

Motor cortex

Sensory cortex

Broca's area
(in inferior
frontal gyrus)

Occipital lobe
(vision)

Lateral sulcus or
Sylvian fissure

Inferior parietal lobule

Temporal lobe
(audition)

Wernicke's area
(in posterior portion of
inferior temporal gyrus)

Auditory area

FIGURE 4-1 Major surface features and language-related areas of the left hemisphere.

easily demonstrable or testable than articulation deficits, and many (e.g., Zurif, 1980) argue that Broca's aphasics do not have the relatively intact comprehension long ascribed to them. Zurif claims that they have problems comprehending complex syntax. They normally understand a sentence by inferring what makes factual sense from a sampling of its major lexical items (e.g., nouns and verbs) independently of the sentence's syntactic structure. They do this even for written presentations, suggesting that their deficit is not exclusively phonological. Be this as it may, the most obvious clinical characteristic of Broca's aphasics is that they typically produce little speech and do so slowly, nonfluently, and with effort and poor articulation. Speech is telegraphic or agrammatic; articles, connective words, auxiliaries, and inflections tend to be omitted; and there is a corresponding reliance on nouns and to a lesser extent on verbs. A typical example, elicited in response to a picture showing a boy hiding, a broken window, and an angry householder threatening a surprised girl who was passing by, might be: "Window . . . break. Boy, man, anger . . . girl what, boy hide, do it."

In Broca's aphasia ability to name objects is poor, but prompting helps, further indicating that the deficit is not solely at the articulation level, though the fact that the more encoded consonants seem to cause more difficulty than vowels and long words more than short suggests the presence of a motor component as well, which is to be expected in this frontal syndrome. Other evidence that Broca's aphasia is not due to partial paralysis of the articulators comes from the finding that right hemisphere lesions can induce the partial paralysis without the Broca component and that singing may be preserved in cases of Broca's aphasia. These aspects, and the frequent occurrence of phonemic paraphasias (deformed utterances where incorrect sounds are substituted for the correct ones in a word) are taken as evidence for the disorder's involving disorganization of the processor whereby phonological units are encoded (Benson, 1979a; Dimond, 1980; Hécaen & Albert, 1978; Walsh, 1978; Zurif, 1980). Dimond (1980) argues that the frontal lobe, where Broca's area is located, is a sort of drive mechanism for language, thus accounting for the fact that frontal lobe lesions outside the classical limits of Broca's area result in loss of verbal fluency, production, and spontaneous verbal activity (Benton, 1968). He therefore believes that Broca's area may extend a good deal further forward than was originally thought, with subcortical regions (e.g., the thalamus; discussed later in this chapter) also being involved in the generation, sequencing, and control of speech. The actual language generator may lie posterior to Broca's area, in the vicinity of what we shall see is normally regarded as the flow-through system for the echoic repetition of heard speech, from Wernicke's area (see the following section). Dimond therefore speculates whether an anteriorly enlarged Broca's area represents the homunculus or phonation map of articulation, where language elements for speech are laid down and which the brain can call upon to have its instructions realized in actual words. The output mechanism then smooths, shapes, and forms what it receives into a flowing sequence of articulated activity. Zangwill (1978) also speculates whether an area anterior to Broca's classical speech area may be involved in the more subtle aspects of linguistic activity and cautions against placing too great an emphasis on the localization of highly circumscribed aspects of language. He further cautions that lesions in Broca's area may result in permanent aphasia only if the subadjacent white matter is involved; otherwise, circumscribed cortical lesions in Broca's area itself perhaps only produce relatively transient motor aphasia.

Wernicke's aphasia (also known as sensory, receptive, or jargon aphasia). A few years after Broca first described the expressive form of aphasia that we have just discussed, the German Carl Wernicke in 1874 described a patient who had apparently lost his memory for the "auditory images" of words. This receptive aphasia was apparently the result of damage to the posterior portion of the superior temporal convolution, the first temporal gyrus on the parietal-temporal junction of the left hemisphere, which lies adjacent to Heschl's gyrus, the primary projection zone for hearing. Bogen and Bogen (1976) however, discuss the confusion as to the exact limits of Wernicke's area. The comprehension of speech is greatly affected, leaving the prosody and superficial form of expression unaffected, with apparently intact grammar and syntax, but with the actual content curiously devoid of meaning. Typical utterances, therefore, of a Wernicke's aphasic are fluent, rapid, effortless, but meaningless jargon, syntactically and prosodically well formed, but irrelevant and empty of content. Dimond (1980) gives the following example. The patient, when asked how he was, replied, "I felt worse because I can no longer keep in my mind from the mind of the minds to keep me from my mind and up to the ear which can be to find among ourselves."

Generally, there may be frequent semantic paraphasias (e.g., substituting *telescope* for *spectacles*), poor ability to name objects (without prompting), and grossly disturbed abilities to repeat or to read (Dimond, 1980; Hécaen & Albert, 1978; Walsh, 1978). Wernicke's aphasia should perhaps be seen in the context of the general effect of damage to wider areas of the left temporal lobe. Coughlan and Warrington (1978) thus found in such cases impaired (verbal) semantic memory in complex tasks of language comprehension and expression, word definition, word retrieval, object naming, naming from descriptions, word comprehension, and vocabulary, and where complex instructions had to be carried out. Since phoneme discrimination and articulation were relatively unimpaired, they concluded that temporal lobe damage affects the verbal memory store rather than the phonological, syntactic, and articulatory mechanisms that are involved with frontal lesions. Dimond (1980) appears to hold similar views when he argues that Wernicke's area contains the cortical map, or receptive template, for the analysis of spoken speech, a sensory dictionary. He also argues (just as he did for Broca's area) that Wernicke's area extends further back (occipitally) and upwards (parietally) than was classically thought.

Conduction aphasia. A major theoretical advance made by Wernicke at the time of his description of the aphasia that bears his name was the postulation of an as yet undescribed form of aphasia. Based on what he already knew about the two existing types, Wernicke predicted that patients would be found with a lesion that interrupted the (subcortical) connections between the two areas that subserved speech comprehension and speech production. A break in this conducting pathway should, he argued, interrupt a patient's ability to transmit what he had heard to the motor speech centers; in other words, it should disrupt his ability to repeat aloud what had been heard. Such a syndrome, known as conduction aphasia for obvious reasons, was subsequently described. Where the arcuate fasciculus, the connecting tract between Broca's and Wernicke's areas, is damaged or destroyed, there is typically a syndrome that may include some spontaneous speech abnormalities and that always includes loss of repetition ability and poor naming ability, with preserved comprehension of written and spoken speech, and inability to carry out verbal commands since the pathway forward to the motor areas is now destroyed.

Dimond (1980) however, argues that not only the arcuate fasciculus (the cortical pathway between the two major speech areas) but also the thalamus (a subcortical forebrain structure) is involved in integrating the input and the output aspects of speech. He wonders whether the arcuate fasciculus may even be part of the neural locus for the *generation* of language (it cannot be the *entire* locus, since spontaneous speech is not *entirely* destroyed or even necessarily *grossly* affected by fascicular damage). Somewhere in this region may lie the mental lexicon, for it would seem curious to argue that speech is received in Wernicke's area and produced in Broca's unless somewhere between them is the main semantic and phonological storehouse and generative area. This, however, is still speculation; we are as yet nowhere near knowing where (or how) speech is assembled and generated. The only conclusion that can be reached is that the left hemisphere is uniquely specialized more in terms of its anterior (expressive) rather than its posterior (comprehensional) aspects of speech (see Chapter Eight), though even in this respect severe damage to Broca's area may on occasion have surprisingly little apparent effect on motor speech (Mohr, 1973).

The localizationist (connectionist) versus holist debate. We have just seen that, according to Wernicke, the representation of language in the cortex involves the discrete operation of anatomically discernible interconnected areas, centers that involve the breaking down of language not simply in terms of linguistic categories (e.g., phonology versus semantics), but rather into the linguistic faculties of speaking versus listening. Broca's area is said to contain the rules for coding language into articulatory form, and Wernicke's area is said to be critical for the recognition of spoken language, with transfer of information in some sort of auditory form taking place between the two; a specific syndrome (conduction aphasia) is assumed to result if this connecting pathway is cut. A consequence of this localizationist-connectionist approach is that other linguistic faculties such as reading and writing, and their associated syndromes consequent upon focal brain damage, may be accommodated by identifying them with additional interconnected cortical regions. This approach, initiated by Wernicke (who opposed both the doctrine of the equipotentiality of the brain and the phrenological viewpoint of the brain as a mosaic of innumerable discrete centers) and further extended in modern times by such workers as Geschwind (1972) results in the formal typology of aphasia. This typology can predict the site of lesions in the case of previously undescribed constellations of symptoms (Zurif, 1980). Thus the condition known as *transcortical aphasia* is said to result if the two primary areas (Broca's and Wernicke's) are spared, though isolated from the rest of the brain, with consequent impaired speech production and comprehension, but intact repetition, of spoken words. In some ways it is the logical converse of conduction aphasia. Similarly, if the left visual cortex is damaged along with the splenium of the corpus callosum (the posterior portion interconnecting the visual areas), the patient, although still able to see in the left visual field, cannot *read*, because information received by the intact right occipital lobe cannot be transmitted to the left language area (Walsh, 1978). Consequently the patient, while unable to comprehend *written* language, can, if both Broca's and Wernicke's areas remain intact, both comprehend speech and speak spontaneously. We shall discuss this condition, known variously as pure, or agnosic, alexia, or alexia without agraphia, in more detail later.

Therefore, according to the neolocalizationist viewpoint as exemplified by Geschwind (1970, 1972), we can identify those parts of the brain that are implicated in the exercise of language, in that we know that when such regions are damaged, language becomes disrupted in predictable and selective ways. As Zurif (1980) observes, while pinpointing the source of symptoms is not the same as locating the functions involved, the selective manner in which language breaks down as a result of circumscribed lesions does bear some relationship to the manner in which language is organized in the brain.

However, even before the end of the last century the localizationist position was under attack, led by Pierre Marie in France and Hughlings Jackson in England. A typical argument was that Wernicke's area is the one true center for thought and that all aphasia is associated with defective comprehension. In contrast to the localizationists, who sought to place important functions in discrete cerebral structures, the holists conceived of the brain as a self-regulating total system of information flow with many redundant interconnections and saw language as a dynamic process derived from the integrated function of the entire brain, a view that has still not lost its adherents (Goldstein, 1948). It is certainly true that none of the speech areas is totally indispensible and that surviving speech functions often depend more on the amount of a given area left, rather than just the locus of a lesion (one example of the principle of mass action). Consequently, while there is *largely* a comprehension deficit after damage to Wernicke's area, and there is *largely* a difficulty with expression after damage to Broca's area, both decrements may appear, to varying degrees, after damage to either area. Zurif (1980) reviews the evidence for a moderately severe comprehensional deficit in Broca's aphasia, especially for the more complex syntactic forms, with Broca's aphasics seeming to be agrammatic not only in their speech production but also in their comprehension. Moreover, Broca's area may on occasion be totally destroyed *without* permanent aphasia (Mohr, 1973), while damage to another speech area that we have not yet mentioned and about which comparatively little seems to be known, the supplementary motor area (on the medial surface of the left hemisphere), invariably permits subsequent recovery. The suddenness of the lesion seems to be very important, as is the age at onset, with progressive damage in a child being far less serious than abrupt total onset in an older person (Finger, Walbran, & Stein, 1973).

The holists therefore criticize the localizationists (associationists) as providing an incomplete and insufficiently dynamic viewpoint, as giving too much emphasis to a collection of more or less independent components interconnected by tracts. Their arguments are cogent, as Marshall (1980) observes, in that the connectionist viewpoint, while describing symptoms well, does not satisfactorily capture the rich complexity of psycholinguistic organization. Marshall sees danger in "gluing" psychological flow charts, black boxes, arrows, and so on for hypothetical language elaboration to the surface of the brain and identifying the black boxes and arrows of the former with the centers and tracts of the latter. The alternative, he says, is a brain viewed as four-dimensional dynamic patterns of activities, undergoing moment-to-moment transitions from one steady state to another, with aphasia-producing damage merely leading to new, simpler, developmentally more primitive steady states. Conversely, with ontogenetic maturation the child's brain is seen as progressing up through a hierarchy of increasingly complex configurational steady states.

This is exactly the viewpoint of Brown (1980): The brain is built up of a series of successive layers, through both evolutionary and maturational growth, and after brain damage, speech descends to an ontogenetically simpler steady state. He discards the view of Broca's and Wernicke's areas as being depots in a cortical language circuit and regards the neocortical language zones and their adjacent perceptual (posterior) and motor (anterior) regions as being like the tips of an iceberg. These "tips," both in brain evolution and in brain function, are seen as being the latest evolved, as well as being activated from below. (We shall shortly discuss the possible role of the thalamus in the context of subcortical activation of language mechanisms.) Brown views the recovery from aphasia as a form of recapitulation of original language acquisition, mutism leading to agrammatism, which in turn gives way to phonemic and articulatory errors, and so on. Brown's position is one of an emergent rather than a flow system, with lesions not interrupting flow but producing a qualitative disruption that points to a particular level of representation. He does not view language as generated posteriorly and conveyed to the anterior for articulation, via pathways and tracts, or even via the thalamus; rather, he views the two areas as homologous, with the intervening pathways merely serving to time phase relationships, resulting in simultaneous realization of speech in both areas. He does not, however, say why we need both areas, except perhaps merely to increase, in a mass action sense, the overall processing capacity of the brain. As Marshall (1980) observes, while the associationist theory may eventually be proved wrong, it has proved supremely fruitful, and the holist (gestalt) view, while perhaps having a lot to say for itself, may be impossible to fully validate. Likewise, as Zurif (1980) observes, at some level of neural organization the effect of focal damage on language is selective. Connectionist (associationist, localizationist) theory is still too useful to be abandoned. We believe the final compromise is likely to involve discrete localization of function *between* certain areas, with a predominantly mass action effect *within* such areas, except perhaps for the primary projection areas of the senses where topographical organization is of fundamental importance.

Typologies of aphasia. We have not dealt so far with the typology of aphasia, except to point out the three major classifications that emerged from the localizationist–associationist approach (Broca's, Wernicke's, and conduction aphasia), and the single-mode, sensory aphasia, which the holists say underlies all others. But as Gaddes (1980) and Benson (1979a) observe, there are a vast number of classifications as a consequence of the number of neurologists, psychologists, speech pathologists, linguists, and psycholinguists who each have their own individual barrows to push, along with those of their disciplines. As the holists point out, no one aphasia fails to have elements of the others. Benson (1979a) suggests that to the above three major aphasias, which all involve disturbance of repetition ability, can be added four others where repetition is always intact. The first is mixed transcortical aphasia, where Broca's and Wernicke's areas are intact and still interlinked but isolated from surrounding tissue. This isolation of the speech areas results in very poor comprehension and no spontaneous speech. Repetition may be preserved in the extreme form of echolalia, where the patient merely echoes everything said to him or her. The second, transcortical motor aphasia, is somewhat similar to the above syndrome, but with prominent motor disturbance. The third, transcortical sensory aphasia, again resembles the first, but with fluent output, badly damaged comprehension, gross paraphasia, anomia (difficulty in finding and naming words), alexia (inability to read), and agraphia (inability to write). It involves lesions around but sparing Wernicke's area. Finally, in anomic (amnesic or amnestic) aphasia, comprehension is preserved, as of course is repetition, with fluent speech and little or no paraphasia, but there are problems in naming and difficulty in word finding, especially in conversational speech, leading to frequent "tip-of-the-tongue" states, which can result in lengthy circumlocutions. Although we seem to be contacting the site of the mental lexicon and the semantic associative network with these lesions, losses are rarely discrete for certain classes or categories of words or concepts. We are still a long way from understanding how words, concepts, and ideas are topographically represented in the brain.

Alexia

Reading is of course a complex learned activity, requiring a more deliberate participation by the learner than the initial acquisition of the first language. Consequently, it demands participation from several different anatomical areas. In this chapter we are only concerned with "acquired" disabilities, those that result from trauma after the patient had fully developed his or her linguistic (or other) skill. Developmental dyslexia (when the child does not acquire reading skill or acquires it only with great difficulty or incompletely) will be the subject of Chapter Thirteen. Acquired dyslexia was first reported in A.D. 30 by Valerius Maximus, who mentioned a man who was hit on the head by an axe and lost his memory for letters but experienced no other problem (see Benton, 1964). Mercuriale in 1588 first reported a case of alexia without agraphia: "A truly astonishing thing; this man (following a seizure) would write but could not read what he had written" (Albert, 1979).

As Albert (1979) and Hécaen and Albert (1978) observe, the alexias, like the aphasias, may be further subdivided: for example, pure alexia (without agraphia), alexia with agraphia, and pure agraphia (without alexia). The angular gyrus in the inferior parietal lobule (which lies at the confluence of the parietal, temporal, and occipital lobes and therefore integrates the various sensory systems of the body) seems to be of fundamental importance for reading. All the different classifications, moreover, boil down to a general agreement of two main types, alexia without agraphia and alexia with agraphia. Alexia with agraphia is fairly straightforward, involving a damaged or destroyed angular gyrus (the reading and writing center) with consequent loss of both faculties, usually with some aphasia. We have already mentioned alexia without agraphia in the context of connectionist theory as originally proposed by Déjerine and adopted by Geschwind: as a result of localized damage to the left occipital lobe and the splenium of the corpus callosum, which would otherwise link the (preserved) right occipital lobe to the angular gyrus, only the ability to read is lost because the latter reading center cannot receive visual input. Usually, the only symptom is a discrete loss of the ability to read (but not to write).

Albert (1979), however, further subdivides alexia without agraphia into three subtypes: literal alexia, verbal alexia, and global alexia, which is a combination of the other two. In literal alexia the ability to read letters is lost, but the ability to read whole words, especially common and concrete ones, may be preserved, though there may be paralexias (e.g., reading *stone* for *rock*). Low-frequency, abstract, and grammatical function words fare worst, and the patient cannot read nonsense words (e.g., *jife, zole,* etc.). Literal alexia seems to have much in common with a recently described acquired dyslexia known as deep dyslexia (see, e.g., Coltheart, Patterson, & Marshall, 1980), though Albert does not make this equation. We shall discuss deep dyslexia in greater detail in Chapter Eight, since many of the symptoms of the latter disorder seem to be the product of minor hemisphere reading mechanisms.

Albert's (1979) second form of alexia without agraphia, verbal alexia, is the opposite of literal alexia: the patient cannot grasp words globally but can read them letter-by-letter, synthesizing them into words (even with nonsense words), though with increasing difficulty in long words.

In Japanese, as we shall discuss further in Chapter Eight, there are two forms of script—*kanji* (ideograms, derived from Chinese and having no phonological values) and *kana* (representing syllabic sounds). Clinical studies with Japanese acquired dyslexics (see, e.g., Sasanuma, 1975; Sasanuma & Fujimura, 1971) demonstrated the independent functioning of the two systems of processing (semantic and phonological) and the two different anatomical loci that subserve them. Thus, as we shall see later, it is perhaps the phonological aspect of reading that is largely represented in the left hemisphere, while the right may retain the ability to obtain direct semantic information from a written word independently of grapheme-to-phoneme (phonological) recoding.

Brain Stimulation

In the introductory sections of this chapter we mentioned, as an alternative to lesion mapping of the language areas, the technique of brain stimulation, pioneered by Penfield (1958). This technique uses an exploring electrode on the exposed brain of a conscious patient to search out the epileptic focus, which can then be removed, terminating the disabling seizure activity. Penfield describes the effect of electrode stimulation on speech activity (usually arrest, sometimes perseveration, rarely the eliciting of true speech). The technique has since been further studied by Ojemann and his colleagues. Ojemann and Whitaker (1978b) found that the overall topographic extent of the language cortex is wider than that proposed in the classical (lesion) maps, though only a narrow band of the posterior-inferior frontal lobe, immediately anterior to the motor strip, showed speech involvement in *all* their patients. This motor area constitutes only a small portion of the frontal language area. Other inferofrontal, parietal, and posterotemporal sites showed considerable variability, some of this variability possibly being correlated with the individual's language experience as shaped by education and socioeconomic status. Ojemann and Mateer (1979) likewise performed stimulation mapping of the human peri-Sylvian language cortex during craniotomies under local anaesthesia. They tested naming, reading, short-term verbal memory, single and sequential orofacial movements, and phoneme identification. They found that orofacial movements and phoneme identification were altered by stimulation from the same sites, thus identifying a common system for language production and understanding. This finding supports the motor theory of speech perception, whereby from an analysis of errors, it is said that we comprehend speech more immediately in terms of the requisite motor movements that would be required to *reproduce* the heard speech sounds, rather than in terms of the sounds themselves. Ojemann and Mateer found that this common system for language production and understanding surrounds a final motor pathway for speech and is in turn surrounded by a separate short-term verbal memory system. Between the sequential motor-phoneme identification system and the memory system are sites where only naming or reading are altered, including sites related exclusively to syntax.

Ojemann and Whitaker (1978b) concluded that lesion mapping has problems because of the likelihood of plastic recovery. Stimulation mapping acts as a temporary lesion, much like introducing noise, and indicates which areas have *some* role in speech; the study of *stable* deficits after lesions indicates which areas are essential. However, one can ask what the effects of such stimulations really tell us, since it is a little like taking a high-voltage probe blindly to a computer. A positive response merely means that that area is in some way involved (maybe only as a distant access or trigger point), *not* that it is essential. A negative response does not even mean that the area is not involved in that function.

The Role of the Thalamus

So far we have almost exclusively discussed the role of the cortex in mediating language functions. However, as Dimond (1980) points out, the cortex is not the only part of the brain involved in language. He reviews the fairly long history of studies on the effects of thalamic lesions on language in terms of dysnomia, aphasia, loss of verbal fluency, perseveration, and decrements in verbally mediated cognitive performance. As in the cortex, there is a verbal–nonverbal dissociation of the effects of damage to the left and right thalamus (Ojemann, 1976; Riklan & Levita, 1970). Ojemann (1976) reviewed all his previous work on the effects of thalamic lesions on object naming, word finding, calculation, verbal short-term memory, and verbal fluency and concluded that the effects are often transitory, lasting for a few days or weeks, whereas the effects of cortical damage are lengthy or permanent. If the thalamus were an integrating center between the frontal and parietal language areas, one would expect the consequences to be more serious and long-lasting. Consequently, Ojemann speculated that the thalamus (in particular, the ventrolateral thalamus and a corner of the pulvinar) is an alerting mechanism, an attention-directing system for verbal information, retrieval, and so on.

In a subsequent paper, Ojemann (1977) reviewed his work on the effect of thalamic stimulation, performed during stereotaxic operations for the treatment of dyskinesias. Stimulation typically led to speech arrest and/or anomia (inability to name a pictured object) and perseveration of the first syllable of what would have been the correct name, together with repetition of the name of the previous item. There was also slowing, slurring, distortion, and a verbal short-term memory deficit. Ojemann speculated whether the left thalamus normally operates in an alerting capacity to direct attention to verbal information present in the external environment, this being blocked by stimulation, and to partly control the mechanical substrate of speech, respiration, the control of the oral facial muscles, and so on. However, it is difficult to see exactly how the analogous memory, recognition, and identification effects operate for nonverbal shapes with right thalamic stimulation.

Nonverbal Syndromes
Involving the Left and Right Hemispheres

In addition to verbal deficits, left hemisphere lesions are sometimes associated with impairment of learned purposeful movements (Albert, 1979; Hécaen & Albert, 1978), including both ideational apraxia (in which an object is inappropriately manipulated) and ideomotor apraxia (in which an action is incorrectly performed). Although a verbal involvement may underlie some syndromes, many of the problems, whether of perceptual discrimination or performance, seem to lie at a more abstract level of conceptual thought. They may in some cases be consequent on left hemisphere deficits associated with the ability to perform fine temporal discriminations and to perceive—or produce—sequential series of events. We shall discuss in detail left hemisphere mediation of serial, segmental, analytic activity in Chapter Nine.

The ability to find one's way around a building or through city streets—the dynamic topographical sense of oneself moving in the spatial environment—also appears to have a strong left hemisphere component (see Hécaen & Albert, 1978 and Walsh, 1978, for reviews; see De Renzi, 1978, for a contrary opinion), but the ability to form and manipulate static topographical maps and concepts without reference to one's own progression through that space depends more heavily on the right hemisphere. Likewise, left-lesioned patients generally do poorly on Gottschaldt's embedded figures test; those injured on the right do poorly with Street's figure completion test (Orgass, Poeck, Kerschensteiner, & Hartje, 1972).

Although the hemispheres are often not differentiated by either the incidence or the severity of visuoconstructive failures in constructional apraxia (see, e.g., Dimond, 1980; Walsh, 1978), when the patient is required to manipulate or construct shapes, patterns, or blocks, either from memory or from example, the nature of the errors or the inadequacies does often depend on the side of the lesion. With left hemisphere lesions (forcing the patient to rely on the intact right hemisphere), patients tend to draw pictures that show poor discrimination of elements and tend to simplify and to lose detail while preserving spatial relationships, keeping the overall configuration coherent and intact. With right hemisphere damage patients tend to draw pictures with laborious and haphazardly juxtaposed combinations of correctly discriminated features; they include unidentifiable details, superfluous elements, and scattered or fragmented parts. The whole lacks an overall coherent configuration or plan, and proportion and spatial interrelationships are typically faulty (Warrington, 1969).

Nonverbal, Visuospatial Performance and the Minor Hemisphere

During the first fifty years of systematic neurological research, the right hemisphere seemed to be mysteriously silent in all the higher functions of purposeful action, imagination, and reasoning. For most neurologists it was an unconscious automaton, obedient to the dominant hemisphere, a viewpoint that has not yet entirely disappeared (Eccles, 1973). It was not until World War II that the importance of the right hemisphere for nonverbal, visuospatial functions was demonstrated and the idea arose that the hemispheres are complementary (Paterson & Zangwill, 1944). A longstanding problem, however, (see Chapter Nine) has been how to define *nonverbal* and *visuospatial*. Is *nonverbal* defined by exclusion? What is space? How does it relate to personal and extrapersonal space? Can we distinguish the movement of an individual in space and his or her relationship to topography from the spatial relationships of elements relative to each other and to a whole, independent of an observer? Lack of agreement about how *nonverbal* and *visuospatial* are to be used has led to an unfortunate proliferation of contradictory claims and findings in this area; moreover, the more nebulous nonverbal, or visuospatial, deficits have often been more difficult to demonstrate than verbal ones.

Before attempting to systematize the findings in this area, we will briefly list some of the major ones (reviewed by Hécaen & Albert, 1978; Nebes, 1978; Walsh, 1978) so as to give the reader a feel for what is meant by a right hemisphere nonverbal, visuospatial deficit. The first thing to be noted is that while the deficits are by and large nonverbal, the term *visuospatial* is a misnomer in that the auditory and tactile modalities may also be involved. Right hemisphere damage is said to be associated with deficits in the following capacities:

Size discrimination and perception of direction (in both the visual and tactile modalities)

Stereopsis

Appreciation of spatial relationships between and within objects in extrapersonal space

Judgment of the location and orientation of stimuli, both with respect to each other and the observer

Perception of three-dimensional spatial relationships from two-dimensional representations

Ability to select components to complete a partially complete design

Completion of incomplete pictures

Perception of the relationship of parts to wholes

Recognition of objects portrayed by line drawings when much of the contour is missing

Recognition of objects from incomplete pictorial representations

Accurate perception, memory, and recognition of abstract or nonsense patterns that are too complex for verbal specification

Recognition of anomalies in paintings

Ability to correctly arrange pictures to tell a story

Ability to recognize objects when viewed from unusual angles

Ability to copy geometrical shapes and to perform block-design subtests of the WAIS

Facial recognition

De Renzi (1978) has attempted with some success to bring order into this somewhat confused picture, but perhaps the clearest and simplest account is that of Benton (1979). Both authors agree that bihemispheric involvement is most apparent with the more complex tasks; the more elementary the spatial ability tested, the more it is represented unilaterally in the right hemisphere. According to Benton, at the visuoconstructive level (whether the patient is required to synthesize components into a single entity as in block construction, to copy line drawings, or to draw objects from command) both the left and the right hemisphere may be involved, though in different ways, with different patterns of errors, and depending on whether the whole configuration or the component elements are emphasized to the patient. At the visuoperceptual level (which includes recognizing objects by separating figure from ground or on the basis of incomplete, inadequate, or mutilated figures; recognizing familiar faces and discriminating unfamiliar ones; perceiving colors and associating them with common objects), right hemisphere involvement is more pronounced, though as we shall see in the next section the situation is by no means clear-cut in face processing. Moreover, although the matching of color patches to each other is apparently largely mediated by the right hemisphere, when they have to be paired with the most appropriate achromatic line drawings of common objects, left hemisphere damage seems to be the more disabling, despite the apparent lack of verbal mediation. This is in accord with left hemisphere mediation of abstract conceptual thought. As we saw, Warrington and Taylor (1978) found that a left hemisphere injury was the more detrimental when a patient had to decide whether, for example, pictures of a deck chair and a wheelchair both represented a common superordinate category (chairs). We shall encounter in the next chapter exactly similar findings in a study that employed commissurotomized subjects (Levy & Trevarthen, 1976).

Finally, at the simple visuospatial level (e.g., matching of dot patterns and judgments of line orientation and of depth), Benton argues that clinical studies show that the right hemisphere is almost exclusively involved. The same seems

effect polar opposites. In verbal alexia patients are unable to grasp written words globally but are able to spell them out laboriously, letter by letter. With literal alexia the patient, while unable to sound out a word letter by letter or to identify it in terms of its phonology, can nevertheless read whole words, especially if they are common, concrete, high-frequency, high-imageable nouns (though such para-lexic substitutions as *rock* for *stone* are frequent). However, the ability to read low-frequency, abstract, non-imageable, grammatical, or function words (even if high-frequency) is impaired. There is also clinical evidence that the two forms of Japanese script—ideographic, non-phonological *kanji* and syllabic or phonological *kana*—are processed independently, the latter being much more clearly lateralized to the left hemisphere.

Brain stimulation has proved to be a valuable recent alternative and comple-ment to lesion mapping. Both approaches have recently demonstrated a lateralized role of the thalamus in the mediation of verbal and nonverbal functions. Thalamic effects are more transitory than those involving the cortex, and the thalamus may play an alerting role.

The left hemisphere is involved in ideational and ideomotor apraxia, disorders of learned purposeful movements. It also appears to play some role both in the dynamic topographic sense of the self moving in a spatial environment and in such visuospatial tasks as disembedding Gottschaldt's embedded figures. The right hemi-sphere appears to be responsible for the ability to form and manipulate static topo-graphic maps and concepts and to perceive Street's incomplete figures. In drawing and block-construction tasks, left hemisphere lesions result in compositions with poor discrimination of elements and oversimplification, though a pattern's overall configuration, or gestalt, remains intact. Damage to the right hemisphere, on the other hand, is typically associated with patient drawings showing a haphazard jux-taposition of correctly discriminated features and elements, superfluous elements, scattered or fragmented parts, and a whole lacking in an overall coherent configura-tion, plan, or proportion.

Visuospatial processing disabilities associated with right hemisphere damage include deficits in the recognition of objects, in the separation of figure from ground, in recognition on the basis of incomplete, inadequate or mutilated figures, in the matching of simple dot or line patterns, and in judgments of line orienta-tion and depth. Unilateral hemineglect is predominantly left-sided (after right hemisphere damage), while left hemisphere damage does not usually produce a complementary right-sided neglect.

Face recognition does not seem to be an exclusively right hemisphere func-tion, despite the fact that faces are typically recognized by global, holistic, or rela-tional rather than by piecemeal processes. Prosopagnosics, however, may be forced to rely on the feature-by-feature processing strategies. Deficits in face processing may take two forms: The first is true prosopagnosia, or agnosia for familiar faces, which, while largely mediated by the right hemisphere, nevertheless has some bilateral involvement; the second is defective discrimination of unfamiliar faces, which is almost exclusively a right hemisphere phenomenon. The question of whether there is something special about the recognition of faces compared with other complex monoorientational configurations is still unresolved.

A right hemisphere involvement may be demonstrated in certain aspects of music and singing, but clinical evidence shows that bilateral functions are often also involved. The clinical neurology of music is only beginning as an independent study, and the component elements of music are only now being isolated.

FURTHER READING

ALBERT, M. L. Alexia. In K. M. Heilman & E. Valenstein (Eds.), *Clinical neuropsychology*. Oxford: Oxford University Press, 1979.

BENSON, D. F. Aphasia. In K. M. Heilman & E. Valenstein (Eds.), *Clinical neuropsychology*. Oxford: Oxford University Press, 1979.

BENTON, A. Visuoperceptive, visuospatial and visuoconstructive disorders. In K. M. Heilman & E. Valenstein (Eds.), *Clinical neuropsychology*. Oxford: Oxford University Press, 1979.

BENTON, A. The neuropsychology of facial recognition. *American Psychologist*, 1980, *2*, 176–186.

DE RENZI, E. Hemispheric asymmetry as evidenced by spatial disorders. In M. Kinsbourne (Ed.), *Asymmetrical function of the brain*. Cambridge: Cambridge University Press, 1978.

DIMOND, S. J. *Neuropsychology: A textbook of systems and psychological functions of the brain*. London: Butterworths, 1980.

HÉCAEN, H., & ALBERT, M. L. *Human neuropsychology*. New York: John Wiley, 1978.

WALSH, K. W. *Neuropsychology: A clinical approach*. Edinburgh: Churchill-Livingstone, 1978.

ZURIF, E. Language mechanisms: A neuropsychological perspective. *American Scientist*, 1980, *68*, 305–311.

CHAPTER FIVE
Evidence from Commissurotomized (Split-Brain) Patients

In this chapter we shall be less concerned with the effect on verbal and nonverbal performance of localized or massive damage to one hemisphere and more concerned with the effect of disconnection of the otherwise relatively intact hemispheres. Severing some or all of the connecting fibers or commissures that run between these hemispheres disconnects them. Such surgery is usually performed to control or relieve otherwise intractable epilepsy. As we shall see, with suitably subtle testing this can result in a number of dramatic and unexpected manifestations of what is frequently described as a dividing or doubling of the state of consciousness.

It is only in the last few decades that, as a consequence of the commissurotomy operation, such questions as the unity of conscious awareness have been amenable to empirical investigation. However, speculation on such issues goes back to the middle of the last century. Harris (1980a) notes that Holland wrote a chapter in 1840 entitled "On the brain as a double organ," and Wigan developed an elaborate theory and claimed that "each cerebrum is a distinct and perfect whole as an organ of thought," and that "a separate and distinct process of thinking or ratiocination may be carried on in each cerebrum simultaneously. . . . In the healthy brain one of the cerebra is almost always superior in power to the other and capable of exercising control over the volitions of its fellow" (1844, p. 26). Fechner (1860) also pondered the brain's duplex structure; according to Zangwill he argued that if it were possible to divide the brain longitudinally in the midline (which he thought to be impossible in practice), something like the duplication of a human being would be brought about: "The two cerebral hemispheres, while beginning with the same moods, predispositions, knowledge and memories, indeed the same consciousness generally, will thereafter develop differently according to the external relations into which each will enter" (Zangwill, 1976, p. 537). McDougall (1911), however, disagreed that the stream of consciousness would be divided. He even bargained with Sherrington that if ever he (McDougall) should become incurably ill, Sherrington should sever McDougall's commissures to resolve the issue. As we shall see, the issue is not yet satisfactorily resolved: Although sophisticated and artificial procedures can demonstrate a division of consciousness, to casual observation the commissurotomized patient is surprisingly normal. As recently as 1957, Tomasch wrote that in consequence the corpus callosum, the most important of the forebrain commissures, is hardly connected with psychological functions at all. According to Bogen (1979) McCullough is reputed to have said at about the same time that the only function of the corpus callosum appeared to be to transmit seizure activity from one hemisphere to the other, and Lashley (1960), in jocular despair, declared that the corpus callosum served only to keep the hemispheres from sagging. This last remark is reminiscent of that of Vesalius who in 1543 argued that the corpus callosum does indeed serve as a mechanical support, its role as an intercommunicating nerve trunk not being recognized until the time of Viq d'Azyr in 1784 (Bogen, 1979).

The Forebrain Commissures

Of the three forebrain commissures—the corpus callosum and the anterior and hippocampal commissures—the first is by far the largest, interconnecting almost every part of the two cortices (see Figure 5-1). The genu and anterior third of the body interconnect the frontal lobes, the middle third is concerned with parietal and temporal lobe activity (somatosensory representation), and the posterior third of the body and the splenium interconnect the occipital lobes and deal with visual information (Gazzaniga & LeDoux, 1978; Walsh, 1978). The anterior commissure has mainly temporal interconnections but seems able to mediate the transfer of visual information in the absence (surgically induced or naturally occurring) of the corpus

FIGURE 5-1 The forebrain commissures (corpus callosum and anterior commissure), shown from a medial view of the right hemisphere, and the lobes that they interconnect.

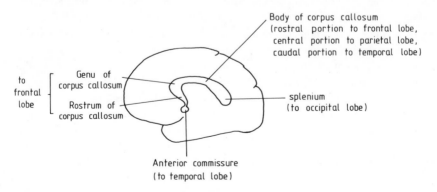

callosum. The hippocampal commissure interconnects the fornix. In addition to the above forebrain commissures, there is present in some human brains the massa intermedia, which, since it consists of grey rather than white matter, is not a true commissure; its role is uncertain. Midbrain connections that cannot be divided include the posterior and habenular commissures and, further back, the commissures of the brainstem and spinal cord (Bogen, 1979).

Sensory and Motor Representation:
Ipsilateral and Contralateral Pathways

For all senses except olfaction (which is predominantly ipsilateral), each half of the brain has dominant responsibility for the opposite half of the body. For vision, basically the left visual field (LVF) projects to the right side of the brain, in both midbrain and forebrain routes. In nonmammals the general rule is for the optic nerves from each laterally located eye to go to opposite sides of the brain, and in mammals partial decussation at the optic chiasm ensures that the LVF from both frontally located eyes reaches the right side of the brain, while the RVF projects to the left side of the brain. Thus, fibers from the nasal (inside) and temporal (outside) halves of each eye split up, fibers from the temporal hemiretinae projecting ipsilaterally and those from the nasal hemiretinae crossing at the chiasm to the opposite hemispheres (see Figure 5-2).

FIGURE 5-2   The visual system in man. The geniculo-striate system is arranged such that fibers from the nasal hemiretinae decussate, and the temporal fibers project to their ipsilateral cortices. This pattern of partial decussation ensures that stimuli falling in the left visual field project to the right hemisphere and vice versa.

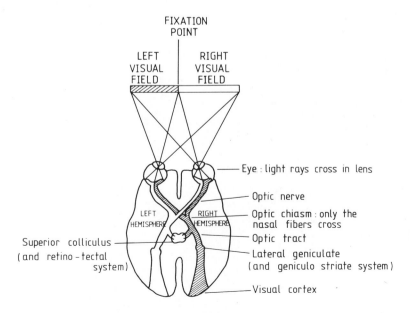

FIXATION
POINT

LEFT
VISUAL
FIELD

RIGHT
VISUAL
FIELD

LEFT
HEMISPHERE

RIGHT
HEMISPHERE

Eye : light rays cross in lens

Optic nerve

Optic chiasm : only the
nasal fibers cross

Optic tract

Lateral geniculate
(and geniculo striate system)

Visual cortex

Superior colliculus
(and retino-tectal
system)

With hearing, there is a greater degree of duplication of hemisphere function in mammals; each ear projects to both sides of the brain, due to a variety of decussations and commissures starting in the medulla (Pearson & Pearson, 1976; Seitz, Weber, Jacobson, & Morehouse, 1980). The contralateral auditory projection is, however, the more direct, and when information received from the two ears conflicts, the ipsilateral channel may be actively suppressed (Aitkin & Webster, 1972). Thus, visual input is much more strictly lateralized to the opposite side of the brain than is auditory input (see Figure 5-3).

The somatosensory (skin senses) organization is also predominantly contralateral: The dorsal column-medial lemniscal system, which mediates such functions as active exploratory touch and stereognosis, is completely crossed; passive touch, pain, and temperature, which are mediated by the spinothalamic system (see, e.g., Gazzaniga & LeDoux, 1978), have both contralateral and ipsilateral components.

Finally, motor control, like somatosensory organization, is predominantly contralateral, at least for the pyramidal motor system, though there is also a weaker ipsilateral route. The extrapyramidal system may act as a fail-safe auxiliary alternative, coming into use if the pyramidal system is damaged. Certainly the extrapyramidal system seems to be involved in the gradual restoration of motor function after extensive damage to the pyramidal system. It is also involved when in a com-

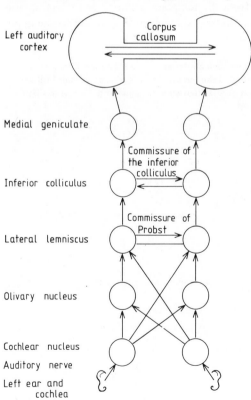

FIGURE 5-3 The auditory pathways. Note that each ear projects to both sides of the brain due to a variety of decussations and commissures, such that auditory input is less strictly lateralized than vision.

missurotomized subject a hemisphere is called upon to control its ipsilateral limb and cannot use the pyramidal system directly because it is contralaterally organized, or indirectly via the commissures (which are cut) and the opposite hemisphere. The pyramidal system dominates the weaker extrapyramidal system, otherwise synkinesis could result, rendering the individual unable to refrain from making bilaterally symmetrical movements when attempting to make a unilateral response. The pyramidal system, the most important motor system in primates, is responsible for fine, skilled movements of the distal musculature (e.g., fingers); the extrapyramidal system can initiate gross, coarser movements of the more proximal musculature (see, e.g., Brinkman & Kuypers, 1973).

Interhemispheric Learning and Memory Transfer in Animals

We have just seen that the LVF of either eye in mammals, especially those with medial eyes and forward vision, projects to the right hemisphere and the RVF of either eye projects to the left hemisphere. If we could be sure that the animal would maintain fixation, we could easily send visual information to one hemisphere by displaying it to the contralateral visual field. Since procedures to insure fixation are impractical, one solution is to cut the chiasm so that the nasal pathways (which cross at the chiasm) are destroyed, and each eye projects to the brain exclusively via the temporal, ipsilateral pathways. If this is done and one eye is covered, all visual input to the open eye will project to the ipsilateral hemisphere (see Figure 5-4).

In interhemispheric learning experiments, a chiasm-sectioned cat could have one eye covered while it learned a visual discrimination through the other. The

FIGURE 5-4 In normal animals, information from either eye reaches either hemisphere. When the chiasm is divided, this continues to hold true as long as the commissures are intact. When these are severed, information fed to the left eye reaches only the left hemisphere and that fed to the right eye goes no further than its ipsilateral hemisphere.

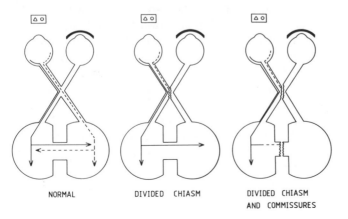

NORMAL   DIVIDED CHIASM   DIVIDED CHIASM
                                         AND COMMISSURES

occluded eye could then be uncovered, and the training eye in turn occluded. With intact commissures, the animal shows total interocular (i.e., interhemispheric) transfer of learning (Myers, 1955). However, when Myers (1956) cut the corpus callosum in cats prior to such training, he found that transfer did not take place. Similar findings were extended to the monkey and chimpanzee. Surgery *after* training seemed possibly to lead to slightly better performance (though still inferior to performance in unoperated cats) than surgery *before* training, suggesting that *some* information is transmitted without a learning test, though others dispute this (see, e.g., Guiard, 1980, for a review). However, in primates, unilateral training of one hemisphere prior to surgery apparently always results in the formation of bilateral engrams.

Although the interocular transfer of pattern discrimination in the cat was disrupted by commissurotomy, simple (perhaps subcortically mediated) brightness discriminations were unaffected (Meikle & Sechzer, 1960); however, deeper mid-sagittal section down to the commissure of the superior colliculus prevented transfer. It is even possible to teach commissure- and chiasm-sectioned monkeys to simultaneously make two mutually contradictory responses (Trevarthen, 1962, 1965). One hemisphere learns to respond positively to a circle and negatively to a cross, and the other hemisphere learns the opposite response. The response emitted at any one moment depends on which eye is open. Under these circumstances one hemisphere usually learns quicker and better than the other, suggesting midbrain attentional or inhibitory mechanisms of the sort that Trevarthen would refer to as involving metacontrol. Using the technique of spreading depression, whereby potassium chloride placed on one cortex can temporarily suppress its activity, Russell and Ochs (1963) found that with such unilateral training stored information is not transferred between the hemispheres, even if the animals are left to recover for long periods. If, however, the untrained hemisphere is given a few trials, an active "carbon-copy engram" is apparently transferred. Gazzaniga and LeDoux (1978) question whether it is engrams or sensory information that transfer (i.e., with intact commissures the trained hemisphere learns by direct sensory exposure and the naive one by *transcommissural* sensory exposure: in both cases it would be sensory information that is important and that transfers, rather than the engrams). They also criticize the cortical-spreading depression technique (which was said to prove the existence of mobile engrams) as being methodologically unsound. As proof of their thesis that sensory information rather than engrams transfer, they cite an experiment by Risse and Gazzaniga (1976) in which a human subject had his left hemisphere inactivated by intracarotid sodium amytal while the right acquired the engram of a spoon by palpating it, unseen, with the left hand. The left hemisphere, when it recovered, was unable to say what had been presented, but the right hemisphere could still pick out the unseen spoon from among other objects using the left hand. This suggests that engrams remain localized to the hemisphere that originally acquired them, do not transfer, and remain inaccessible to the other side. In answer to the question of why the commissures should transfer sensory but not mnemonic information, they argue that the commissural connections are largely homotopic, the fibers arising and terminating in the same general location in opposite hemispheres, in the *sensory* (and motor) but not the association (*memory*) areas.

The Psychological Consequences
of the Commissurotomy Operation in Humans

A number of problems of interpretation are associated with the otherwise often dramatic observations of the consequences of commissurotomy. Relatively few such subjects are available for study, and they vary greatly in their age at the time of original brain damage, age at operation, severity of their preexisting illness, educational attainment, and so on. Prior to surgery many of them have had long-standing epilepsy, which can lead to functional reorganization of the brain. The surgery itself is fairly traumatic, involving manipulation of brain tissue and the disruption of blood supply.

Moreover, since it is obviously impractical and undesirable also to divide the optic chiasm in humans, special highly artificial techniques are usually required to demonstrate the effects of dividing the forebrain. One such technique is to tachistoscopically flash visual information to one or the other visual field for shorter durations than would permit a fixational eye movement toward the stimulus. Such durations, typically around 150 msec, do not permit much visual information to be presented. Zaidel's scleral contact lens system, an alternative technique that occludes one or other hemifield (see p. 68), also has disadvantages. Dichotic presentation, whereby two competing messages are simultaneously presented, one to each ear, results in almost total occlusion of the ipsilateral auditory pathways by the contralateral auditory pathways in commissurotomy patients (Milner, Taylor, & Sperry, 1968; Sparks & Geschwind, 1968) and the unilateral reception of an auditory signal (but see Chapters Six and Seven for recent contrary views). Again, however, dichotic presentation is an artificial technique requiring precise temporal alignment of items matched for length.

Other interpretive problems are the possibility of interhemispheric transmission by other midbrain commissures and the fact that the disconnected hemispheres are not subject to the mutual facilitation and inhibition of the normal brain, with the result that their functioning must in some sense inevitably be abnormal. Finally, there is the problem of cross cueing (see p. 64), whereby one hemisphere may learn (consciously or unconsciously) how to transmit information extracallosally to the other by initiating bodily gestures, orienting responses, or even vocalizations, which the other can pick up and act on.

We can perhaps divide research on the psychological effects of the commissurotomy operation into four historical periods (see, e.g., Zaidel, 1978a). The first of these, in the 1940s, involved the subjects of Akelaitis, and for them no observable psychological effects were reported—as we now know, because insufficiently subtle testing procedures were available and possibly also because the anterior commissure was often spared (see Gazzaniga & LeDoux, 1978). This commissure can transmit much of the visual information that otherwise would be handled by the corpus callosum.

The next three periods all involved the patients of P. J. Vogel and J. E. Bogen, who were studied by R. W. Sperry from the early 1960s. His early work (1964) demonstrated the often dramatic effects of splitting the hemispheres into two independent cognitive systems, with verbal processes the major responsibility of the left hemisphere and the disconnected right hemisphere being mute but not unthinking. Later work (around 1968 to 1972) elaborated and extended Sperry's findings, in particular demonstrating the right hemisphere's complementary superiority in a number of nonverbal, visuospatial tasks that emphasized the gestalt, holistic aspects of stimulus processing. The most recent work, which has extended over the last ten years, is noteworthy for the development of new and more sophisticated testing procedures, such as the use of chimeric stimulation (discussed later in this chapter) and Zaidel's scleral contact lens technique. This technique permits free ocular scanning by one hemisphere at a time and circumvents the problems associated with brief tachistoscopic exposures to one or the other hemifield. It has extended the concept of cerebral dominance from one of unilateral competence to one of unilateral control, in which the nature of the task and the subject's expectancies, rather than the verbal-nonverbal nature of the stimuli, the modality of input, or the hemisphere stimulated, determine which hemisphere assumes control over the whole behaving organism ("metacontrol"). This, as we shall see in Chapter Nine, has led to the concept of the left hemisphere as operating largely in terms of analytic, sequential, segmental, and logical strategies while the right adopts largely synthetic, gestalt, and holistic approaches. The development of Zaidel's free ocular scanning device has also made it possible to survey the limits of hemispheric competence, from perception to intelligence, language, and personality structure in general, untrammelled by the constraints of the tachistoscopic procedure.

In the early 1960s, when the results of studies performed by Sperry's group were first reported (see, e.g., Sperry, 1964), it appeared that while the commissurotomy patients were well able to report words and pictures flashed to the RVF (left hemisphere), they could not express in words or in writing verbal or pictorial stimuli presented to the LVF. The right hemisphere apparently had a complete expressive aphasia, although it did recognize such LVF (right hemisphere) input, as evidenced by the ability of the left hand to point to a matching stimulus or even in some cases to select the name of the object from a list. If pictures of two objects were simultaneously flashed, one in each hemifield, a patient could only select the LVF object with the left hand and the RVF object with the right hand (in either case from a grab bag containing an assortment of unseen objects) and could only name the RVF (right-hand) object and would often confabulate if asked to name the LVF (left-hand) object. If the pictures of the two objects flashed to the two visual fields were identical, this could not be reported by the patient. Nor could the patient execute with the right hand or foot spatial or pictorial instructions flashed to the LVF (right hemisphere) or obey with the left hand verbal commands presented to the right ear under conditions of competing dichotic input.

Often these apraxias gradually resolved, suggesting that either hemisphere gradually acquired control over the ipsilateral as well as the contralateral motor pathways. Indeed, the only observable deficit of the left hemisphere, a mild constructional apraxia of the right hand for drawing (but not writing) and for building block designs, was itself also transient, passing in a few months as the right hemisphere obtained better control of the right hand.

At the somesthetic level, unseen objects held in the right hand were manipulated, named, and described correctly, while such objects held in the left hand, though correctly manipulated and identified by pointing, selection, or retrieval, could not be named; that is, there was an apparent unilateral tactile anomia. Objects discriminated by palpation by one hand could not be recognized by the other, though there was no difficulty in recognition when the original hand was retested. If, however, the patients knew that there was only a limited number of possible objects for discrimination, and if the objects greatly differed qualitatively and quantitatively from each other, one perhaps being a soft, round, light ball and the other a hard, rectangular, heavy block, intermanual discriminations and verbal identification of objects held in the left hand were sometimes possible. Presumably, this was because ipsilateral (spinothalamic) projection systems for somesthesis can with time develop the capacity to convey these gross aspects of information (Gazzaniga & LeDoux, 1978). Fine tactile details of the sort that can only be mediated by exploratory touch, stereognosis, or such seem, however, to be transmitted more or less exclusively via the contralateral lemniscal system. Similarly, when an examiner imposes a specific position on one hand of a blindfolded patient, the patient cannot mimic it with the opposite hand. Pictures of hand positions flashed to one visual field can be copied by the ipsilateral hand but not by the contralateral one. The patient cannot name exact points stimulated on the left side of the body, particularly in the case of the fingers, less so for the face, nor can the patient touch thumb to finger of one hand to indicate which finger has been touched by the examiner on the other hand (Bogen, 1979). Interestingly, children also have difficulty in cross-matching tactile information *between* (but not within) hands (Galin, Johnstone, Nakell, & Herron, 1979). Galin et al. (1979) claim this is due to the slow rate of maturation and myelination of the corpus callosum, which is not complete until puberty (see, e.g., Lecours, 1975; Selnes, 1974; Yakovlev & Lecours, 1967). Thus, the late-developing corpus callosum probably subserves late-developing functions.

The fact that the left hand can nevertheless obey *verbally* given instructions, as long as they are not too complex, and can retrieve named objects or even objects described by their functions indicates that the right hemisphere can comprehend simple speech. It can also read simple names, as indicated by the left hand's ability to select an appropriate item, even though it cannot *say* what the objects (or names) flashed to the LVF are. Similarly, commissurotomy patients cannot name smells presented to the right nostril (unilateral verbal anosmia), though they can identify them nonverbally by pointing to the correct associated objects, and they have no difficulty with smells presented to the left nostril. This follows from the fact that the olfactory pathways transmit ipsilaterally, to the same side of the brain, unlike the other senses, which are largely contralateral in their projections.

The Phenomenon of Cross Cueing

As we saw in the previous section, early reports emphasized the lack of any evidence for expressive language from the right hemisphere; subjects were unable to name, verbally or in writing, objects seen in the LVF or felt by the left hand, though nonverbal testing showed comprehension was unimpaired. Later, however, it became apparent that with practice the patients became able to report verbally whether a light flashed in the LVF was in the upper or lower quadrant. Upward or downward eye movements were apparently read off by the left hemisphere (as revealed by cinematography), which initiated the appropriate verbal response. Similarly, the patient can come to report verbally whether a light flashed in the LVF is red or green (if these are the only two possibilities). The right hemisphere, knowing the answer, emits a motor response (e.g., a flinch, sigh, groan, frown, or grimace) whenever the left hemisphere emits an incorrect response (Gazzaniga, 1970). These somesthetic cues are picked up by the left hemisphere and a correction is made. This cross cueing may not necessarily be conscious and deliberate, though when, as we shall see in a later section, the left hand is observed tracing letters on the back of the right hand, enabling the left hemisphere to name something flashed to the LVF, one wonders about the possibility of deliberate, independent initiation of informative actions by the right hemisphere for the benefit of the left. We shall discuss the question of two separate and independent volitional systems and streams of consciousness in a later section of this chapter.

A further example of what appears to be deliberate cross cueing is reported by Nebes (1978). Some patients became able to name numbers flashed to the LVF, apparently by subvocal counting (in the left hemisphere); the right hemisphere, when it perceived that the correct number had been reached, initiated a bodily movement of some sort, which signaled the left hemisphere to stop counting and to call out the number that had been reached. That this was happening became evident from the fact that the LVF response time was a function of the magnitude of the digit (0-9) flashed, but the RVF response time was not. While this cross-cueing explanation accounts for some, though perhaps not all, manifestations of apparent expressive powers in the right hemisphere, it also points to the need to determine what the *left* hemisphere knows when the capacity of the right is being tested.

The Right Hemisphere's Visuospatial Superiority

While the right hand in the commissurotomy patient, as in normal subjects, continues to be superior for writing, the left hand generally appears to be superior (unlike before surgery) for tasks such as drawing and copying (Bogen, 1969a). In tasks that call for construction of patterns (e.g., Koh's blocks), the left hand is generally quick and accurate, while the right is slow and spatially disorganized. Indeed, the left hand often reaches out and attempts to correct mistakes made by the right hand (Nebes, 1978), something that does not seem to happen with the right hand when the left hand attempts writing. In fact, as we shall see, the right hemisphere often seems to be aware of the existence and cognitive potential of the left, while the verbal left hemisphere seems far more often to be unaware of or to ignore or neglect the right. The general picture of the right hemisphere readily producing drawings whose general outline and spatial interrelationships are preserved, at the expense of detail, and the left hemisphere producing labored, detailed constructions with an inaccurate overall configuration or pattern of interrelationships between the elements is one we have already met in the clinical context (Chapter Four).

Levy-Agresti and Sperry (1968) devised a task where the commissurotomy patient was required to choose the two-dimensional representation that, when (mentally) folded into three-dimensional form would produce the solid shape that the patient was currently feeling, unseen, with the left or right hand. The test objects each had a unique shape and pattern of textural surfaces. The left hand was generally greatly superior, though the two hands seemed to employ different perceptual strategies in terms of the observed pattern of errors: The right hand (left hemisphere) adopted an analytic approach, concentrating on specific features or details, and the left hand (right hemisphere) seemed to fold up the two-dimensional layout mentally and to visualize the solid form as a whole.

Zaidel and Sperry (1973) devised a tactile version of Raven's Progressive Matrices, a nonverbal, visuospatial task where the subject is required to identify and select the component that would complete an otherwise incomplete pattern. The subject was shown a pattern with a piece missing, while he felt around behind a screen to select a plate with the raised pattern of lines that would complete the visual design. Again the left hand (right hemisphere) proved far superior, and again it seemed to perform its examination in a different style from the right hand (left hemisphere). The left hand seemed to operate primarily in terms of spatial wholes, while the right hand (left hemisphere) put a higher priority on such details and isolated features as the number of elements, the length of the lines, the size of the angles, and so on.

Using tactile and visual appreciation of forms to be matched, Franco and Sperry (1977) found that the hemispheres differed in their recognition of geometric similarity in a manner that is related to the mathematical rules for space by which the forms were constructed. While all forms were perceived or understood better by the right hemisphere, there was a gradient for this lateralization. Topological similarities were perceived better than all others by the right hemisphere; the more rule-bound and more verbalizable Euclidean forms were relatively better understood by the left hemisphere. Projective and affine groups were intermediate. Thus, the mathematical groups seemed to engage different intuitive analyses, even in subjects with no experience in the relevant geometries.

Nebes (1978) reviews three experiments of his own, which are in the same tradition. In the first (Nebes, 1971a) the commissurotomy patients were required to choose, from among three different-sized circles, the one to which a given arc would belong. Either arcs or the circles or both were examined haptically by either the left or the right hand. Subjects were better at matching arcs to appropriate-sized circles when using the left hand, though the hands did not differ in ability when matching circles to circles or arcs to arcs. These findings suggested that the right hemisphere, once more, was better at matching parts to wholes, at generating the concept of the whole stimulus from partial information. In his second study, Nebes (1972) again required his commissurotomy subjects to conceive of the whole from its parts by showing them a series of line drawings, each depicting a geometrical shape that had been cut up and the pieces moved apart, though the pieces still maintained their original orientation and relative positions, as in the "exploded" diagrams of workshop manuals. For each visual stimulus the subject had to reach behind a screen, feel three solid forms, and select the one that the fragmented figure would constitute if reunited. Again the left hand (right hemisphere) proved superior. In his last experiment, Nebes (1973) confirmed that the left hand was superior at discerning patterns inherent in an array of raised dots.

Such experiments seem to suggest that the right hemisphere is superior at perceiving the overall stimulus configuration inherent in the spatial organization of its parts, and that it functions more efficiently where a configurational synthesis must be formed from fragmentary or incomplete information. Conversely, as we shall see in more detail in Chapter Nine, the left hemisphere appears to be superior for performing an analytic, serial, or segmental breakdown of a whole into its component elements. This characterization may often cut across the general verbal-nonverbal or verbal-visuospatial dichotomy, though we believe that the latter two dichotomies are dependent on, and are largely special cases of, the analytic-holistic distinction.

Gazzaniga and LeDoux (1978) argue from their studies of commissurotomy cases that the left hemisphere is deficient in tasks requiring *active touch* for the recognition of unfamiliar objects or complex patterns; the right hemisphere's advantage is strongest for active manual exploration, being merely "small and statistical" for purely visuospatial (i.e., nontactile) discriminations. We agree that effects may be strongest when there is motor involvement (and see also Harris, 1980b, and Harris & Carr, 1981), just as the right hemisphere is most deficient in *expressive* verbal processes, although it possesses considerable powers for *comprehending* language. Nevertheless, we believe that there is now a vast body of research in the clinical literature (see Chapter Four), in the commissurotomy literature (cited in this chapter), and in the work on normal subjects (in Chapter Six) indicating that the right hemisphere is superior on visuospatial tasks in general and tasks involving holistic, gestalt apprehension in particular, whether or not there is motor or tactile involvement. In fact, we strongly disagree that visuospatial differences between the hemispheres are merely "small and statistical" (Gazzaniga & LeDoux, 1978, p. 68).

Ambient Vision and Focal Vision

Trevarthen (1974a, b) describes a number of his studies that employed point-source shadow casting of apparently three-dimensional images on a back projection system that filled most of his subjects' visual field. It gave subjects the impression of objects or space moving around them and permitted the exploration of long-lasting moving stimuli and contours in the peripheral visual field. Trevarthen found that bars moving together on each side of a fixation point generated the perception of a single inclined plane sloping up or down in front of the subject, despite the fact that the two elements went separately to the two (*divided*) hemispheres. Subjects were able also to judge whether two moving lines on each side of the fixation point were colinear or not, or equidistant or not, or moving in the same or opposite directions. He explains the survival of such an ability, despite hemispheric deconnection, as depending on an alternative, undivided midbrain visual system, analogous to the second (extrapyramidal) motor system described earlier in this chapter. Thus, while we rely on the classical geniculostriate projection system (focal vision, which is divided in commissurotomy) for fine detailed vision and for the recognition and identification of specific objects viewed in the fovea, there is also a phylogenetically older, undivided midbrain system. This latter retinotectal system ("ambient" vision) is still important in higher vertebrates for the detection of movement, of "where" rather than "what," and for signaling to the geniculostriate system that there is an event in the periphery that requires foveal fixation for its identification (see, e.g., Schneider, 1969). It may account for the paradoxical reported capacity of some people blinded by damage to the striate cortex to be able under forced choice conditions to detect the presence of moving and flashing objects whose very existence they nevertheless deny seeing (Weiskrantz, 1980). Be that as it may, Trevarthen certainly found that his subjects could not identify patterned objects in this way; they could report only on orientations, relative positions, and relative movements, and then only if they were careful not to try to describe or reach out with the right hand toward the stimuli. If they did so, the LVF component would typically tend to disappear, presumably as focal vision was "switched in" (see also Trevarthen & Sperry, 1973).

Chimeric Stimulation

Trevarthen together with Levy was also responsible for the pioneering of another technique for determining the limits of cognitive abilities in the disconnected hemisphere, that of chimeric stimulation. Just as the Greek chimera was a mythical composite beast, part lion, part goat, with a dragon's tail, so chimeric stimuli in these experiments consisted of pictures of two halves of separate objects (faces, line drawings), the right half of one object abutted to the left half of the other. These pictures were flashed so that the junction of the composite fell on the retinal

meridian. The phenomenon of completion across the midline, present both in commissurotomy patients and hemianopics, meant that each hemisphere perceived a
different complete whole object, rather than either two separate halves or a composite made of two disparate halves juxtaposed. Levy, Trevarthen, and Sperry
(1972) noted that this completion process (as indexed by the subject's being asked
either to describe what he or she had seen or to point to it from among an array of
alternatives) was particularly strong to the left when verbal report was used; that is,
the subject selected the object corresponding to the RVF half of the chimera. Conversely, it was particularly strong to the right (the subject selected an object corresponding to the LVF half of the chimera) when the subject instead was asked to
point to it or draw it.

Thus, under chimeric stimulation both hemispheres operated simultaneously
on the conflicting information, in their own preferred modes of operation, and the
preferred side depended on the response asked of the subject and the hemispheric
strategy that was most proficient. When the subjects pointed to the picture of an
object whose name rhymed with the name of the seen (chimeric) object, the right
half of the chimera predominated; when they picked from an array the line drawing
of a common object that was similar to the chimeric item, the right hemisphere
(i.e., left half predominating) made *structurally* similar matches while the left
hemisphere (right half predominating) made *conceptually* or *functionally* similar
matches (Levy & Trevarthen, 1976). These effects occurred either as a result of
specific instructions to the subjects (e.g., match items that *look alike,* or that *go
together*), or when the instructions were deliberately left vague and ambiguous
(e.g., match items that are similar *in some way*). In the latter ambiguous condition,
sometimes the left hemisphere predominated (employing a conceptual matching
strategy), and sometimes the right hemisphere predominated (employing a structural or similarity matching strategy). This suggests that hemispheric dominance
is not just due to a speed or skill contest between the hemispheres, but rather that
it depends on expectations as to the cognitive requirements, regardless of whether
these cognitive specialties are actually utilized or optimal. Levy and Trevarthen
describe this phenomenon as *metacontrol,* whereby expectancy may determine
moment-to-moment hemispheric supremacy, perhaps via brain stem activating
mechanisms. We have already seen (Trevarthen, 1962, 1965) another instance of
this metacontrol concept, in split-brain monkeys who have learned two mutually
contradictory discriminations, one in each hemisphere: One hemisphere usually
wins out when both are exposed simultaneously to the conflicting stimuli; which
is the winner is often determined by, for example, the hand available for responding.

Getting Away from the Limitations of the Tachistoscope:
A Device to Permit Ocular Scanning by a Single Hemisphere

Up to this point we have considered only situations where visual information is
briefly flashed, usually for about 150 msec to avoid fixational eye movements, to
one or the other visual field and in consequence to the contralateral hemisphere.
Zaidel (1976, 1978a, b) reported the development of a technique for presenting

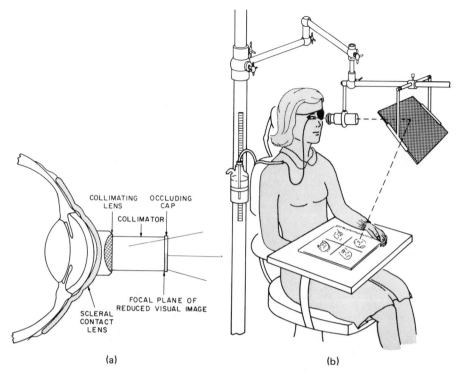

(a)   (b)

FIGURE 5-5 (a) Zaidel's scleral contact lens with mounted collimator and occluding screen for prolonged, lateralized visual presentations. (b) His experimental set-up. (From E. Zaidel, "Auditory Language Comprehension in the Right Hemisphere Following Cerebral Commissurotomy," Figures 12.1 and 12.2, pages 232 and 233, in A. Caramazza and E. B. Zurif, eds., *Language Acquisition and Language Breakdown: Parallels and Divergencies.* Baltimore, Maryland: The Johns Hopkins University Press, 1978. Courtesy of the publisher and author.)

continuously lateralized visual stimuli to a single hemisphere, therefore permitting free ocular scanning. The commissurotomized subjects are fitted with a scleral contact lens on one eye (the other is covered). On the lens is mounted a small screen in the system's focal plane, half of which is opaque, blocking out vision in one half field. Thus, it blocks out the desired half field of vision wherever the gaze is directed. This technique is a variation on the collimator method for presenting stabilized retinal images; the main difference is that the half-field occluder rather than the viewed image itself is stabilized. In this way free ocular scanning and manual manipulation of the lateralized stimuli are possible (see Figure 5-5).

Using this technique, Zaidel (1978a) employed a tactile version of a visual sequential memory test, which required subjects to reorder from memory a sequence of nonmeaningful but probably verbalizable geometric figures, and found that the left hemisphere was superior. The right hemisphere was superior for short retention intervals in a task that simply required the memorization of geometric figures, but with longer retention intervals this gave way to a left hemisphere superiority as the subjects were forced to employ verbal recoding. When embedded figures were to be disembedded from larger, more complex figures (Zaidel, 1973) a left hemisphere superiority emerged, the left hemisphere having the better analytic ability at discovering an element or pattern within an irrelevant background.

At the level of language, Zaidel (1978b) found that the disconnected right hemisphere can form both upper and lower case writing and has an elaborate awareness of meaning, but it is normally blocked from vocal responding by the left hemisphere, presumably via brain stem motor systems. The right hemisphere's auditory comprehension is less for low-frequency, abstract words or for more complex or lengthy instructions, perhaps because it has a short-lasting verbal memory. This in turn may be due to its lack of a constructive phonemic rehearsal mechanism. The right hemisphere is consistently poorer at reading than at auditory comprehension, and its visual vocabulary is smaller than its auditory one. It appears to possess no grapheme-to-phoneme translation rules and so may read words ideographically, as visual gestalts (Zaidel, personal communication). Earlier attempts (see Gazzaniga, 1970, and Chapter Eight) to demonstrate right hemisphere comprehension of written verbs and adjectives, tense, number, active or passive, and syntactic relationships may well have been unsuccessful because of the brief duration of the tachistoscopically exposed stimuli. This would penalize the slower right hemisphere processes. They might also have been unsuccessful because inappropriate "acting out" motor responses were used, which would have been subject to left hemisphere blocking. Zaidel's use of Socratic questioning techniques (requiring yes or no answers) and pointing obviated these difficulties.

We can therefore conclude, contrary to all the earlier reports in the literature, that the isolated right hemisphere can arrange letters into words and even perform some limited writing and can recognize a wide range of written words, not just concrete nouns as earlier claimed (Gazzaniga, 1970). Syntactically inferior to the left, the right hemisphere in Zaidel's studies is shown to be able to recognize and select objects on the basis of abstract descriptions or definitions of their usage, given aurally. It behaves like a nominal aphasic, knowing an object's use and qualities, but not its name, which is then often provided, incorrectly, by the left hemisphere's guessing. Indeed, while the right hemisphere is directing writing responses of the left hand, the left hemisphere may assume control, via the ipsilateral pathways, halfway through, and incorrectly complete the word, also verbally supplying its guess, which corresponds to the incorrectly completed ending of the word. Inadequate writing performance by the right hemisphere, however, is likely to be more a cause than a consequence of left hemisphere interference under these circumstances. We shall discuss later (in Chapter Nine) why the right hemisphere may be better at written than at vocal expression, though we should note at this stage that speech is an older (phylogenetically and ontogenetically) and more automatic capacity than writing; the speech apparatus, unlike the limbs, is unpaired and may therefore require unilateral control to avoid competition for output.

It is misleading to conclude that language is lateralized to the left hemisphere; this may be true for *expressive* speech since the right hemisphere is indeed almost entirely mute except, occasionally, for single word or phrase clichés, automatisms, or oaths that can be uttered as discrete units and can briefly escape left hemisphere inhibition. However, writing, though still very strongly lateralized, is less lateralized, and comprehension is the least lateralized. The right hemisphere has a surprisingly rich aural lexicon but is poor at the phrase, sentence, and syntax level. The left hemisphere retains its lead in semantic association. As we shall see in Chapter Eight the linguistic mental age profile for the isolated right hemisphere, as tested by Zaidel's technique, does not correspond to any particular stage in first language acquisition. Interestingly, the isolated left hemisphere also is found to have some deficits, such as in reading speed and richness of spoken vocabulary, perhaps partly attributable to the lack of a normal right hemisphere contribution (Zaidel, 1978a).

Employing versions of standard intelligence tests, Zaidel (1978a) found that the two hemispheres may reach approximately the same levels of competence, suggesting that the tests tap bilateral components but often via different strategies and with a different preferred style of performance. Thus, an error analysis once again revealed that the left hemisphere operates via a feature analytic approach, while the right adopts a more holistic strategy of pattern recognition; using these two strategies the two isolated hemispheres can often attain the same general level of competence. Zaidel concludes that hemispheric specialization therefore falls on a continuum, being a matter of degree rather than an all-or-none qualitative difference. Each hemisphere has a wide range of cognitive competence that is sufficient to support diverse behaviors, including some that in some circumstances would be better performed by the other hemisphere. Indeed, even where the left hemisphere is inferior, it seems more likely than the right to assume overall control. Also, it seems to have better functional use than the right of ipsilateral projection systems, sensory and motor. Thus, to use the concept of metacontrol, the left hemisphere seems more likely to neglect or deny right hemisphere experiences than vice versa.

At the level of awareness of events, situations, emotional states, personal relationships, and social activities, the right hemisphere seems to operate in a characteristically human fashion. This is the case as long as, under Zaidel's technique, it is interrogated appropriately—by, for example, being required to nod or shake the head or, occasionally, to spell out answers with the left hand using cut-out letters. The right hemisphere seems to have largely the same likes, dislikes, preferences, and ambitions as the left (Gazzaniga & LeDoux, 1978). Thus Sperry, Zaidel, and Zaidel (1979) found that the right hemisphere was able to locate pictures of the patient, his or her relatives, friends, pets, belongings, household scenes, and well-known political, historical, religious, or entertainment figures or personalities from among an assortment of pictures. It was able to make appropriate evaluative judgments, even while the left hemisphere was verbally querying what was happening and attempting to produce intrusive confabulations of its own. Interestingly, emotional reactions seemed to cross rapidly, presumably via the brain stem, to the left hemisphere and to color its speech, sometimes enough for the left hemisphere to be able to identify correctly what had been shown to the right. Sometimes the right hemisphere was seen to cross cue the left by tracing letters with the left hand on the back of the right. Other implicit movements and subvocal responses may also have cued the left, but there did seem to be evidence of information, perhaps in the form of emotional and mental "auras" spreading through brain-stem connecting systems to the left hemisphere. These were sufficient even for it to be able to perform categorical distinctions, for example, between private and social life, political and personal events, family and friends, domestic and foreign, historical and entertainment. Sperry, Zaidel, and Zaidel note that such emotive and conative auras may play an important orientational role in *normal* brain functions, as in mnemonic retrieval. However, while the subject could often verbalize (with the left hemisphere) the presence of a family member in the LVF (right hemisphere), it could not describe the visual details of the scene or, usually, the *identity* of the particular person. Consequently, connotative, affective, and semantically diffuse information may "diffuse" across, but specifically denotative information does not. Still, it is surprising that such subcortical routes can carry such detailed information.

Two Streams of Consciousness, Two Wills?

Considerations of the sort discussed in the previous section inevitably bring us back to the questions raised at the beginning of this chapter by philosophers and physiologists over the last hundred years. The general questions, of course, of consciousness, free will, and the interface between mind and brain are the biggest issues in the neurosciences; moreover, they involve the capacities most treasured by us mortals (Sperry, 1979). There seems to be little doubt that the right hemisphere, when tested in isolation, performs and operates in a thoroughly human way. Such a view, which is certainly that of a majority, is quite contrary to that, for example, of Eccles (1973), who argues that consciousness and selfhood are the exclusive property of the dominant, verbal hemisphere; the minor hemisphere acts more like an automaton or a superior animal brain. The latter viewpoint would relegate all global aphasics, left hemispherectomies, and deaf mutes to the limbo of the unconscious (Nebes, 1978).

Does the fact that each disconnected hemisphere has independent perceptual, memory, and cognitive capacities mean that commissurotomy patients in all other circumstances of everyday life are like Siamese twins, two minds within a single head? While at a gross level few signs of the callosal syndrome are evident, even without subtle testing there are reports (see, e.g., Dimond, 1980) of personality changes, negativism, apathy, a tendency to disregard requests or commands, and a reduction of reported dreaming. With subtle testing, as with Zaidel's technique, the left hemisphere confabulates answers to requests made to the right hemisphere, rationalizes actions initiated by the right, and may even counteract its responses, as when one hand unfastens buttons just fastened by the other.

Puccetti (1981), however, takes the extreme viewpoint that even without section of the commissures we possess two independent streams of consciousness, two minds and volitions, but we are not simultaneously aware of them (as if by a superordinate mind) any more than the commissurotomy patients are. Such a viewpoint, rather than considering that section of the commissures desynchronizes the hemispheres and frees them to act independently, would hold that commissurotomy is merely a maneuver that makes it possible to demonstrate a preexisting duality. Thus Puccetti argues that if hemispherectomy leaves a single, conscious, volitional being, there must have been two to start with. We believe that the fallacy in this argument can be demonstrated by reference to holography, the photographic process that stores every part of a reconstitutable image in a distributed fashion throughout every part of the hologram. If the hologram is torn in two, we are left with two slightly degraded holograms, each containing the same general information as before. This process can be continued more or less indefinitely, with a cumulative loss of definition. That one hologram can be divided into many does *not* mean that there were many preexisting holograms in existence prior to section. Moreover, if we accept Puccetti's argument of a preexisting duality, why stop at two? The interconnecting commissures are not qualitatively different from other *intrahemispheric* tracts. One can make a good case for a whole *mosaic* of personalities. We are frequently unsure of the reasons for our actions or even for our emotional responses. Psychoanalysis and even hypnosis abounds with descriptions of well-intentioned, self-deceptive, confabulatory accounts of actions and emotional states. Is there really any reason why we should not all have a number of nonverbal, cognitive, emotional, and memory systems, a mosaic of subconscious processors, each vying for momentary awareness and loosely intercoordinated like a colony of cells in a sponge? We are often a battleground of competing desires, whims, and drives, part of us wanting to do one thing, part wanting another. This is a view of the mind not as a psychological but as a sociological entity (cf. Dimond, 1980).

There is debate as to whether commissural section augments or decreases the overall capacity of the brain to carry out more than one task simultaneously. Sperry (1968) and Selnes (1974) support the idea of total hemispheric independence, with commissural section effectively increasing the brain's capacity to deal independently with two parallel streams of information. Gazzaniga and Sperry (1966) compared the performance of normal and split-brain subjects on a double discrimination task, a red–green discrimination in the RVF requiring a right-hand response and a light–dark discrimination in the LVF requiring a left-hand response. Reaction times were lengthened for normal subjects and preoperative patients when the second task was added to the first, but not for postoperative commissurotomy patients. Ellenberg and Sperry (1980) review and report similar findings whereby commissurotomy patients were able to employ both hands independently in two simultaneous sorting tasks. Normal subjects were able to achieve skill in performing two simultaneous tasks only after very extensive practice, only at the cost of automatic, unmonitored, and inflexible performance by one hand, and only when the sensory and/or response modalities were separate and dissimilar and the tasks easy and familiar. Consequently, Ellenberg and Sperry conclude that one of the functions of the corpus callosum, separate from its information-transmission role, is allocating attention to insure its focal unity. Trevarthen (1974a), although less certain about the ability of such patients to carry out two separate tasks in true independence, agrees that commissural section leads to problems in the unilateral allocation of attention and results in an overall decrease in processing capacity. Indeed Sperry, Gazzaniga, and Bogen (1969) admit that, overall, the split brain is probably not more efficient than the unified; the two parallel functions required of the two hemispheres must be relatively simple and such that they can be performed from a common posture and with a common mental set. Moreover, bimanual coordination is often grossly disturbed after commissural section (Kreuter, Kinsbourne, & Trevarthen, 1972; Preilowski, 1972; Zaidel & Sperry, 1977).

It is perhaps best to regard commissurotomy patients as behaving *as if,* under certain artificial circumstances, they possess a potential duality of consciousness, without an actual *doubling* of cognitive processing capacity. Indeed, there is little evidence of a substantial *reduction* in general cognitive capacity as a consequence of *hemispherectomy.* Our two hemispheres serve sensory-motor control in a two-sided world, and the commissures link sensory-motor rather than cognitive brain areas. Although functions can take place in each hemisphere separately and independently in commissurotomized patients, at any one moment subcortical meta-control processes almost certainly lead to the relative suppression of activity in one or the other hemisphere, with a possible reduction in overall capacity and, probably, a fluctuating cognitive style (Preilowski, 1979; Trevarthen, 1974a). Normally, although they may have separate momentary awarenesses, memory traces, and so on, commissurotomy patients retain a high degree of unity of purpose, attention, and motive. The body normally remains fully coordinated in acts of attending, orienting, locomoting, and praxis, except under unusual testing conditions. The two hemispheres generally have the same experiences, memories, motivations, and emotions and are carried around in the single body. All of these factors, along with an undivided subcortical arousing and coordinating system, will act as powerful factors for unification.

Thus, the two hemispheres act to complement each other, even after surgical separation, though perhaps with reduced efficiency. As Levy and Trevarthen (1976) observed, metacontrol processes tend to switch in one or the other hemisphere to a dominant processing position (even in circumstances where its specialized strategies may not best fit it for the particular circumstances). It seems more often than not to be the left hemisphere: The commissurotomy subject tends to express surprise at the wayward doings of the left hand more often than the right and may seek ways to restrain it, or may even deny it, in a manner analogous to left hemineglect in brain-damaged patients (see Chapter Four).

Humans are, of course, verbal animals, which may partly explain why the part which is speaking may be seen as the single unique source and locus of the self. Perhaps whatever neural subsystem currently has access to response or output processes automatically attains a level of conscious self-awareness. Studies of reaction time for choices made within the framework of information theory suggest that response uncertainty (i.e., response selection) is more important than stimulus uncertainty (i.e., stimulus identification) in determining response times (see, e.g., Keele, 1973). While, with practice, we can come to process a number of discrete *inputs* simultaneously, though often preconsciously and incompletely, we generally cannot simultaneously initiate two different sets of *responses,* unless they can somehow be integrated into a single, composite, higher-order movement.

Agenesis of the Corpus Callosum

As a consequence of faulty development at a critical stage of ontogeny, a very small percentage of the population is born without the corpus callosum. Usually the anterior commissure is still present and may even be enlarged, possibly in compensation. Described as an "experiment of nature" (Chiarello, 1980), since it is a form of prenatal commissurotomy, it provides the maximum opportunity for neural and behavioral compensation. Thus, deficits shared by surgical and congenital acallosals reflect functions that cannot be compensated. Agenesis cases permit review of claims that the corpus callosum is critical for the development of lateralization and localization of language functions to the left hemisphere (see, e.g., Chiarello, 1980).

The condition has recently been critically reviewed by Chiarello (1980), Ferriss and Dorsen (1975), Field, Ashton, and White (1978), Jeeves (1979), and Milner and Jeeves (1979) from various standpoints, including the ontogeny and development of forebrain commissures, the timetable for pathological events to interrupt, partially or completely, the growth of commissures, the presence or absence of other brain abnormalities, the presence or absence of acallosal and other clinical or behavioral symptoms, possible bilateralization of language, and possible compensatory mechanisms such as enlargement of the anterior commissure, use of ipsilateral sensory and motor pathways, cross-cueing strategies, and bilateralization of function.

The condition, when diagnosed, is never pure; there is always some other brain abnormality present that could account for or, conversely, mask any apparent acallosal or other syndrome. Not only is the anterior commissure frequently enlarged, possibly in compensation, but there are usually other neural modifications. Probst's bundle, a longitudinal tract of fibers seen in the medial walls of the hemispheres, is usually present (Chiarello, 1980). These fibers are thought to represent the decussating axons that normally cross the midline to connect heterotopic structures, but with callosal agenesis they terminate ipsilaterally, possibly in a random manner. According to this view callosal agenesis represents a failure to achieve interhemispheric connections rather than a total lack of requisite fibers. There is often also an abnormal pattern of sulci and shape of the lateral ventricles, possibly also with a reduction in number of cortical cells.

It is frequently claimed that callosal agenesis is conspicuous for its lack of symptoms. When the condition is first determined on routine autopsy, one must rely on the unsophisticated judgment of friends and relatives to reconstruct possible symptomatology in life. When diagnosed during neurological examination, routine or otherwise, obviously *some* clinical symptoms must have been present. However, it does seem that visual field and ear superiorities are often comparatively normal. While the right ear and RVF are superior, nonetheless congenital acallosals have few problems in identifying verbal material presented to the left ear or the LVF. Intermanual tactile matching usually is little different from that of normal subjects, though there are occasional reports of inferior bimanual manipulation, coordination, and integration and deficits in interhemispheric transfer of kinesthetic learning. These would be expected in the absence of forebrain commissures. For detailed reviews of all cases reported to date, see Chiarello (1980) and Milner and Jeeves (1979). Although there are two reports of congenital acallosals being unable to perceive the join in chimeric face stimuli, unlike surgical commissurotomy patients they never fail to see the incompleteness of partial pictures or words cut off at the visual midline and so never experience total perceptual completion, as do the surgical patients. Congenital acallosals usually have no problems in reading words spanning the midline, in adding numerals presented separately to the two visual fields, in perceiving simultaneity and succession of events occurring in the two visual fields, in experiencing the ϕ phenomenon (apparent movement) to light flashes occurring in the two fields, in naming objects palpated out of sight by the left hand, in cross matching hand-held objects, in retrieving with either hand objects whose pictures were flashed to either visual field, or in locating one hand (passively positioned in space) by means of the other.

However, in spite of a surprising lack of the expected symptoms, congenital acallosals do not perform quite normally. Apart from the occasional deficits in bimanual manipulation, coordination, and integration and difficulties in transfer of kinesthetic learning, there are consistent reports of poor intellectual, spatial, and/or motor functioning, with large discrepancies between verbal performance IQs (see e.g., Ferriss & Dorsen, 1975; Field, Ashton, & White, 1978; Nottebohm, 1979; and Weber & Bradshaw, 1981). One possible explanation for this is the reported existence of bilaterally represented speech in congenital acallosals. Clinical (i.e., brain-damaged) patients with major hemisphere pathology of very early onset are frequently said to be liable to develop speech in both hemispheres (see Chapters Four and Eight; Gazzaniga & LeDoux, 1978; and Smith & Sugar, 1975). It could be argued that such bilateral speech representation, if present at a motor level, could conceivably be thought of as leading to competition for access to the unpaired speech apparatus and thus to an increase in the probability of stuttering. According to Jeeves (personal communication) this has in fact been observed. Bilateral speech could also lead to cognitive "crowding" of nonverbal, spatial right-hemisphere functions, to their detriment, and thus account for the above-mentioned spatial and performance IQ deficits (see, e.g., Sperry, Gazzaniga, & Bogen, 1969). On the other hand it is not uncommon to find RVF superiorities and right ear advantages for verbal stimuli to be normal in congenital acallosals. Moreover, as Chiarello (1980) points out, the absence of visual field and ear asymmetries is also not uncommon with *normal* subjects. These techniques are not very reliable for determining the locus of language lateralization, particularly at the *expressive* level, and in any case language *comprehension* is often fairly bilateral for most of us.

The relative absence of the acallosal syndrome in congenital acallosals may well reflect the operation of maximal neural and behavioral plasticity to compensate for early-onset abnormalities, as suggested at the beginning of this section. Indeed, as Bogen (1979) observes, even in surgical patients the callosal syndrome tends to decrease over time. As we noted above, the anterior commissure is frequently found to be enlarged, and this structure can stand in for the corpus callosum for many visual functions. In addition, the midbrain (retinotectal) visual system may also partly compensate. Greater use of ipsilateral auditory, somatosensory, and motor pathways has also been implicated as a further possible compensatory mechanism, though such an explanation is obviously inappropriate with respect to vision. Indeed, reliance on ipsilateral motor pathways could possibly account for the reported tendency to synkinetic movements, the inability to suppress completely mirror-symmetrical movements of the opposite limb when making voluntary movements of one limb. These in turn could also partly account for impaired bimanual manipulatory performance and motor control. Synkinesis, however, seems to have been reported only for one patient (Dennis, 1976). Nevertheless, the possible role of the corpus callosum as an *inhibitory* mechanism, to inhibit synkinetic movements and the development of language in the right hemisphere, as well as its other communicatory roles should still be borne in mind.

A final mechanism of compensation to account for the near-normal performance of congenital acallosals, this time operating at the behavioral level, is the possible development of sophisticated cross-cueing strategies, which could have taken place over the subject's entire developmental lifetime. Jeeves (1979), however, argues against this possibility, finding no evidence of any increase in compensation over a fifteen-year interval between initial testing and retest. Moreover, everyday experiences, unlike those of artificial laboratory situations, are unlikely to demand cross-cueing strategies.

Summary and Conclusions

For over a hundred years people have speculated on the unity or duality of conscious awareness in view of the brain's duplex structure. This issue has not yet been satisfactorily resolved. Of the forebrain commissures that interconnect the two cerebral hemispheres, the corpus callosum and the anterior commissure are the most important, with the posterior third and the splenium of the corpus callosum and the anterior commissure particularly involved in the interhemispheric transfer of visual information.

Apart from olfaction, which is ipsilaterally mediated, all sensory functions, especially the visual and tactile ones, are largely contralateral. In vision the LVF (right hemiretinae) of both eyes projects to the right hemisphere, the RVF (left hemiretinae) to the left. The decussating nasal fibers cross at the optic chiasm. With hearing there is a relatively greater degree of bilateral representation from each ear, though the contralateral component is stronger, especially with dichotic stimulation. The pyramidal motor system, which exerts fine control over the distal musculature of the extremities, is almost entirely contralaterally organized. The extrapyramidal system involves a relatively bilateral control of the proximal musculature for gross movements.

In nonhuman studies of the effects of commissurotomy, the optic chiasm may be cut so that only the ipsilaterally projecting temporal pathways of the visual system are preserved. Thus, if one eye is covered, a single hemisphere (ipsilateral to the training eye) can then be stimulated. If the eye cover is then switched to the training eye, interocular (and, by implication, interhemispheric) transfer of learned habits can be tested. Total transfer takes place with intact commissures, though this is largely abolished if the forebrain commissures are cut prior to training. Under these circumstances it is even possible to train two mutually contradictory responses, one in each hemisphere. There is currently some dispute as to whether it is *sensory* information or *engrams* that transfer with intact commissures. The results of studies involving sodium amytal suppression of single hemispheres in humans support the former hypothesis.

In humans the commissurotomy operation is performed to relieve otherwise intractable epilepsy. A large number of methodological and theoretical problems arise in interpreting the results of human commissurotomy studies. Subtle testing (e.g., use of tachistoscopic or dichotic procedures) is often necessary to demonstrate the predicted effects. This is one reason why the early (1940s) studies of Akelaitis failed to reveal any obvious psychological consequences of the commissurotomy operation. It was not until the 1960s that Sperry's group demonstrated the often dramatic consequences, showing that the hemispheres may be split into two independent cognitive systems, with the left hemisphere largely mediating verbal and analytic functions and the right subserving nonverbal, visuospatial, and gestalt or holistic aspects.

Commissurotomy patients can verbally report words or pictures flashed to the RVF or objects palpated by the right hand; they usually cannot verbally report such stimuli flashed to the LVF or explored by the left hand, and a confabulatory response may be initiated by the left hemisphere. That the nonverbal right hemisphere can nevertheless correctly identify such presentations is revealed by its successful identification via a pointing or selection response by the left hand. The patient is unable to report (verbally or otherwise) the identity of two pictures (or words) flashed one to each visual field, or of two objects placed one in each hand. Patients may occasionally show some ability to employ ipsilateral (spinothalamic) projection systems for somesthetically discriminating between two very different objects, such as a hard, heavy, square item and a soft, light, round item. The isolated right hemisphere may comprehend spoken material and some fairly simple written material.

The verbal left hemisphere becomes adept at reading off voluntarily or involuntarily initiated responses (by the right hemisphere) that involve posture or expression. In this way it may interpret a stimulus presented to the right hemisphere and correctly respond to it. Occasionally such cross cueing may even be possible at a surprisingly complex level; sophisticated techniques may be required to demonstrate its occurrence.

While the right hand maintains its superiority in writing, the left hand (right hemisphere) may become superior in drawing, copying, block construction, and interpreting spatial relationships, often at the expense of detail. The right hand tends to adopt an analytic approach, concentrating on specific features or details in tactile interpretations; the left treats objects as spatial wholes. Thus, the right hemisphere is superior at perceiving overall stimulus configurations and performing a configurational synthesis from fragmentary or incomplete information; the left excels in performing an analytic, serial, or segmental breakdown of a whole into its component elements.

There is dispute as to whether the left hemisphere is deficient in visuospatial functions per se, or simply in tasks requiring active exploratory touch. Laterality differences are certainly stronger at a *motor* than at a *sensory* level in both verbal and nonverbal situations.

Trevarthen distinguishes ambient from focal vision; the former (retinotectal) system is undivided by the commissurotomy operation and at a midbrain level mediates perception of "where" rather than "what." Actual stimulus identification (what) is performed by the (divided) focal, or geniculostriate, system. With ambient vision commissurotomy patients are able to judge colinearity, equidistance, and relative movement of two moving lines, even when they are in opposite visual fields.

Tests using chimeric stimulation showed visual completion to be very strong to the left (subjects subsequently selecting an item corresponding to the RVF half of the chimera) when phonological processing or verbal reporting was required; the opposite happened when attention to physical features was required. The right hemisphere was shown able to match structurally similar items; the left to match conceptually or functionally similar items. In the phenomenon of metacontrol, one hemisphere predominates as a result of expectations about subsequent cognitive requirements, whether or not such cognitive specializations are indeed actually utilized. This phenomenon may be mediated via brain-stem controlling and activating mechanisms.

Using a scleral contact lens system that permitted prolonged lateralized viewing in one or the other visual field, Zaidel studied the analytic and holistic processing capacities of both hemispheres and the verbal capacities of the right. The latter was shown to be able to form both upper and lower case writing, to have a fairly extensive auditory and visual lexicon, but to have no phonological or articulatory capacity; its syntactic competence was inferior to the left's. The right hemisphere may recognize written words ideographically, and it can identify objects on the basis of abstract descriptions or definitions of usage given aurally. It behaves like a nominal aphasic, knowing an object's use and qualities but is unable to utter its name, which is often provided in a confabulatory manner by the left hemisphere. Comprehension is thus the least lateralized verbal function, articulation the most. The two hemispheres may reach approximately the same level of measured intelligence, but as an analysis of errors reveals, they do so via different strategies. However, this analytic–holistic processing distinction is relative rather than absolute. The isolated right hemisphere operates in a characteristically human way at a level of awareness of events, situations, emotional states, personal relationships, and social, political, and historical occurrences as long as its interrogation requires nonverbal responding. It has the same likes, tastes, and ambitions as the left. Apart from the possibility of cross-cueing strategies, there is some evidence of emotional and mental "auras" spreading slowly through brain-stem connecting systems from the right hemisphere to the verbal left hemisphere, often sufficient for the latter to be able to broadly categorize input to the former.

The as yet unresolved question arises as to whether there are two simultaneous, coexisting streams of consciousness in the divided brain, two wills and two volitions. Is this duality found in the *normal* brain, the commissurotomy operation merely serving to highlight a preexisting condition? It is sometimes argued that if *hemispherectomy* leaves a single conscious volitional being, then there must have been two to start with. The fallacy of this argument is demonstrated with an analogy to the hologram. A hologram can be successively split n times with a loss only in the degree of resolution, without there ever having been n preexisting copies. The possibility still remains that we are all mosaics of competing nonverbal, cognitive, emotional, and memory systems, the human mind being a sociological entity. Nevertheless, there are powerful factors for unification present even in the divided brain; only under exceptional testing procedures can anything approximating a true duality of consciousness ever be demonstrated, and even then it may be little different from what is found in normal subjects under equally artificial conditions of hypnosis and training to perform more than one task at once. Perhaps whatever neural subsystem currently has access to response or output processes automatically attains a level of conscious self-awareness, with response selection perhaps more important than stimulus identification in these respects.

In cases of callosal agenesis there is surprisingly little evidence of the disconnection syndrome. This may be due to compensation by the frequently enlarged anterior commissure and the use of ipsilateral sensory and motor routes and cross-cueing strategies. Other concomitant brain abnormalities may account for or mask any acallosal syndrome. However, such individuals do not perform quite normally, exhibiting occasional deficits in bimanual manipulation, coordination, and integration and poor intellectual, spatial, and/or motor functioning. These may be due to bilateral representation of language, with the subsequent cognitive crowding detrimental to nonverbal right hemisphere functions. However REAs and RVF superiorities are generally normal, with no real evidence of bilateral language representation.

FURTHER READING

BOGEN, J. E. The callosal syndrome. In K. M. Heilman & E. Valenstein (Eds.), *Clinical neuropsychology.* Oxford: Oxford University Press, 1979.

CHIARELLO, C. A house divided? Cognitive functioning with callosal agenesis. *Brain and Language,* 1980, *11,* 128–158.

GAZZANIGA, M. S., & LEDOUX, J. E. *The integrated mind.* New York: Plenum, 1978.

LEVY, J., & TREVARTHEN, C. Metacontrol of hemispheric function in human split brain patients. *Journal of Experimental Psychology: Human Perception and Performance,* 1976, *3,* 299–312.

MILNER, A. D., & JEEVES, M. A. A review of behavioural studies of agenesis of the corpus callosum. In I. Steele Russell, M. W. Hof, & G. Berlucchi (Eds.), *Structure and function of cerebral commissures.* London: Macmillan, 1979.

NEBES, R. D. Direct examination of cognitive function in the right and left hemispheres. In M. Kinsbourne (Ed.), *Asymmetrical function of the brain.* Cambridge: Cambridge University Press, 1978.

PUCCETTI, R. The case for mental duality: Evidence from split brain data and other considerations. *Behavioral and Brain Sciences,* 1981, *4,* 93–123.

SPERRY, R. W. Lateral specialization in the surgically separated hemispheres. In F. O. Schmitt & F. G. Worden (Eds.), *The neurosciences: Third study program.* Cambridge, Mass.: MIT Press, 1974.

SPERRY, R. W., ZAIDEL, E., & ZAIDEL, D. Self recognition and social awareness in the deconnected minor hemisphere. *Neuropsychologia,* 1979, *17,* 153–166.

ZAIDEL, E. Concepts of cerebral dominance in the split brain. In P. A. Buser & A. Rougeul-Buser (Eds.), *Cerebral correlates of conscious experience.* Amsterdam: North Holland, 1978.

CHAPTER SIX
Evidence from Normal Subjects

Although the hemispheres after commissurotomy are truly independent, at least with respect to cortico-cortical influences, preexisting morbidity and surgical trauma raises questions about the extent to which the findings from studies on commissurotomized subjects can be considered typical of the functions of otherwise intact isolated hemispheres. In normal human subjects the morbidity and trauma are presumed absent, but the hemispheres cannot be said under any circumstances to operate truly independently. However laterality differences, as we shall see in this chapter, can be demonstrated in normal people, and the findings complement those obtained from studies of clinical and commissurotomy patients. Indeed, the same general procedures are typically employed as with commissurotomy patients—that is, tachistoscopic and dichotic presentations and, to a lesser extent, tactile stimulation. Attempts have recently been made to lateralize continuously presented visual information in such a way as to permit scanning within a hemifield. However, it must again be emphasized that the commissures are now present and functional, operating in both a facilitative and inhibitory fashion and mediating the transfer of sensory, perceptual, or mnemonic information. Consequently, reaction time and other differences between visual fields, ears, and hands may be variously interpreted in terms of delay in interhemispheric transmission times, signal degradation during such transfer, relative functional superiority of one hemisphere for a particular mode of operation, or attentional biases. We shall discuss these issues further in Chapter Seven.

Visual Studies

As with commissurotomized subjects, visual studies with normal subjects have relied on central fixation with tachistoscopic stimulation. To avoid scanning eye movements, exposures of 150 msec or less are usually employed (see A. W. Young, 1981a, for review of work on latency of saccades). Each visual half field projects first to the contralateral hemisphere; the optic fibers from the nasal hemiretinae cross at the optic chiasm and project contralaterally, and those from the temporal hemiretinae project ipsilaterally to the hemisphere on the same side. Since the image of a laterally presented object falls on the nasal hemiretina of one eye and the temporal hemiretina of the other, information is initially projected to one hemisphere only (see Figure 5-2).

In the visual studies the two basic measures are speed and accuracy, the former perhaps being the more sensitive in that it is obviously far less subject to floor and ceiling effects. Vocal naming latencies or manual response times are collected over an appropriate number of trials, and condition means (or sometimes medians, to avoid the problem of bias arising from the occasional and inadvertent long reaction time) are calculated. For differences that may typically be of only a few milliseconds, it is obviously important to have enough trials to counterbalance all possible conditions and to pseudorandomize all sequences. There is no single truly satisfactory way of coping with errors and long reaction times. The latter are sometimes dropped from analysis, replaced with further trials (still obeying the sequencing constraints), or replaced with an arbitrary cut-off value used to define a long reaction time. The value of the last again varies from study to study: Sometimes two standard deviations from the series mean is employed; sometimes a more subjectively based figure is used. Nor is there agreement on how long an experimental sequence should be, though in our experience (and see also Hamsher & Benton, 1977) there should be a *minimum* of thirty-two trials in each limb of the simplest possible contrast (e.g., thirty-two LVF and thirty-two RVF trials where nothing else is being compared). However, as we shall see in Chapter Seven, we can then run into fresh problems of practice, fatigue, changes in strategy, and so on.

With manual responses, a unimanual or a bimanual paradigm may be employed. With unimanual responding, experimenters have all too often used only one hand throughout, or one hand for one response and the other hand for the other. A bimanual response (where, e.g., the forefingers of both hands respond "target" or "same," and the two middle fingers make the opposite response) is one satisfactory solution as it is likely to involve both hemispheres equally in response organization (see, e.g., Patterson & Bradshaw, 1975). The results of Geffen, Bradshaw, and Wallace (1971) and Moscovitch, Scullion, and Christie (1976) indicate that the responding hand does not normally interact with visual field of presentation in cognitive tasks (see Chapter Seven). A less satisfactory technique requires half the subjects to make one response with one hand and the other half to use the opposite hand. If instead a go-no-go paradigm is employed, while half of the potential data is sacrificed, subjects can respond with one hand for half of the trials, switching to the other for the remainder.

One reason for the often contradictory findings in laterality research with normal subjects is the great diversity of experimental techniques available for use. These may involve reaction time or accuracy measures; a speed or an accuracy set imposed on the subject; vocal or manual responding; go-no-go or target-nontarget responding; identity, similarity, or category (e.g., male-female) matches or discriminations; perceptual matching between two simultaneously presented stimuli versus matching a test item to a previously memorized target (with long or short retention intervals); constant or single target versus continuously changing or multiple targets. Moreover, the task material itself may be familiar or unfamiliar, easy or difficult, practiced or unpracticed, accompanied by another easy or difficult secondary task, of a verbal or nonverbal nature, or entirely on its own. It may be easily verbalized, subject to verbal recoding, or impossible to verbalize. It may be treatable as a unitary integrated configuration, or it may be loosely organized as a collection of isolated features or elements. These factors do not constitute a comprehensive list, nor probably are they independent of each other in their effects, and all may well affect the replicability of laterality studies. Even the employment of extrafoveal tachistoscopic exposures of brief duration (to ensure fixation) may *itself* affect laterality patterns. Thus Rizzolatti and Buchtel (1977) found that LVF superiorities for face recognition were greater for exposures of very brief duration.

The hemiretinal division.   If exposure durations can affect laterality patterns, can the degree of retinal eccentricity do likewise, either for anatomical reasons or simply because gradients of decreasing perceptual acuity affect cognitive processing strategies? More important, there is the possibility (see Gazzaniga & LeDoux, 1978, for review) that while the contralateral visual field is fully represented in each hemisphere, the ipsilateral field is also represented by the splenium of the corpus callosum, equivalent to a narrow slit of a few degrees of arc down the visual midline. The functional significance of this ipsilateral representation may be limited purely to stereopsis in foveal vision. Stone, Leicester, and Sherman (1973) claim that the central strip is (in monkeys) 1° wide, as do Bunt, Minckler, and Johanson (1977), who also note that the strip may possibly widen a little in the vicinity of the fovea. This may account for the reported phenomenon of macular sparing in humans (see, e.g., Koerner & Teuber, 1973), though as A. W. Young (1981a) observes, this phenomenon is not established beyond doubt (see also Haun, 1978). Others (e.g., McIlwain, 1972; Thorson, Lange, & Biederman-Thorson, 1969; Westheimer & Mitchell, 1969) claim that the degree of nasotemporal hemiretinal overlap is hairline or at most a few minutes of arc and that, apart possibly from stereopsis, it has no functional significance (see also Harvey, 1978).

The nasal and temporal hemiretinae: Acuity differences and pathway strength.
Two reviews (Maddess, 1975; White, 1969; see also Osaka, 1978) conclude that normally the contralateral pathways (i.e., those leading from the nasal hemiretinae)

are somewhat more efficient than the ipsilateral pathways (projecting from the temporal hemiretinae), particularly under normal binocular viewing or under conditions of dichoptic viewing, when separate information is simultaneously fed to the two eyes. One possible reason why the crossed nasal pathways dominate in binocular viewing is that the far periphery is only projected onto the *nasal* hemiretinae; the temporal hemiretinae are blind for these spatial regions. It would therefore make adaptive sense for an organism to be more sensitive to distant objects. With monocular noncompetitive stimulation, on the other hand, temporal superiority may result (see Carmon, Kleiner, & Nachshon, 1975; Markowitz & Weitzman, 1969; Neill, Sampson, & Gribben, 1971; Overton & Weiner, 1966). Given these factors, it is obviously important in visual laterality research to employ binocular viewing and subjects without marked eye dominance (see, e.g., Hayashi & Bryden, 1967; Wyke & Ettlinger, 1961).

Letter and digit stimuli. With accuracy of recall as the dependent variable, there is now a long history of reports of RVF superiority for lateralized single-letter presentations (Bryden, 1965, 1966; Bryden & Rainey, 1963; Heron, 1957; Zurif & Bryden, 1969). Schmuller (1979) found that while there was either a faster loss from storage or slower processing in the right hemisphere, nevertheless the pattern of errors between the hemispheres was very similar in terms of multidimensional scaling, hierarchical clustering, and correlation analyses. With the potentially more sensitive reaction-time measures to the presence of a target letter or digit, again a RVF superiority is found, whether for English material (see, e.g., Geffen, Bradshaw, & Wallace, 1971; Rizzolatti, Umiltà, & Berlucchi, 1971), or for Hebrew letters with Israeli subjects (Carmon, Nachshon, Isseroff, & Kleiner, 1972). With vocal naming latencies again a RVF superiority is found (Geffen et al., 1971; Moscovitch & Catlin, 1970), though only when a *discriminative* response is required, as opposed to a meaningless ("bonk") vocalization for *any* digit (Geffen et al., 1971), and perhaps only when the subject knows in advance the possible alternatives (G. Cohen, 1975a). Curiously, RVF superiorities may be larger for consonants than for vowels (Umiltà, Frost, & Hyman, 1972) and for stop consonants than for fricatives (Klisz, 1980), exactly as in dichotic studies, suggesting perhaps a common type of left hemisphere specialization for auditory and visual information-processing systems.

When pairs of letters are simultaneously presented to the same visual field, for matching same and different, a RVF superiority is typically reported when the letter pairs are *nominally* identical (e.g., *Aa, Bb, Dd, Gg*, etc.); a LVF superiority may occur with *physically* identical letter pairs (*AA, bb, dd, GG*, etc.; see, e.g., G. Cohen, 1972; R. Davis & V. Schmit, 1973; Geffen, Bradshaw, & Nettleton, 1972).

Strings of random letters have also been presented to one or the other visual field or occasionally to both. RVF superiorities are typically obtained with unilateral presentations, and LVF superiorities with bilateral presentations, except perhaps where there is a gap at the midline. However, such findings are largely determined by factors other than those pertaining to cerebral asymmetry—for example, foveal acuity gradients, directional scanning during perceptual processing, serial report order, lateral masking or inhibition, and so on—and will not be discussed further here (see, e.g., J. L. Bradshaw, Nettleton, & Taylor, 1981b).

Unilaterally presented words. With both recall accuracy and manual reaction times, a RVF superiority is typically found, even for bilaterally presented words (for review see J. L. Bradshaw et al., 1981b). It is also found with vocal naming latencies (J. L. Bradshaw & Gates, 1978; J. L. Bradshaw & Taylor, 1979; G. Cohen, 1975a). Leiber (1976) found RVF superiorities only for word and not for nonword stimuli (whether pronounceable, as in GOZE, or not, GRZK) in a lexical decision task where subjects were timed in deciding whether or not a letter string constituted a real word, but Bradshaw, Gates, & Nettleton (1977) obtained an equally strong RVF superiority for all these classes of stimulus. Bradshaw and Gates (1978), in addition to finding a RVF superiority for both words and pronounceable nonwords as above, also found a RVF superiority when subjects decided whether nonwords were or were not homophonic with (nonpresented) real words, for example, *gurl, caip, cote* in the former (pseudohomophone) category and *cipe, goap, sern* in the latter. G. Cohen and Freeman (1978) employed a lexical decision task where half of the nonwords were pseudohomophones and half were not. Only for presentations in the RVF (left hemisphere) did it take longer to reject the pseudohomophones as nonwords. This confirmed that phonological processing is likely to be an exclusive prerogative of the left hemisphere; the automatic phonological recoding by the left hemisphere of these nonwords that sounded like real words slowed down their rejection as nonwords. Indeed, as we shall see in Chapter Eight, deep dyslexics, who are thought to rely on right hemisphere mechanisms for preserved reading functions, also fail to be slowed by pseudohomophones when performing lexical (word-nonword) decision tasks. Other evidence from normal subjects of extreme inferiority of the right hemisphere in phonological processing comes from the work of Klatzky and Atkinson (1971). Subjects memorized a set of letters and were then shown a picture tachistoscopically in either the left or right visual field; they had to decide whether or not its name began with one of the letters. The magnitude of the RVF superiority remained constant, regardless of the number of stored letters. Had the degree of right hemisphere inferiority increased with memory set size, this would have indicated an inferiority of the right hemisphere relative to the left in phonological processing, with an incremental response-time effect for each successive comparison. That the response-time difference remained constant is compatible with an explanation that suggests all phonological information is transferred to the left hemisphere for processing.

Left hemisphere verbal superiority is certainly more pronounced at the level of expressive speech, and for phonological processing at the level of comprehension (see Chapters Four, Five, and Eight). With respect to the extraction of semantic information, J. L. Bradshaw (1974) found that subjects' interpretation of the meaning of an ambiguous centrally located homograph (e.g., *palm, box, bank*) was more often influenced, consciously or unconsciously, by a flanking word in the RVF than one in the LVF, though the simultaneous presence of three words could have induced this effect as a result of directional scanning. Martin (1978) found no RVF superiority for processing words at a semantic level (e.g., in terms of plant or animal categories), only for processing in terms of orthographic or phonological aspects. Saffran, Bogyo, Schwartz, and Marin (1980) likewise failed to get a consistent RVF superiority when subjects were asked to judge whether laterally presented first names were male or female, a finding that we also have independently made in our own laboratory (unpublished). On the other hand, with a *small* ensemble of names simultaneously presented in unilateral pairs for matching same-opposite with respect to sex, J. L. Bradshaw, Gates, and Nettleton (1977) did find a RVF reaction-time superiority. Similarly, Gross (1972) also found a RVF superiority with category matching (i.e., whether both words were members of the same category, such as animal names or body parts).

The possible contribution of directional scanning to RVF superiorities with word stimuli. The experimental strategy to determine whether RVF superiorities with words is wholly or in part due to directional scanning mechanisms has long relied on determining whether RVF superiorities are reduced or reversed under certain conditions. These include left–right mirror-reversed stimuli (which, if words *are* directionally scanned in reading, would have to be scanned in the reverse direction and should generate LVF superiorities), Hebrew words (which are written right to left), and vertically organized words, for example, $\begin{smallmatrix}W\\O\\R\\D\end{smallmatrix}$, which obviously cannot be scanned horizontally. As we have pointed out (J. L. Bradshaw, Nettleton, & Taylor, 1981b) studies prior to the 1960s have all been deficient in some aspects. They have employed long and/or uncontrolled exposure durations, long or regularly alternating sequences of presentations to the same visual field (both of which would lead to lack of control over stimulus lateralization), large format and/or polysyllabic words, letter-by-letter responding and/or scoring, admixture of nonwords and/or mirror-reversed or part-reversed words (all leading to a fragmentary, letter-by-letter approach by the subject), ceiling and/or floor effects, uncontrolled handedness of subjects, and small number of subjects and/or stimuli. These problems have all led to a plethora of inconsistent results. However, after the mid 1960s, experimental control improved and a clear picture has emerged, indicating that left-to-right directional processing has little or no effect on RVF superiorities. This suggests that field differences reflect cerebral rather than any other factors and that the use of vertically organized words to avoid scanning artifacts is unnecessary and probably even counterproductive.

Isseroff, Carmon, and Nachshon (1974) found that the RVF superiority for left–right mirror-reversed words was no less than that for normal words. With respect to Hebrew, while Orbach (1967) found that only dextrals gave a RVF superiority, Carmon, Nachshon, and Starinsky (1976) found a RVF superiority for both Arabic number sequences (sequenced left-to-right) and Hebrew words (sequenced right-to-left) for children of all ages and totally rejected a scanning explanation. With respect to vertically organized words, only one study (McKeever

& Gill, 1972) found a smaller RVF superiority for vertical than for horizontal stimuli, and they used a bilateral exposure paradigm with a central fixation digit. Under these circumstances there could have been a right hemisphere contribution with the vertically organized words for preprocessing unfamiliar stimuli (see below). All other studies (Bryden, 1970; H. D. Ellis & Young, 1977; MacKavey, Curcio, & Rosen, 1975; Turner & Miller, 1975) have obtained a RVF superiority for vertical words of the same magnitude as for horizontal ones. Barton, Goodglass, and Shai (1965) obtained a consistent and equally strong RVF superiority for vertical Hebrew and English words, as did Kershner and Jeng (1972) for (the normally horizontal) English and (the normally vertical) Chinese words. In a series of target-detection studies with manual response-time measures, J. L. Bradshaw, Bradley, Gates, and Patterson (1977) and J. L. Bradshaw and Mapp (1982) used laterally presented single-syllable four-letter words with nontargets differing from targets by a single letter change at any one of the four letter positions. The RVF superiority was stronger for targets, for changed letters in the two middle positions in nontargets, and for both upper and lower case letters. There was a weak, nonsignificant RVF superiority with cursive script, and where word shape (in terms of ascender letters such as *b, d, h, k, l,* and *t* and descender letters such as *g, j, p, q,* and *y*) was changed between targets and nontargets. A change at the first letter position was always detected fastest, followed, usually, by a change at the last letter, with no difference between the others. This argues against the operation of a serial left-to-right scan. Thus, we cannot support the idea of short single-syllable words being processed as single, unitary, global entities even in the right hemisphere, since the letter-position functions were essentially similar for the two visual fields. Rather, we believe that words are apprehended largely by a parallel letter-processing strategy, with ends-first advantages (see J. L. Bradshaw, Nettleton, & Taylor, 1981b). Sex and handedness effects in word processing tasks are in the expected direction of weaker field asymmetries for females (see Chapter Eleven) and for sinistrals, who also have weaker and more variable asymmetries (see Chapter Ten; also J. L. Bradshaw, Gates, & Nettleton, 1977; J. L. Bradshaw & Gates, 1978; J. L. Bradshaw & Taylor, 1979; J. L. Bradshaw, Nettleton, & Taylor, 1981a; Bryden, 1965; McKeever, Gill, & Van Deventer, 1975; McKeever, Van Deventer, & Suberi, 1973). These facts, together with the findings from mirror and vertical English, Hebrew, and Chinese words all argue in support of a thesis appealing to mechanisms of cerebral dominance underlying RVF superiorities with word stimuli. They also argue against the employment of an unnatural vertical format. The only indication that reading Hebrew has a consequence relevant for laterality research is the finding (Rayner, Well, & Pollatsek, 1980) that bilingual Israeli readers of Hebrew have effective visual fields that extend further to the right while reading English and further to the left while reading Hebrew. This finding, however, probably relates to inter*word* rather than inter*letter* phenomena.

The Stroop paradigm.   When color words (*red, green, blue*) are themselves written in colored dyes, and the subject's task is to name the dyes (and to ignore the words), a congruent color-word–dye relationship (e.g., *red* written in a red dye) facilitates performance, and an incongruent color relationship (e.g., *blue* written in green dye) interferes with performance, relative to a baseline control condition when subjects name the dye of a meaningless letter string. Schmit and Davis (1974); Tsao, Feustel, and Soseos (1979); and Warren and Marsh (1979) all found, as might be expected, that greater interference was produced when incompatible color and name information was presented to the left hemisphere.

A right hemisphere contribution for the preprocessing of unfamiliar or de-graded verbal stimuli. We have seen that for letter and word stimuli, a RVF superiority usually appears, whether the subject is detecting the presence or absence of prespecified targets or is engaged in phonological or lexical processing or even, in certain instances, in semantic categorization. Sometimes, however, a LVF superiority may emerge, for example, when subjects perform physical matches (*AA, bb*) of letter pairs. J. L. Bradshaw, Bradley, and Patterson (1976) found that the usual RVF superiority for the detection of target letters was reduced or reversed when left–right mirror-reversed letters were presented, possibly because now a right hemisphere-mediated spatial transformation was required to recognize the stimuli. G. Cohen (1975b) also employed normal and mirror-image digits and letters, presented at varying angles to the upright. Again, when subjects were asked to decide whether the stimulus was normal or a mirror image, a LVF superiority appeared. Moscovitch (1972) found that a RVF superiority appeared only with a relatively large target set of letters (six), which presumably required a verbal or phonological strategy; with fewer targets, a physically based strategy might have operated, at least in part, leading to nonsignificant or LVF superiorities. Umiltà, Frost, and Hyman (1972) obtained a RVF superiority for target letters grouped into an *acoustically* matched set and a LVF superiority for target letters grouped into a *visually* matched set. Moscovitch (1976) gave his subjects their target letters verbally and then laterally flashed a test letter, which was either the same letter as the target or was a letter with the same or a different terminal phoneme (e.g., *b* and *t* versus *b* and *k*). The subject was required to respond in terms of the identity of the terminal phoneme. While a RVF superiority appeared when test and target item shared the terminal phoneme, indicating left hemisphere mediation of phonological processing, when the stimuli were identical a LVF superiority emerged. This was presumably a consequence of a right hemisphere physical match, even though it would seem likely that under these circumstances the right hemisphere would have had to *generate* an *image* of the (verbally given) target. Jonides (1979) obtained a LVF superiority for a difficult letter-detection task (target and test letters were visually confusable) and the ("normal") RVF superiority when they were easily discriminated visually. Wilkins and Stewart (1974) obtained the expected RVF (left hemisphere) superiorities in a letter-matching task when target and test stimuli were separated by a "long" interval (990 msec), which presumably permitted and probably required phonological recoding. However, when the retention interval was "short" (50 msec), a LVF (right hemisphere) visuospatial match sufficed. Bryden and Allard (1976) obtained the usual RVF superiorities in letter processing when normal type fonts were employed and a LVF superiority when an unusual, florid, or Gothic style of type was used, which again presumably demanded right hemisphere visuospatial mechanisms. Gordon and Carmon (1976) obtained an essentially similar result: An initial LVF superiority with unfamiliar scripts gave way later to RVF superiorities; materials in a conventional format gave a RVF superiority from the beginning. Hellige and Webster (1979) found that single letters were better recognized in the RVF; however, when perceptually degraded by an overlapping mask, a LVF superiority emerged. This LVF superiority persisted for about 40 msec on either side of stimulus presentation (i.e., the effect occurred whenever the mask was presented ± 40 msec from letter presentation). The authors concluded that the right hemisphere is better at extracting the relevant visual features of a letter when it is perceptually degraded, despite the fact that *verbal* stimuli were employed. On the other hand, several studies (G. Cohen, 1976; McKeever & Gill, 1972b; Oscar-Berman, Goodglass, & Cherlow, 1973) have found that letters or words presented to the RVF are less vulnerable to disruption by backward-masking stimuli or are read out faster from iconic storage. Others have also reported that the time required to escape backward masking is shorter for RVF presentations (Ward & Ross, 1977; McKeever & Suberi, 1974).

With *words,* G. J. Bradshaw and Hicks (1977) and G. J. Bradshaw, Hicks, and Rose (1979) obtained a LVF superiority in a lexical decision task when exposure durations were too short to permit categorical identification of the word (though long enough to permit its acceptance or rejection as a word, presumably in terms of lower-level orthographic features). At longer exposures, when the words could also be identified, the "normal" RVF superiorities emerged. Pirozzolo and Rayner (1977), while obtaining an overall RVF superiority for word recognition, nevertheless found that subjects made more visual than acoustic confusions (the response alternatives contained both types of word), especially with LVF (right hemisphere) presentations. As we saw above, J. L. Bradshaw and Mapp (1982) found that with target judgments for word stimuli, RVF superiorities were weakest for cursive script and where word envelope shape could be used as a cue.

As we shall demonstrate in Chapter Seven, this all shows that levels of coding, perceptual difficulty, and stimulus familiarity are important determinants of the extent and direction of laterality effects (Moscovitch, 1979). We can also conclude that it is not so much the verbal–nonverbal nature of the stimuli that determines the direction of laterality differences but *how* they are processed or encoded. This conclusion, though denied by some (e.g., Simion, Bagnara, Bisiachi, Roncato, & Umiltà, 1980), was reached by Seamon and Gazzaniga (1973) and reiterated by Metzger and Antes (1976). They required their subjects to remember nouns either by relational imagery or by subvocal rehearsal and then presented lateralized picture probes. A LVF superiority appeared when relational imagery was used, a RVF superiority when verbal rehearsal was used. As we saw previously, Klatzky and Atkinson (1971) flashed pictures of common objects to one or the other field; the subjects were required to determine the initial letter of the object's name and compare it to a set of previously memorized letters. Despite the visuospatial nature of the pictures, the demands of verbal coding generated a RVF superiority. While Simion et al. (1980) reject such conclusions and find a RVF superiority in a letter matching task, whether the letters were physically identical, nominally identical, or analogue-matched (e.g., *Cc, Oo*), we feel that their findings and conclusions run against the tide of current research.

Left-field superiorities for nonverbal visual stimuli. A LVF (right hemisphere) superiority has been reported for processing simple nonverbal stimuli, ranging from the discrimination of lightness (Davidoff, 1975) and color (Davidoff, 1976; Hannay, 1979; Pennal, 1977), dot detection (Davidoff, 1977; Umiltà, Salmaso, Bagnara, & Simion, 1979) and localization (Bryden, 1976; Kimura, 1969), perception of line orientation (Atkinson & Egeth, 1973; Umiltà, Rizzolatti, Marzi, Zamboni, Franzini, Camarda, & Berlucchi, 1974) and curvature (Longden, Ellis, & Iversen, 1976), matching arcs to circles (Hatta, 1977a), the McCullough effect (G. E. Meyer, 1976), stereopsis (Carmon & Bechtoldt, 1969), and depth perception (Kimura & Durnford, 1974). Umiltà et al. (1974) found that for the perception of line orientation and slant, the LVF was superior only for values that could not be easily coded in verbal terms (i.e., the RVF proved superior when lines were horizontal, vertical, and at a 45° slope). However, it should also be noted that Brizzolara, Umiltà, Marzi, Berlucchi, and Rizzolatti (1975) still obtained a LVF superiority for the task of telling time from an unnumbered clock face, even with verbal responses.

It has proved more difficult to demonstrate a LVF superiority with more complex patterns and shapes than with either simple perceptual discriminations or face processing (see following section), both of which have themselves proved to be associated with weaker and more labile right hemisphere superiorities than the left hemisphere superiorities found with verbal stimuli. If we can anticipate and risk generalizations, a RVF superiority seems to be more likely for familiar patterns and simple shapes, and a LVF superiority more likely for more complex items, for target ("same") judgments that require *memory* rather than simple *perceptual* matching (see, e.g., J. L. Bradshaw, Gates, & Patterson, 1976; M. J. White & White, 1975), and for longer retention intervals, especially where the interval is varied rather than kept constant. Under these circumstances subjects may develop a set to attend to the more difficult or unfamiliar stimuli, and the coding strategies they adopt for these, especially where different types of stimuli are intermingled, may also determine what happens for the easier or more familiar items. Thus, even where exactly similar stimuli have been employed (though with quite different conditions of stimulus randomization), variable results have been reported. Fontenot (1973) obtained a LVF superiority for high-complexity random forms and no field differences for simple ones; Hannay, Rogers, and Durant (1976) obtained a RVF superiority for both levels of complexity. Using different stimuli, Umiltà, Bagnara, and Simion (1978) essentially replicated Fontenot's results, finding a LVF superiority in the matching of simultaneously presented, complex, multisided polygons and a RVF superiority in matching simple geometric shapes or nonsense patterns. Bryden and Rainey (1963) reported essentially similar findings. Dee and Fontenot (1973) obtained a LVF superiority for complex random forms only when retention intervals longer than 10 sec were employed. Similar results were reported by Hatta (1976). A LVF superiority has been reported for *speed* in matching simultaneously presented checkerboard patterns (M. M. Gross, 1972), but not for *accuracy* (Kimura & Durnford, 1974). With verbal report of (bilaterally presented) line drawings of common objects, the first-to-be-reported drawing being cued to the subject at the time of presentation, A. W. Young and Bion (1981a) found that differences (a small RVF superiority) only appeared for the second-reported item. They concluded that the right hemisphere is less able to effect the temporary storage needed when a drawing is to be reported second. It is possible that the right hemisphere cannot so readily store a verbal name as it can a visual code, while the left can store both.

   Studies with faces.   A LVF superiority in terms of recognition accuracy has been reported with photographed faces (Hilliard, 1973) and cartoon line drawings (Ley & Bryden, 1977). Similarly face stimuli are recognized faster when presented to the LVF than to the RVF, whether the stimuli are identikit constructions (Geffen et al., 1971), photographs (Berlucchi, Brizzolara, Marzi, Rizzolatti, & Umiltà, 1974; Rizzolatti, Umiltà, & Berlucchi, 1971; Suberi & McKeever, 1977) or schematic drawings (Patterson & Bradshaw, 1975). Geffen et al. (1971) found that this (26 msec) LVF superiority with discriminatory manual reaction times disappeared when subjects were instead timed in making yes or no vocal judgments to target and nontarget faces. This finding seemed to suggest that the differences between the hemispheres are relative or quantitative rather than absolute or qualitative; the right hemisphere is quicker at processing the faces and slower at initiating a vocal response than the left, the two effects canceling. Were faces exclusively processed by the right hemisphere and the simple yes or no discriminatory vocal responses initiated solely by the left, the LVF superiority should have been preserved. However, when subjects are required to *name* lateralized drawings of common objects, hues, or such (McKeever & Jackson, 1979), rather than utter simple yes or no vocal responses (which may lie within the limits of right hemisphere capacities), a large RVF superiority for vocal latencies is maintained. The same authors (McKeever, Gill, & Van Deventer, 1975) also failed to obtain RVF superiorities with simple yes or no vocal responses in a dot-detection task. A RVF superiority for naming hues is of course uncontaminated by scanning artifacts.
   Bertelson, Vanhaelen, and Morais (1979) presented pairs of faces successively, the first at fixation and the second (test item) in either the LVF or RVF. The second face was physically identical to the first, or quite different, or of the same person viewed from another angle (cf. nominal identity, *Aa,* in letter-pair judgments). The biggest LVF superiority appeared for this last category, leading the authors to suggest that the right hemisphere mechanisms of face recognition operate in terms of "physiognomic invariants," extracting feature information that is independent of orientation, expression, and possibly aging. Moscovitch, Scullion,

and Christie (1976) likewise found that LVF superiorities were stronger when subjects matched sketched caricatures to target photographs. Such considerations have led to the claim (see Chapter Four) that the right hemisphere has a specialist mechanism dedicated to the processing of faces, over and above its general superiority in mediating visuospatial material in general or complex meaningful configurations in particular. Yin (1969, 1970) and Carey and Diamond (1977) make this claim partly on the basis that inverted faces do not generate the LVF superiorities typical of upright faces (S. Leehey, Carey, Diamond, & Cahn, 1978; Rapaczynki & Ehrlichman, 1979), though others dispute both the findings and the conclusion (Ellis & Shepherd, 1975; Phillips & Rawles, 1979; Phillips, 1979; J. L. Bradshaw, Taylor, Patterson, & Nettleton, 1980). Still others argue that the LVF superiority with faces stems at least in part from right hemisphere involvement in emotional affect (Suberi & McKeever, 1977; see also Chapter Seven), though the findings of Ley and Bryden (1977) argue for a true independence, with both functions being separately mediated by the right hemisphere.

Some studies have reported a RVF superiority for familiar faces (Marzi & Berlucchi, 1977; Marzi, Brizzolara, Rizzolatti, Umiltà, & Berlucchi, 1974). This effect seems not to be a consequence of (possibly covert) verbal naming or identification, since Umiltà, Brizzolara, Tabossi, and Fairweather (1978) found that after days of practice and increasing familiarity, unfamiliar faces (which originally gave the normal LVF superiority) reversed to give a RVF superiority. Familiarity seemed to induce a shift from right hemisphere processing (for initially novel stimuli) to left hemisphere processing. Not everyone, however, has obtained a RVF superiority with familiar faces (e.g., S. C. Leehey & Cahn, 1979; Moscovitch, Scullion, & Christie, 1976).

A RVF superiority, independent of both naming and familiarity, was found when nontarget schematic faces were very similar to targets, differing from them only by a single feature, thus requiring detailed analytic processing (K. Patterson & Bradshaw, 1975; see also Chapter Nine). It was also found (B. Jones, 1979) when subjects classified faces as male or female, again confirming our earlier suggestion that while the right hemisphere may be superior for operations on particular configurations, the left is better at classification or categorization.

Three studies employing normal subjects have presented chimeric face stimuli (as used with commissurotomy patients; see Chapter Five), with left and right halves of the composite drawn from two different faces and abutted at the midline. Milner and Dunne (1977) found that if a narrow strip was pasted over the join, normal subjects were generally unaware that the (centrally presented) stimuli were chimeric, the left and right halves not matching (commissurotomy patients, of course, did not need such a strip, since the $2°$ to $3°$ of central vision that are possibly cross connected by the commissures are now separated). Thus normal subjects, like the commissurotomy patients, experienced perceptual completion under these conditions and demonstrated a LVF superiority for identification by pointing, but only when the left hand was employed. Campbell (1978), using chimeric face stimuli, found that the left half of such faces was normally preferred, and

M. Schwartz and M. L. Smith (1980) found that the LVF was superior in recognition tasks.

Target and nontarget stimuli. In most experiments of this sort, target judgments are usually faster than nontarget judgments. Nickerson (1978) reviews a number of possible explanations and concludes that none is entirely satisfactory. One possibility (see also Krueger, 1978; Hellige, 1980b) is that the configuration must be thoroughly checked before a nontarget response is emitted, with the associated possibility that perceptual noise produced by an aberrant nontarget item in a display slows down processing. This idea is in accord with Sternberg's (1975) claim that target superiority occurs at the *decision* rather than the *comparison* stage of information processing.

Regardless of whether targets are or are not faster than nontargets, a very general finding is that visual field superiorities in the predicted direction are stronger or more consistent for target stimuli (for reviews see J. L. Bradshaw, Gates, & Patterson, 1976; Hellige, Cox, & Litvac, 1979). Suberi and McKeever (1977) suggest that subjects adopt a set to respond to targets, responding to nontargets with little awareness of what was presented. Moscovitch (1972) suggests that there is a bias to check information in both hemispheres before responding "different" to nontargets but not before responding "same" to targets. Finally, Hellige et al. (1979) suggest a response bias: When in doubt respond "different" since there are more possible ways that a stimulus can be different than it can be the same. Consequently, there may be more correct guesses among correct responses on nontarget trials than on target trials. Response times of correct responses on target trials may be more sensitive to the relatively small differences caused by visual field and hemisphere. Possible support for such a conclusion comes from the finding of J. L. Bradshaw, Taylor, Patterson, and Nettleton (1980) that visual field differences were stronger for nontargets than for targets when the former were designed to be maximally different from the latter and considerably less different from each other.

Bilateral presentations. We have assumed until now that visually presented stimuli are unilaterally flashed to one or the other visual field. McKeever and Huling (1971a) attempted to simulate the dichotic technique in audition, which independently channels two simultaneous and competing messages, one to each ear, by simultaneously flashing pairs of stimuli, one to each visual field. It had previously been found that when random letter strings were flashed across fixation, letters to the left were better reported than those to the right (see M. White, 1969, for review). Bryden and Rainey (1963) ascribed this to a postexposural scan of a rapidly fading visual trace, proceeding from left to right in accordance with reading habits, where the right half decayed before it could be reported. Subsequently, in a paradigm even closer to that of dichotic stimulation, Hines, Satz, Schell, and Schmidlin (1969) presented four digit pairs successively, one letter of each pair in each visual field, and obtained a LVF superiority. However Zurif and Bryden (1969), using letters in a similar design, obtained a significant RVF superiority for dextrals, but nonsignificant RVF superiority for sinistrals. Reasons for the difference between the two studies are not clear, though the fact that handedness affected the results supports an involvement of cerebral asymmetry (see also Schmuller & Goodman, 1979). Moreover, a RVF superiority with bilateral presentation seems to depend on the presence of a gap between the two elements of the display, perhaps reducing scanning tendencies (Hirata & Bryden, 1976).

Recent studies have usually noted a large RVF superiority under conditions of bilateral presentation of a pair of letters or words, frequently larger than that obtained under unilateral presentation (Hines, 1972a; McKeever, 1971; McKeever & Huling, 1971a; but see Hines, 1976). This has been ascribed to the competitive nature of the stimulation, which forces both hemispheres to process independently, whereas with unilateral presentations the right is free to refer its input to the left hemisphere.

With unilateral presentations, unless the subject fixates on the fixation point, he or she is likely to miss half the stimuli. With bilateral presentations the subject can consciously fixate or unconsciously attend to one side and be sure of always receiving foveal input. For this reason a new control measure was adopted with bilateral presentations, a fixation stimulus that the subject has to report before or after responding to the lateralized stimulus. This measure introduces a new set of problems, which we shall deal with in the next section. For now we should note that it cannot satisfactorily eliminate those other problems in bilateral presentation alluded to earlier—directional scanning and biases of report order. The biases can be partly avoided if reaction time rather than report accuracy measures are employed, and both can be further reduced, though in theory never completely eliminated, by cueing the subject on which field to report first. Thus, McKeever (1971) and Rosen, Curcio, MacKavey, and Herbert (1975) found no diminution of the RVF superiority, even if the subject was cued to report one or the other field first. Similar effects with nouns are reported by A. W. Young and Bion (1981a) and A. W. Young, Bion, and Ellis (1980), though these authors also note that when their subjects named line drawings, field differences (RVF superiority) only emerged for the second-reported items, emphasizing the relative disability of the right hemisphere to store verbal codes. Schmuller and Goodman (1980) with cued (from a directional arrow at fixation) order of report of bilaterally presented line drawings, nevertheless obtained a significant *LVF* superiority, which was strongest for the *first* reported item. Obviously, the situation with drawings awaits resolution. With words, however, a large RVF superiority appears to be a stable phenomenon, whether measured from first or second item reported, and even where items in the LVF are given a 20-msec temporal advantage, by being presented ahead of those in the RVF by that amount (McKeever & Huling, 1971b).

Use of fixation control stimuli. In the previous section we mentioned that bilateral presentation necessitated the use of fixation controls. Many methods have been tried, from direct or video monitoring of fixation before and during stimulus presentation, with elimination of trials where an eye movement occurred, to electro-oculography or infrared monitoring devices, but to many experimenters such techniques have seemed costly and inconvenient. Generally, where such measures have been made, undesirable eye movements seem to have occurred in less than 1 or 2 percent of trials (Geffen, Bradshaw, & Nettleton, 1972; B. Jones & Santi, 1978).

Consequently, a practice has developed with bilateral presentations of employing a fixation stimulus such as a digit or letter to be reported before or after responding to the laterally presented materials. Such a procedure is obviously somewhat less practical when reaction times are being measured, though it is sometimes still used. The technique was pioneered by McKeever and his colleagues (see, e.g., McKeever & Gill, 1972a; McKeever et al., 1975), and substantial RVF superiorities were reported. According to Hines (1972a) these effects were simply the result of directional scanning, the subjects continuing to scan to the right after processing the fixation digit. In support of this claim he found a significant RVF superiority in one group of subjects required to report the fixation digit prior to word recall and a nonsignificant LVF superiority in another group not so required. However, Hines (1972b) modified this view when McKeever, Suberi, and Van Deventer (1972) demonstrated that randomly omitting the fixation digit on half the trials had no significant effect on RVF superiority (and see also MacKavey, Curcio, & Rosen, 1975). Hines concluded that the fixation digit ensured fixation and prevented subjects from adopting fixation biases that favor the LVF.

A possibly more serious objection to the technique is the question of whether its verbal or nonverbal nature might modify the hemispheric set for processing the lateralized stimuli. This would follow from Kinsbourne's attentional hypothesis, which we shall discuss in more detail in Chapter Seven and which would predict that visual field superiorities may be biased by an established verbal or nonverbal processing set as a result of hemispheric activation. Kershner, Thomae, and Callaway (1977) and Carter and Kinsbourne (1979) make such a claim. In the former study, children showed a LVF superiority in a digit-reporting task when the fixation stimuli were geometric shapes and a normal RVF superiority when they were letters. Mancuso, Lawrence, Hintze, and White (1979) also showed that altering the nature of the fixation stimulus affected the outcome of peripheral recognition and concluded that the central fixation stimuli serve as more than a simple fixation anchor. They warned against their use. Similar conclusions were reached by Hellige and Cox (1976). On the other hand, Hines (1978) and Duda and Kirby (1980) found that the verbal or spatial nature of the fixation control stimulus did *not* affect the magnitude or direction of obtained asymmetries. The issue is obviously still unresolved (the studies differ on the codeability of the fixation stimuli, nature of the lateralized stimuli, and other task requirements), but it seems safer to avoid the technique. One version, however, which may have much to recommend it, was developed by Schmuller and Goodman (1979, 1980). The fixation stimulus consists of an arrow pointing towards one or the other lateralized stimulus, indicating which requires prior (or only) processing. With this technique the authors have demonstrated LVF superiorities for outline drawings and RVF superiorities for words; the effects are reduced or reversed with sinistral subjects. This seems to be a fairly convincing demonstration that the technique taps cerebral asymmetry.

Other techniques for laterally presenting visual stimuli. The tachistoscopic techniques we have reviewed so far all rely on very brief exposures, limiting the amount of information that can be presented and probably also constraining or altering the way the information is processed. Attempts have been made to develop systems that would permit scanning, over lengthy periods, of lateralized stimuli. In Chapter Five we described E. Zaidel's technique of a collimating system mounted on a scleral contact lens. This technique, though highly successful, is complicated, unwieldly, and uncomfortable and has only been employed with a handful of commissurotomy patients since individual lenses must be molded for each subject.

Dimond and Farrington (1977) used opaque contact lenses with a small slit to channel information into one or the other hemiretina. We had tried a similar technique in our own laboratory and found that refraction around the edge of the slit, slippage, and discomfort to the subjects severely limited applicability of the technique. Dimond and his colleagues appear themselves not to have followed it up further.

Rayner and his colleagues (see, e.g., Rayner, 1979) have linked eye-monitoring devices to a computer display so that they can alter certain parts of the display in response to fixational positions. Although they were not generally working in the field of cerebral asymmetry or even nonverbal pattern processing, their technique has obvious implications for the problems we have described, and we have currently established a somewhat similar system in our own laboratory and are now making preliminary observations. We feel that, at least in the visual modality, this is likely to be the direction in which future research will go.

Auditory Studies with Normal Subjects: Dichotic Stimulation

In this section we shall review the findings under conditions of dichotic stimulation of a right-ear advantage (REA) for verbal stimuli and a left-ear advantage (LEA) for nonverbal materials. It will be recalled (Chapter Five) that dichotic stimulation involves the simultaneous presentation of paired materials, one to each ear. The paradigm was originally developed to study processes of selective attention, and it is perhaps curious that the two fields, laterality research and selective attention, have since then continued more or less independently, though employing the same basic technique. In the laterality context a list of three items is typically presented to the left ear while a second sequence, temporally aligned with the first, is presented to the right ear. Obviously intensities are very important; with verbal material a 15dB difference in favor of the left ear is needed for it to outperform the right, on a baseline level of 80dB. This asymmetry in favor of the right ear drops to 5dB at 50dB (Berlin, 1977). The two signals should also be synchronous, though if they are asynchronous the second one is better perceived (perhaps because it masks the first), within the time-separation range of 0 to 500 msec; beyond that the first is better (Berlin, 1977).

Kimura's direct-access account of dichotic ear differences. The finding of opposing ear superiorities for verbal and nonverbal stimuli, initially only under conditions of simultaneous, competing, dichotic stimulation, led Kimura (1967, 1973a) to propose that in addition to hemispheric specialization (the left for verbal and the right for nonverbal processing), there is a perceptual advantage for information transmitted via the contralateral auditory pathways; the ipsilateral routes are said to be partially or completely suppressed by contralateral activation. In addition, she argued that verbal information fed to the left ear suffers degradation either in the right hemisphere or during transcallosal transmission to the left hemisphere, where it is processed. There is neurophysiological evidence that the contralateral auditory pathway has more fibers and that contralateral stimulation produces larger cortical activity (Brugge & Merzenich, 1973; Hall & Goldstein, 1968; Majkowski, Bochenek, Bochenek, Knapik-Fijalkowska, & Kopec, 1971; Rosenzweig, 1951, 1954; see also Berlin, 1977, for review of findings concerning the auditory pathways). However, as we have already seen, the *manner* in which stimuli are processed may well be more important than the nature (verbal or nonverbal) of the stimuli *per se* (see, e.g., Metzger & Antes, 1976; Seamon & Gazzaniga, 1973; and Chapter Nine). Moreover, as we shall discuss shortly, the *nature* of the competition (e.g., the extent to which the two inputs may centrally compete for the same kind of processing) may be as important as the fact of peripheral competition (Teng, 1980) and even that may be unnecessary, given that ear differences may be demonstrable under certain conditions with monaural presentations. Presumably in the latter instance the contralateral pathways still predominate.

Perceptual and memory effects and order of report. The REA with recall of dichotically presented digits was first reported by Kimura (1961a, b). It is typically small and rather unstable. As with the directional scan problem for letter strings and words in the visual modality, with dichotic listening there is also the problem of order of report. Most subjects choose to report from the right ear first, giving all the items presented to that ear, then all the items presented to the left ear. As Inglis (1962) and Inglis and Sykes (1967) observed, first-reported items have a short-term memory advantage, since while they are being reported the stored items presented to the left ear may be lost; however, the REA, though sometimes reduced, is not eliminated when order of report is controlled (Bryden, 1978). Thus, the REA cannot be just an order-of-report artifact; a REA still appears even if the left ear is cued for first report (Bryden, 1963, 1965) or if the subjects, instead of recalling as many items as possible, are tested for recognition by a test probe (Broadbent & Gregory, 1964). Nor can the REA be purely a memory rather than a perceptual phenomenon, as the REA persists whether analyzed over the first or the second reported channel (Borkowski, Spreen, & Stutz, 1965).

It does seem likely that two independent mechanisms may be operating in the dichotic recall procedure, first-ear reports reflecting a perceptual processing advantage and second-ear reports reflecting a contribution from memory. As is frequently found in other contexts (see Chapter Seven), laterality effects may be stronger at the level of memory storage than pure perception, with second-ear reports often giving a greater REA than first (see, e.g., Oscar-Berman, Rehbein, Porfert, & Goodglass, 1978, for review). Thus, larger laterality effects may be observed for material that is more difficult to store briefly in echoic memory (Darwin & Baddeley, 1974; Yeni-Komshian & Gordon, 1974). Conversely, since overall accuracy is higher on first-reported items, ceiling effects may reduce the possible magnitude of any REA for such items. Notwithstanding these considerations, the fact that REAs can be demonstrated with recognition probes, as we saw, or with reaction-time measures for target detection (see following section) argues against the *necessary* involvement of memory. Nor are attentional factors preeminent; Bryden (1969) found that regardless of instructions to attend more to one ear than the other, or to both equally, the REA persisted.

Consonants, vowels, and fricatives. Reviewed in detail by Krashen (1976, 1977), the general findings of the dichotic listening paradigm with verbal stimuli are as follows: Dirks (1964) obtained a REA with words, Curry (1967) with nonsense sounds, and Kimura and Folb (1968) with speech played backwards. The effect was then extended to consonant-vowel (CV) syllables (Shankweiler & Studdert-Kennedy, 1967) that contrasted in the consonant segments alone, such as *ba* and *ga,* suggesting that phonology was an important determinant. These same authors (Shankweiler & Studdert-Kennedy, 1967; Studdert-Kennedy & Shankweiler, 1970) then found that while encoded (i.e., perceptually complex) stop consonants gave a REA, the effect did not extend to the perceptually simpler, more invariant, and steady-state vowel sounds. The fact that stop consonants are of brief duration and require a great deal of restructuring and phonetic processing for identification, perhaps involving a specialist phonological processor in the left hemisphere, seemed to account for their associated REA. Indeed, a REA could be produced with vowels if their perception was made more difficult by embedding them in noise (Weiss & House, 1973) and/or shortening their duration (Godfrey, 1974; Studdert-Kennedy, 1972). Darwin (1971) found that synthetic vowels *do* give a REA when the listener is uncertain about the effective vocal tract size, and the left hemisphere is presumably required to perform the normalization necessary for the accurate perception of speech, regardless of the speaker's age or sex. Haggard (1971) also obtained a REA for vowels when there was contextual uncertainty as to voice pitch. Whether or not a REA is found for vowels seems to depend on the complexity of the required discrimination; vowels normally convey relatively little information to listeners, whereas the highly encoded stop consonants are acoustically very complex. Vowels are also of longer duration and are more easily discriminated than consonants; thus, consonants are more vulnerable to distortion or loss than vowels if initially transmitted to the wrong hemisphere;

vowels, if presented under unfavorable listening conditions, may generate the "expected" REA.

Darwin (1971) also obtained a REA for synthetic fricatives (e.g., /f/) only when formant transitions (which require complex analysis and decoding) were included in the signal, not when the other cue sufficient for their perception (the noise burst produced at the point of constriction in the articulators) alone was present. Cutting (1973) observed that the REA for initial stop consonants (e.g., /g/) is greater than for less encoded liquids (e.g., /l/) and semivowels (/y/ and /w/), which are in turn greater than for the still less encoded vowels. Spellacy and Blumstein (1970) obtained a REA for vowels when the subject expected to hear them in a language context and a LEA for the same material heard out of a language context when the subjects were expecting to hear nonspeech sounds. A LEA was also obtained by Blumstein and Cooper (1974) for the identification of intonation contours corresponding to the intonation used to convey information on declarative, imperative, conditional, and interrogative sentences in English, even when such contours were superimposed on short nonsense syllables. On the other hand, Van Lancker and Fromkin (1973) found a REA with Thai speakers discriminating Thai words that differed only by pitch; in the tonal Thai language, pitch is a phonological cue to meaning. The same tones presented in a nonlinguistic context gave no REA.

At the sentence level, Zurif and Sait (1969) and Zurif and Mendelsohn (1972) obtained a REA for nonsense words that follow the morphemic structures of English (i.e., are syntactically regular and are presented with the correct prosody, intonation, and stress, like Lewis Carroll's "Jabberwocky," rather than being read out like a laundry list).

The REA and its relationship to cerebral dominance. In one of the first studies employing the dichotic technique, Kimura (1961b) observed that variations in the direction of ear superiority were associated, at least in statistical terms, with differences in hemispheric lateralization, as determined by the Wada amytal test (see Chapter Four). Subjects with left hemisphere speech generally demonstrated a REA; those with right hemisphere speech showed a reversed asymmetry. Geffen, Traub, and Stierman (1978) validated their version of the dichotic monitoring test (i.e., manual reaction times to the detection of prespecified targets embedded in dichotic sequences) against another invasive clinical test for hemispheric specialization, unilateral ECT (see Chapter Four). All patients who were shown to be left speech dominant by unilateral ECT also showed REAs; four out of five patients with right hemisphere speech showed LEAs; two patients with bilateral speech had no ear asymmetry. They concluded that the ear contralateral to the hemisphere dominant for speech, as determined by unilateral ECT, was superior in hit rate and/or reaction time in their dichotic monitoring test.

Further confirmation of the utility of the dichotic technique comes from the findings of reduced or reversed ear asymmetries with females or sinistrals (Bryden,

1965, 1970; Curry, 1967; Satz, Achenbach, & Fennell, 1967; Zurif & Bryden, 1969; see also Chapters Ten and Eleven). Shankweiler and Studdert-Kennedy (1975) obtained a significant positive correlation in dextrals between strength of dextrality and magnitude of the REA. They concluded that cerebral lateralization for speech perception and for manual praxis are both best viewed as gradients and, being correlated, are derived from a common source. However, since ear asymmetries may switch with practice (see Chapter Seven) and far fewer (70 to 80 percent) of normal dextrals typically demonstrate REAs than are believed on clinical grounds to have speech in the left hemisphere (maybe 95 percent; see Chapter Eight), Berlin (1977) believes that the REA is merely a correlate of lateralization for speech and language functions. The REA is not, however, an *index* of the magnitude of lateralization, any more than the noise emitted by a motor vehicle is a direct index of its speed. Indeed, why do tachistoscopic and dichotic techniques invariably indicate a much smaller percentage of normal dextrals with "left hemisphere language" than would be predicted from clinical studies? One possibility is that the behavioral tests are unreliable; certainly the newer target-monitoring reaction-time techniques (to be discussed later in this chapter) do give far more consistent and reliable results. Another possibility is that the tests are assessing dominance for language comprehension, not production. Language production, as assessed by typical clinical procedures, is known to be far more lateralized (see Chapter Eight) than comprehension, where practice and strategy effects can cause directional shifts (see Chapter Seven).

Indices of the REA. A major problem with the traditional dichotic technique of comparing ear superiorities in terms of accuracy of recall is that ear differences will depend on overall performance levels and accuracy. Consequently, subjects within a study and different studies cannot easily be compared. Marshall, Caplan, and Holmes (1975) discuss the relative merits of four possible measures in this context (R and L refer to right and left; c and e to correct and error scores):

1. The traditional ear-difference score of percentage correct-right minus percentage correct-left,

    $$Rc - Lc$$

2. Percent of correct, POC: correct scores on right divided by total correct scores

    $$\frac{Rc}{Rc + Lc}$$

3. Percent of error, POE: errors on left divided by total errors

    $$\frac{Le}{Re + Le}$$

4. A double-barrelled laterality coefficient

    (a) when accuracy $< 50\%$, $\dfrac{Rc - Lc}{Rc + Lc}$

    (b) when accuracy $> 50\%$, $\dfrac{Rc - Lc}{Re + Le}$

They point out that the first three measures are all dependent on total accuracy and claim that this problem is minimized with the last. However, Birkett (1977) and Birkett and Wilson (1979) applied all four measures to empirical data, calculating the correlation coefficient between each and their correlation with total accuracy. Finding that all four measures intercorrelated with each other and correlated with total accuracy, they concluded (as does Stone, 1980) that one should be cautious in the use of any of them. Repp (1977) also gives a thorough review of the four measures of Marshall et al., and in addition concludes that Kuhn's (1973) ϕ coefficient

$$\phi = \frac{Rc - Lc}{\sqrt{(Rc + Lc)(2T - Rc - Lc)^{1/2}}}$$

where T equals number of trials or dichotic presentations, is effectively a conjunction of POC and POE, being their geometric mean. J. Levy (1977a) concludes that Kuhn's ϕ function, which, being effectively a correlation coefficient for two independent dichotomously measured dimensions, is related to the X^2 statistic, is *still* not independent of performance level. For such reasons, and because of their generally far greater degree of sensitivity, we have ourselves preferred to use reaction-time measures rather than accuracy scores. In this way floor and ceiling effects may also be circumvented.

Monaural effects. The findings discussed so far have all involved dichotic presentations. Indeed, as we saw, Kimura's functional prepotency model is predicated on the assumption of the need to suppress ipsilateral auditory pathways with simultaneous contralateral stimulation. However, for over ten years it has been apparent that ear differences may appear with monaural stimulation (Bakker, 1970; Bever, 1971; Frankfurter & Honeck, 1973; Harriman & Buxton, 1979; Jarvella & Herman, 1973). These differences generally appear only under conditions of load, difficulty, memorization, or stimulus degradation. Where the two paradigms are directly compared, effects are often stronger with dichotic than monaural presentations (Cohen & Martin, 1975).

Monaural effects, however, are undoubtedly easier to demonstrate with reaction-time measures. First introduced in the auditory modality by Springer (1973) and reviewed by her (1977), this technique taps perceptual processes free of memory factors. It has often involved the use of simultaneous white noise in the other channel as a "lateralizing" device, though there is doubt whether unmodulated white noise can achieve this (J. L. Bradshaw, Nettleton, & Geffen, 1971, 1972). Demonstrations of REAs with monaurally presented verbal materials have been reported by Bever, Hurtig, and Handel (1976); Catlin, Vanderveer, and Teicher (1976); Fry (1974); and Morais (1976). Catlin and Neville (1976) reported that their monaural REAs were no smaller than those obtained with dichotic stimulation; however, since by "dichotic" they meant with competing white noise, we are unconvinced that the latter condition was not simply a variant of their former, monaural presentation. While Kallman and Corballis (1975) reported a LEA for nonverbal stimuli, Kallman (1977, 1978) successfully demonstrated a double dissociation, a REA for verbal and a LEA for nonverbal stimuli.

Teng (1980) employed in a *dichotic* paradigm the following pairings, digit-digit, tone-tone, digit (left ear)-tone (right ear) and tone (left ear)-digit (right ear). Ear differences disappeared when digits were paired with tones, and overall performance was superior, leading her to conclude that there is a capacity limitation and an advantage of the contralateral over the ipsilateral ear only when the inputs from the two ears compete for the same kind of processing. This conclusion (from the *dichotic* paradigm) can also explain our own *monaural* findings (J. L. Bradshaw, Farrelly, & Taylor, 1981). We presented aligned pairs of words with a reaction-time target-detection measure, under conditions either of true dichotic presentation (one word to each ear) or monaural competition (both words simultaneously to one ear). The REA, though significant in the dichotic condition, was vastly greater in the competing monaural condition. This finding argues against the need for occlusion of the ipsilateral by the contralateral pathways and Kimura's functional prepotency model, since competition (between the *same kinds* of material) *within* ears is sufficient. It also suggests that competing monaural stimulation with a reaction-time measure may be the most sensitive technique of all.

Nonverbal materials and LEAs. In the last section we discussed two or three findings with monaural stimulation of a LEA when nonverbal materials were processed. In Chapter Nine we shall discuss in detail the processing of musical and rhythmic materials in the context of the analytic–holistic dichotomy; here we will simply sketch the broad general findings of a LEA. Kimura (1964) reported a LEA for melodies; Spellacy (1970) for melodies but not for timbre, temporal, or frequency patterns; Spreen, Spellacy, and Reid (1970), Goodglass and Calderon (1977), and P. Johnson (1977) for melodies; King and Kimura (1972) for hummed melodies; Gordon (1970) for musical chords; Sidtis and Bryden (1978) for piano tones; Cutting (1974) for synthetic musical tones; and Kallman and Corballis (1975) for notes from musical instruments. With nonmusical sounds, Curry (1967) and Knox and Kimura (1970) reported a LEA for environmental sounds (dishwashing, phones ringing, dogs barking, clocks ticking); Carmon and Nachshon (1973) for nonverbal vocalizations (laughing, shrieking, crying, sighing); Haggard and Parkinson (1971) for emotional tone of speech; Blumstein and Cooper (1974) for intonation patterns; and Chaney and Webster (1966) for sonar signals. With complex tones, Sidtis (1980, 1981) concluded that the right hemisphere is specialized for analyzing steady-state harmonic information of complex tones rather than for music perception *per se,* with discrimination of pure tones bilaterally mediated. Although the LEA for nonverbal stimuli is generally weaker than the REA for verbal (though melody and musical tone do give comparatively large effects), the complex tones of Sidtis (1981) gave LEAs comparable in size to REAs found for verbal materials and the LEAs increased as a function of the number of constituent overtones.

Most importantly, he also found that small changes in the degree and nature of stimulus competition between the dichotically presented signals had a large effect on the magnitude of perceptual asymmetry. Just as Teng (1980) has concluded that the effect depends on competition for the same kind of processing, so Sidtis (1981) believes that the suppression of the ipsilateral by the contralateral pathways is determined not just by physiological factors but also by acoustic aspects.

Finally Deutsch (1974) has reported an unusual "octave illusion." She presented a sequence of two tones (400 and 800 Hz), one to each ear, alternating rapidly between ears. Dextrals tended to hear a single tone oscillating from ear to ear, the pitch oscillating between octaves. Half of the sinistrals reported different, more complex patterns, for example, two alternating pitches in one ear and a third heard intermittently in the other, or two alternating pitches alternating from ear to ear and two further alternating pitches localized at the back of the head. The exact meaning of these curious findings is unclear, and they and others like them are discussed further by Deutsch (1980).

Other auditory techniques: Stroop and delayed auditory feedback (DAF). G. Cohen and Martin (1975) required their subjects to judge the pitch of pure tones (high or low), of two congruent words (the word *high* sung at a high pitch and *low* sung at a low pitch) and of two incongruent words (the word *high* sung low and *low* sung high). Stimuli were either dichotically or monaurally presented. The Stroop effect (a longer mean reaction time for incongruent than for congruent words) was greater for right-ear (left hemisphere) presentations, showing that verbal information was automatically processed, even when this was counterproductive. Effects were slightly stronger with "dichotic" presentations, but since there was no stimulus alignment (the competing signal was a read passage), it is doubtful whether we can place much reliance on such a comparison.

Tsunoda (1966, 1975) claimed to have developed another dichotic method for determining cerebral dominance for speech by using synchronous and delayed auditory feedback and a keytapping task. (Delayed auditory feedback, DAF, which is accomplished by feeding back to a subject the auditory signal emitted by him or her at a critical delay of around 200 msec, is highly disruptive; used with speech, DAF produces slurring and/or repetition of syllables. Similar effects occur with, e.g., keytapping tasks.) Each tap on an electromechanical key triggered an auditory signal that could then be delivered to one ear of the subject in synchrony with the tap or to the other ear after 200 msec delay. The lowest signal intensity to produce disruption was taken as the disruption threshold for that ear. The ear with the lower threshold was taken to be the dominant ear. Tsunoda claimed that for most subjects the left ear proved dominant when the delayed auditory signal was a pure tone, and the right when the key tap triggered release of a vowel sound *a*. Uyehara and Cooper (1980) were quite unable to replicate these findings on two occasions, and in fact strongly questioned many of Tsunoda's assumptions.

When Abbs and Smith (1970) directed a subject's own ongoing speech, delayed, to the right ear and masking white noise to the left, they found that there were more articulatory errors than when the directions were reversed. There were no ear differences for a measure of total speaking time alone. J. L. Bradshaw et al. (1971, 1972) timed subjects reading prose passages with DAF to one ear and simultaneous auditory feedback or some other irrelevant signal to the other. Unlike Abbs and Smith, we found that articulation times were increased by about 6 percent when the DAF was channeled to the right ear, with left ear stimulation producing greater disruption when subjects played a piano, recorder, or electronic organ. The latter device permitted us to manipulate feedback in the absence of *any* simultaneous feedback when we wished to. We found that unmodulated white noise channeled to the other ear was inadequate to produce laterality effects (thus reducing the discrepancy noted above between our results and those of Abbs and Smith, since we measured only speaking time, and Abbs and Smith also got no effects with this measure when using white noise). We concluded that the *nature* of the input to the opposite ear was important (cf. the conclusion of Teng, 1980, that the normal dichotic effect depends on competition for the same kinds of processing). Irrelevant music to the left ear with speech DAF to the right *reduced* the effects of right-ear DAF, presumably because subjects were better able to attend to left-ear music and were distracted from the disruptive effects of right ear DAF. Likewise, distorted DAF to the right ear and nondistorted DAF to the left ear was less disruptive than the opposite condition. In general, changes in the verbal and musical content of the tasks produced changes in the degree of asymmetry, suggesting that the latter is best viewed as a relative rather than an absolute phenomenon.

Roberts and Gregory (1973) required their subjects to repeat tongue-twisting words (*peripatetic, innumerable, balalaika, substitute*—to which we would add *tachistoscope* and *statistical*). They measured the point at which speech breakdown occurred as a function of the intensity of the DAF signal to left or right ears. Intensity levels were lower in the right ear for speech and the left ear for a simple tapping sequence.

Both the DAF and the Stroop technique demonstrate the inability of the dominant hemisphere to refrain from the automatic and often unwanted processing of a speech signal. Thus, DAF was more disruptive even than the complete absence of feedback, achievable with the playing of an electronic organ when the sound to the player's ears was turned off.

The Tactile Modality

It has long been known that in normal subjects the left side of the body (hand, palm, forearm, soles of feet, breasts in females, and many other parts) has a lower absolute pressure sensitivity threshold than the right (see Weinstein, 1978, for review). The left hand is also superior for tactile perception of direction (line slant), according to Benton, Levin, and Varney (1973), though this may be true only for dextrals, without familial sinistrality (Varney & Benton, 1975). It holds whether a cross modal (tactile-visual) or unimodal (tactile-tactile) matching procedure is employed (Benton, Varney, & Hamsher, 1978).

Witelson (1974, 1976a) obtained a left-hand superiority with children using what she termed a dichaptic exploration technique, a tactile analogue of dichotic listening. Subjects actively explored two different nonsense shapes simultaneously presented, one to each hand, and subsequently identified them from a visual array. Nilsson, Glencross, and Geffen (1980) confirmed these findings, though according to Webster and Thurber (1978), who worked with adults, the effect is present only with dichaptic not with monohaptic (single-handed) exploration. This finding is reminiscent of the frequently weaker monaural effects; Dodds (1978), however, was successful with monohaptic stimulation. Moreover, the degree of left-hand superiority found by Webster and Thurber depended on whether subjects were instructed to approach the problems in an analytic or a holistic manner. Gardner, English, Flannery, Hartnett, McCormick, and Wilhelmy (1977) also replicated Webster and Thurber's results with adults, though Hannay and Smith (1979) were unsuccessful. Finally, Flanery and Balling (1979) improved on the Witelson paradigm by using a haptic-haptic rather than a haptic-visual matching task.

Oscar-Berman, Rehbein, Porfert, and Goodglass (1978) extended this dichaptic technique to three-dimensional block letters, digits, and line orientations and required subjects to report the hands in a particular order. They found a right-hand superiority for the letters and a left-hand superiority for the line-orientation task (with no hand differences for digits), but only for reports of the *second* hand. Again analogous to certain auditory findings, tactile *storage* processes would appear to be more sensitive to laterality differences than measures closer in time to the actual perceptual event. Nachshon and Carmon (1975) also successfully demonstrated a double dissociation, a right-hand superiority for a sequential task and a left-hand superiority for a simultaneous one, findings that we shall reconsider later (Chapter Nine) in the context of the analytic–holistic dichotomy.

It has long been known that Braille may be more easily read by the left hand (for review, see Harris, 1980b). Later studies with blind and sighted subjects have confirmed these findings (Harris, 1980b; Hermelin & O'Connor, 1971a, b). It is easy to ascribe these findings to the spatial nature of the Braille character, though written letters, which normally generate a RVF superiority, also are spatial in nature. However, as we saw earlier, difficult, unfamiliar, or masked characters may be associated with LVF superiorities, and such a situation may possibly persist with the reading of Braille. It is also possible that there is some degree of modality specificity (Harris, 1980b), analogous to the now largely discredited idea of a special relationship between the visual modality and the right hemisphere and the auditory modality and the left. Thus, Harris argues that right hemisphere involvement is always greater for tactile stimulation, since the skin senses are poorer in both temporal-resolving power and in spatial resolution. Tactile perception, he says, becomes spatiotemporal, requiring the integration of separate points in space and time. Such ideas, though unconfirmed, are reminiscent of those of LeDoux, Wilson, and Gazzaniga (1977) (discussed in Chapter Five) that right hemisphere advantages depend largely on the active involvement of *manual praxis* rather than on pure visuospatial processing, though we would disagree with the extreme form of their thesis.

Activation Measures

Tachistoscopic, dichotic, monaural, and tactile studies described so far have all measured hemispheric differences in cognitive capacity or proficiency. There are a number of other techniques, such as electroencephalographic, electrodermal, and those involving regional bloodflow and eye and hand movements. These may all be described as activational in that changes in these indices are monitored during ongoing task performance.

Electroencephalographic indices. Space allows only a brief outline of the major findings from EEGs, since this semiautonomous area has now proliferated excessively and a number of very comprehensive reviews are available (Butler & Glass, 1976; Donchin, Kutas, & McCarthy, 1977; Donchin, McCarthy & Kutas, 1977; Galin & Ellis, 1977; Marsh, 1978). Electroencephalographic (EEG) studies in the frequency domain are predicated on the assumption that differential alpha (α) activity in the two hemispheres reflects differential degrees of cortical activation; during conditions of lateralized or generalized attention, concentration, or problem solving, the slow, regular 8–12 Hz α activity is blocked or suppressed. A number of studies (see above reviews; also Goodman, Beatty, & Mulholland, 1980; Rebert, 1978) have obtained evidence of a double dissociation, with greater α blocking over the left hemisphere during verbal tasks and over the right during nonverbal tasks. The Goodman et al. study is of some interest in that it employed a new technique. Words and geometrical patterns were presented by computer to one or the other visual field contingent on the occurrence of α at one of four electrode placements, left or right occipital or temporal. The replicative reliability of α block, and by implication the control of each stimulus type over different cortical sites, was assessed by the α control ratio (the mean α duration divided by the standard deviation of α duration). The α control ratio was significantly greater for α contingent than for random (noncontingent) stimulation, and within the α contingent data alone, cerebral lateralization was demonstrated by the interactions involving visual field and type of stimulus with EEG locus.

Much of the EEG work is necessarily descriptive, with little standardization of measures or methods of quantification, techniques, electrode placements, or nature of tasks (which are rarely validated *independently* with respect to their abilities to address lateralized processing systems). Sex and handedness are often not controlled, though as Butler and Glass (1976) and Donchin, McCarthy, and Kutas (1977) note, the evidence of weaker asymmetries with nondextrals does support the use of these measures as an index of cerebral lateralization. In addition, Butler and Glass found a correlation between EEG asymmetry and cerebral asymmetry as determined by the Wada amytal test. We feel such conclusions counter the claim of Gevins, Zeitlin, Doyle, Yingling, Schaffer, Calloway, and Yeager (1979) that EEG asymmetries are really to be explained in terms of lateralized differences in task-related motor activity—that is, motor artifacts—rather than the differential cognitive engagement of the hemispheres.

Turning now to time domain studies, we must note that cortical evoked responses may be elicited by stimulus events, though these responses are inevitably of smaller magnitude than the ongoing EEG. They can be extracted by recording and averaging (to remove the "random" background EEG component) samples of the EEG time-locked to a repeating stimulus event. This in itself of course is a source of further artifacts, since such regular stimulus repetition is highly abnormal, and laterality effects are easily affected by practice (see Chapter Seven). Typical evoked responses may be quantified and compared in terms of the amplitude (positive and negative) and latency of the waveforms. Although these measures show some evidence of left–right differences to visual flashes or auditory clicks or noise bursts, the most useful and interesting studies have compared evoked potentials over various loci in the two hemispheres to meaningful stimuli of a verbal or nonverbal nature. Although larger responses over the left hemisphere for verbal materials have been reported, together with (less consistently) larger ones over the right for nonverbal stimuli, there have been notable failures to confirm these findings and disagreements over which components of the waveform are significant or important. In addition to the forementioned reviews, Kutas and Hillyard (1980) discuss further methodological and statistical problems with the technique.

Other event-related potentials that are relevant in this context include asymmetries in the contingent negative variation (CNV) and slow potential asymmetries preceding speech production (Butler & Glass, 1976; Donchin, Kutas, & McCarthy, 1977; Donchin, McCarthy, & Kutas, 1977; Marsh, 1978). The CNV is a surface negative potential that develops in the period briefly preceding an expected event, for example, after a warning signal and before a signal to respond. It reflects attentional set, arousal, and expectancy. When the response signal is expected to be verbal or nonverbal, appropriately asymmetrical CNVs may develop over the two hemispheres—larger over the left, for example, when verbal material is awaited. Such findings have not always been confirmed, and eye-movement artifacts may contaminate the measures. The slow potentials that precede speech often show greater negative excursions over the left hemisphere, particularly Broca's area, though again muscle artifacts may make interpretation difficult. However, absence of such an asymmetry when subjects cough or spit argues against this objection. R. Levy (1977) provides a detailed review of these problems.

Regional cerebral bloodflow as an index. It makes good biological sense to hypothesize a feedback circulatory mechanism to supply more blood to those brain areas that are currently under the greatest processing load or level of activation, whether in a sensory, cognitive, or motor capacity. Noninvasive methods have been developed for measuring regional cerebral bloodflow (rCBF), such as the [133] Xenon clearance method. This radioisotope may be injected into a cerebral artery (Lassen, Ingvar, & Skinhøj, 1978) or inhaled (Knopman, Rubens, Klassen, Meyer, & Niccum, 1980; Wood, 1980), and its clearance from the brain measured by sodium iodide crystal emission detectors placed on the subject's head (Gur & Gur, 1980). Risberg, Halsey, Wills, and Wilson (1975) demonstrated differential rCBF responses over the two hemispheres to verbal and spatial task activation, as also have Gur and Reivich (1980) and Knopman et al. (1980). Such local changes in bloodflow reflect local variations in the rate of nerve cell metabolism but are necessarily a rather molar two-dimensional measure of three-dimensional activity, subject to such other processes as generalized arousal with less precise localization. The EEG may be regarded in temporal terms as more resolute and in spatial terms as less resolute than rCBF. New techniques of three-dimensional imaging of localized metabolic activity by emission-computed tomography allow for far greater spatial resolution than rCBF, but again in temporal terms are much less resolute, requiring sustained measurements of more than twenty minutes, a period that in cognitive laterality tasks would be likely to lead to unacceptable practice effects. In these respects, therefore, rCBF may offer a useful compromise.

Other related techniques in this context include that of Shakhnovich, Serbinenko, Razumovsky, Rodionov, and Oskolok (1980), and that of Dabbs and Choo (1980). The former study measured rCBF with a hydrogen polarographic method, and like Lassen et al. (1978) found regularly occurring changes during cognitive tasks (speech, counting, and memory) not only in the left but also in the right hemisphere; the changes occurred as a function of the task complexity and difficulty. Dabbs and Choo in an ingenious design made their subjects drink iced water, which cooled the blood. Thermistors placed on the skin over the ophthalmic branches of the internal carotid arteries measured left–right rCBF differences as a function of the nature of cognitive tasks and the subjects' handedness.

Electrodermal activity as an index. Lacroix and Comper (1979) review the evidence for excitatory and inhibitory centers for electrodermal (skin-conductance) activity at a cortical level, the influence of *inhibitory* centers probably being lateralized, that of excitatory centers probably being bilateral. In their own study, with tasks selected to engage one or the other hemisphere (explaining proverbs, visualizing familiar objects or places), they found electrodermal response amplitudes were substantially smaller in the hand contralateral to the more activated hemisphere than in the ipsilateral hand. These findings with dextral subjects were not replicated with sinistrals, who exhibited no systematic asymmetries of electrodermal response. Such observations support the conclusion that this measure indexes brain lateralization. Other evidence of a double dissociation between side of body and verbal or nonverbal nature of task comes from Myslobodsky and Rattok (1975, 1977).

Diekhoff, Garland, Dansereau, and Walker (1978) recorded surface muscle tension (EMG), skin conductance and finger pulse volume (FPV) from the two sides during left hemisphere tasks (verb memorization and lyric recitation) and right hemisphere tasks (face memorization and humming). While EMG and FPV asymmetries were found in the predicted directions (EMG reducing and FPV increasing on the side contralateral to the hemisphere required for the task-related processing), there were no differences in skin conductance.

Conjugate lateral eye movements as an index.   Trevarthen (1972) claims that an orientation reflex (or its covert homologue, an attentional bias) toward the side of space contralateral to the more activated hemisphere tends to accompany such hemispheric activity. Conjugate lateral eye movements (CLEMs) are a component of this contralateral orienting response, or overflow of cognitive neural activity into the orientation control system within the same hemisphere. They are reviewed in detail by Ehrlichman and Weinberger (1978) and Gur and Gur (1977a, 1980). The direction of eye movements on being questioned is said to be fairly consistent for a given individual (and thus is believed by some to index his or her cognitive style), though much dispute and controversy surrounds this area (see Chapter Nine). More important for our present purposes, the direction of CLEMs is also said to be a function of the verbal or nonverbal nature of the required processing, such as whether a verbal or a spatial imagery problem is posed. Gur and Gur (1980) claim that effects are weaker with sinistrals, thus confirming the fact that they index cerebral lateralization. Many, however, have been quite unable to confirm the effect even with dextrals (see, e.g., Hiscock, 1977; Shevrin, Smokler, & Wolf, 1979; Takeda & Yoshimura, 1979, for recent failures), and Gross, Franko, and Lewin (1978) even claim that gaze direction determines the choice of processing strategies instead.

Ehrlichman and Weinberger (1978) in their sober review say that a conclusion about any relationship between CLEMs and hemispheric activation is at best premature and point out that over half of the published experiments they review have failed empirically to confirm the hypothesis. This may partly be the fault of using otherwise unvalidated tasks and the result of design defects in measuring the eye movements. We must ask, what should count as a CLEM? Any movement, however small or brief? The first movement? The longest lasting fixation? The total number over (what?) interval? Should the eyes be "zeroed" straight ahead before each task, and how should corrections be made if they are not? How are *vertical* CLEMs to be accommodated? What effect may the recorder have on them? One may conclude that despite the attractions of the hypothesis (if it worked it would indeed be an extremely convenient index), support for it is weak. Many other factors obviously help determine ocular behavior during social interactions, and the whole of the presumed neurophysiology involves gross oversimplifications (Ehrlichman & Weinberger, 1978).

Rosenberg (1980) has developed what we believe to be a far more promising variant of the CLEM technique, which avoids many of the measurement problems. He found that the frequency of elicited (by moving stripes) optokinetic nystagmus (OKN) varied with the degree of right hemisphere activity imposed by the task. There was a higher frequency of OKN elicited when the stripes moved in a direction contralateral to the hemisphere presumed to be involved in the imposed mental task. The great advantage of the technique is that rather than looking for "naturally" occurring eye movements, it relies on modification of an *externally* elicited response (OKN).

Hand Movements, Tapping, and Dowel Balancing During Concurrent Tasks

We have reviewed in earlier sections the performance measures that have been adduced as evidence for cerebral lateralization of function, and in the last section such activation measures as the EEG, rCBF, electrodermal responses, and CLEMs. In the same tradition as these activation measures, Kimura (1976) discusses the claims that during speech, dextrals make freer hand movements with the right than with the left hand, while self-touching movements occur equally often with either hand. With sinistrals the pattern of hand movements does not differ between hands. Once again, these findings would be explained in terms of an overflow of activation from cognitive to motor areas of the same hemisphere, a concept in broad agreement with Kinsbourne's attentional theory of lateralization and which we shall discuss in more detail in Chapter Seven. However, at this point we should note that according to Kinsbourne's attentional model an auxiliary or secondary task may prime a hemisphere and facilitate performance of other tasks performed concurrently. But this occurs only under optimal conditions: when the auxiliary task draws a sufficient amount of effort to prime related structures in the same hemisphere, but yet not too much to deprive the other task of its needs. If each of the concurrent tasks requires considerable attention or if they compete for common processing mechanisms, then there will be intertask interference. In this section we shall be concerned with this latter situation—competition for processing space— since in any case as we shall see in Chapter Seven the evidence in favor of Kinsbourne's attentional model is far from unequivocal.

Kinsbourne and Cook (1971) required their subjects to balance a dowel rod on either the left or right index finger, with or without concurrent verbalization (repeating sentences aloud). Verbalization lowered balancing time much more for the right hand (left hemisphere) than for the left hand (right hemisphere). They even claimed that concurrent verbalization *facilitated* left-hand balancing, as compared to the silent condition, due, they said, to a reduction in visual interference between the hemispheres by the distracting task. This last finding and interpretation was not confirmed by R. E. Hicks (1975) and O. Johnson and Kozma (1977), although these authors did successfully replicate the general finding of a verbal task's disrupting right-hand performance. Hicks found this held true only for dextrals, and O. Johnson and Kozma found that the effect did not extend to females. In view of the general finding of reduced cerebral lateralization for sinistrals (Chapter Ten) and females (Chapter Eleven), these observations can be taken as support for a cerebral lateralization account. Other evidence that concurrent verbal tasks interfere more with right- than with left-hand motor skill comes from Hicks,

Provenzano, and Rybstein (1975); Kinsbourne and McMurray (1975); and Hiscock and Kinsbourne (1978, 1980). Several studies have successfully demonstrated the complementary effect, a performance decrement in left-hand dowel balancing or tapping while performing *nonverbal* concurrent tasks, such as remembering faces or shapes or humming a musical theme (Thomson & Clausnitzer, 1980; Piazza, 1977; McFarland & Ashton, 1978a, b). Much of the earlier work (prior to 1977) is reviewed in detail by Kinsbourne and Hicks (1978a, b).

Analogous findings to the tapping and balancing tasks reviewed above have been reported with slightly different experimental paradigms. Botkin, Schmaltz, and Lamb (1977) found that while counting backwards, subjects were better able to hold a stylus at arms' length in a small hole without touching the sides when the left rather than the right hand was used. Rizzolatti, Bertoloni, and Buchtel (1979) found that verbal (mental arithmetic) and praxic (complex patterned finger movements) tasks lengthened simple reaction times to light flashes, especially when in the RVF, while highly automatic finger movements had no such effect. They explained the findings in terms of interference between the activity of mechanisms mediating verbal and praxic behavior, and that of mechanisms responsible for responses initiated to stimuli present in the RVF.

Bowers, Heilman, Satz, and Altman (1978) reported that while verbal tasks interfered more with right- than with left-handed tapping, there was no reverse-flow effect—that is, the cognitive tasks were apparently unaffected by simultaneous digit tapping. For some reason the possibility of such a reverse-flow effect has not received any attention otherwise. According to Lomas (1980) interference must not just occur within the same *hemisphere,* but both tasks must be directed by a system for *nonvisual* control of limb movement; that is, the two tasks must be mediated by *functionally overlapping systems* within that hemisphere. He found no interference effect when limb movement was under visual feedback control, only when such control was absent. He concludes that the left hemisphere contains a system that is specialized for the control of movement transitions made with minimal guidance, and this system is significantly involved in speech control. We find this hypothesis worthy of further investigation but are not sure how compatible it is with some of the earlier work reviewed in this section. However, we do believe that the general findings of interference with right- rather than left-hand performance from a concurrent verbal task are more compatible with a hypothesis appealing to limitations in processing capacity than with one concerned with shifts in attention. Both of these issues will be discussed in more detail in Chapter Seven.

Summary and Conclusions

Although with normal subjects, unlike the clinical and commissurotomy patients of the last two chapters, researchers are working with subjects who are presumed to be free of morbidity, *independent* operation of the hemispheres cannot of course occur.

Visual studies generally employ tachistoscopic presentations of 150 msec or less, which restrict the nature of possible stimuli and impose limitations on the possible types of processing. Alternative procedures such as scleral contact lenses to permit *ad lib* scanning of lateralized stimuli are only just being developed for use with normal subjects, and though they are likely to enjoy popularity in the future, such techniques are not without problems of their own. The tachistoscopic techniques exhibit considerable procedural diversity in terms of exposure durations, speed or accuracy measures, number of trials, methods of dealing with errors and long reaction times, use of vocal or manual responses, unimanual or bimanual responses, same–different or go–no-go responses, nature of matches, discriminations, or processing, perceptual or memory factors, length of any retention interval, number of targets, practice, task difficulty, and so on. This diversity almost certainly accounts for the many failures to replicate. However, it is generally found that target responses are associated with stronger asymmetries in the predicted direction than nontargets, perhaps because subjects adopt a target set.

Two specific theoretical problems with procedural implications relate to the possible bilateral representation of a narrow central strip around the vertical meridian of the fovea and to hemiretinal acuity differences and pathway strength. Apart from stereopsis, however, any bilateral representation close to the center of the fovea appears to be without functional significance and may in any case be functionally hairline. The fact, however, that the nasal hemiretinae may have stronger cortical representation means that studies should employ binocular viewing and subjects free from marked eye dominance.

A RVF superiority is typically found in digit and letter recognition and with nominal matching, though a LVF superiority may occur when matches are based on purely physical attributes. A RVF superiority is found for word recognition and recall, lexical decisions, and phonological discriminations. There is some evidence that phonological effects may be weaker with LVF (right hemisphere) presentations. Bigger RVF superiorities are found for vocal naming latencies, and the smallest of superiorities when processing must take place at a purely semantic level.

Although early experiments suggested that directional scanning played a major role in generating RVF superiorities with words, better designed and controlled studies after the mid-1960s showed that scanning plays little or no part. The magnitude of the RVF superiority is the same whether left–right mirror-reversed words, vertically organized words, or Hebrew or Chinese materials are used. There is little evidence of left-to-right directional processing in word recognition, but there is evidence of a parallel letter-processing strategy with an ends-first advantage.

Lateralized Stroop tasks show that incongruent relationships between a color word and a color dye interfere more with naming the dye color when presentations are to the RVF.

A LVF superiority may appear for letters or words when difficult, unfamiliar, briefly exposed, visually confusing, or perceptually degraded stimuli require pre-processing, demonstrating a right hemisphere superiority in extracting relevant physical features. A LVF superiority may also appear when imagery is used to code verbal material.

With simple nonverbal dimensions such as lightness, hue, dot location, depth perception, and such, a LVF superiority typically appears. This effect may be more difficult to demonstrate with complex patterns, except where memory processes are involved or when longer or variable retention intervals are used. A RVF superiority is more likely for familiar patterns and simple nameable shapes. With faces, a LVF superiority has been reported for photographs, drawings, and schematic figures, especially when deeper levels of processing are required or physiognomic invariants have to be extracted. This has led to questions of whether there is a specialist processor for faces in the right hemisphere, over and above the latter's general mediation of visuospatial—and emotional—processing. A RVF superiority, however, may be found with *familiar* faces, with difficult discriminations where perhaps only a single feature distinguishes faces, and where subjects perform categorical judgments, for example, with respect to sex. The chimeric technique developed for use with commissurotomy patients has also been successfully applied to normal subjects, but a neutral strip must be placed over the central junction of the two halves. Like commissurotomy patients, normal subjects show perceptual completion and a LVF superiority for nonverbal identification.

When bilateral visual presentations are employed in a manner analogous to dichotic procedures in audition, larger asymmetries are often reported. This is possibly due to the competitive nature of the stimulation since both hemispheres may have to perform independent processing operations. This technique, however, brings with it new problems of report order, scanning, and noncentral fixation. The latter problem may be obviated by using a fixation stimulus, which the subject reports after processing the lateralized materials. However, the verbal–nonverbal nature of the fixation stimulus may possibly bias the way the lateralized test stimuli are processed, though this finding is disputed. A satisfactory solution is to employ the fixation stimuli (in this case left- or right-pointing arrows) as cues to indicate which visual field is to be processed. Under these circumstances, opposite asymmetries may be found for verbal and nonverbal materials, with a decrease in the magnitude of the effect among nondextrals, thus supporting an explanation based on cerebral asymmetries.

With the auditory modality, dichotic presentations are most commonly employed, though not everyone has observed the need for careful control of intensities and temporal alignment. While there is evidence that the contralateral auditory pathways do suppress the ipsilateral, the *nature* of the competition (e.g., for the same kind of processing) may be as important as the peripheral competition. Peripheral competition may even be unnecessary in some circumstances, especially where competing monaural stimulation and reaction-time measures are employed. Such findings call into question Kimura's functional prepotency model. This model holds that with dichotic stimulation and ipsilateral suppression a word heard in the left ear can be received only by the left hemisphere after first traveling to the right hemisphere and then across the commissures, during which time it suffers signal degradation.

The dichotic REA is not just a function of order of report or of attentional biases; nor is it nonperceptual, although it is indeed stronger at a memory level. The REA is also larger with encoded stop consonants than with steady-state unencoded vowels, unless the perception of these vowels is made more difficult by superimposed noise, contextual uncertainty, or complex discriminations. That the REA is related to cerebral asymmetry, especially if reaction time measures for target detection are used, is indicated by the sex and handedness effects, and by validation studies employing the Wada amytal test. The REA, however, is a *correlate* rather than an *index* of cerebral dominance, perhaps because it reflects speech *perception* rather than the far more lateralized speech *production*. Many different measures have been proposed to quantify laterality differences in the traditional dichotic-recall paradigm; none are entirely satisfactory, since all to some extent relate to general performance levels. For this reason the use of reaction times is to be preferred.

A LEA is typically found with nonverbal materials, such as melodies, musical chords, piano tones and notes from musical instruments, environmental sounds, intonation patterns, and emotional tones of speech. The right hemisphere may be specialized for the analysis of the steady-state harmonic information of complex tones.

Auditory Stroop effects (pitch judgments of the words *high* and *low* sung at a high or low pitch) demonstrate that Stroop disruption is greater for stimuli presented to the right ear. With delayed auditory feedback (DAF), a subject's delayed speech played to the right ear (with some other lateralizing input, such as synchronous speech, played to the left) causes more speech disruption than when the ear inputs are reversed. The opposite effect is found when playing the piano or electronic organ. The latter instrument permits testing of pure DAF, if required, without *any* other feedback or input. Findings demonstrate that *some* form of competitive input is required to produce ear differences, but again its *nature* is important. Both the Stroop and the DAF technique demonstrate the inability of the left hemisphere to refrain from automatic and unwanted processing of a speech signal.

With tactile laterality, the left side of the body is the more sensitive for a number of measures, including the perception of line slant. A dichaptic stimulation technique has been developed, by analogy with dichotic presentations, which generates possibly stronger effects. With this technique a double dissociation appears for letter and shape stimuli, the effects being stronger at the memory than at the perceptual level. In reading Braille, the left hand is superior, despite the verbal nature of the stimuli. Whether this is due to the spatial characteristics of the stimuli, or to a possibly stronger relationship between the right hemisphere and the tactile modality than any of the other modalities is uncertain.

Turning to *activation* rather than *performance* measures, such as electrophysiological, electrodermal, and other indices, despite many problems of methodology and interpretation, the demonstration of a double dissociation and material specific effects, which are affected by such factors as sex and handedness, supports the conclusion that cerebral laterality is involved, as does the occasional validation by the Wada technique. Differential α activity and evoked responses over the two cortices appear as a function of the type of processing required. Similar effects appear with the contingent negative variation (CNV), which develops just before an expected (verbal or nonverbal) event. Slow potential asymmetries precede speech production. With regional cerebral bloodflow (rCBF) similar material-specific asymmetries appear; though rCBF is a gross two-dimensional measure of three-dimensional activity, it is nevertheless a useful adjunct to electrophysiological measures. Lateralized inhibitory centers appear to control electrodermal activity.

With conjugate lateral eye movements (CLEMs) there is said to be an overflow of cognitive neural activity into motor control systems within the same hemisphere, leading to an attentional bias or an observable orienting reflex (CLEM) to the side of space that is contralateral to the currently more activated hemisphere. Some believe that this procedure indexes individual differences in cognitive style, and reflects the verbal (rightward) or nonverbal (leftward) nature of current processing. Such conclusions may be premature, and many methodological problems remain. Modulation of the optokinetic nystagmus effect (OKN) may possibly be a theoretically and conceptually sounder technique.

Hand movements and performance in tapping and dowel balancing have been observed during concurrent verbal and nonverbal tasks. Again, this is thought to indicate an overflow of cognitive activity to motor areas of the same hemisphere, which may trigger spontaneous hand activity or *interfere* with it when it is to be generated and controlled as part of a concurrent task, if both compete for common processing mechanisms. Thus a concurrent verbal task typically disrupts right-hand tapping, balancing, or fine control, and a nonverbal task may disrupt left-hand performance. These findings appear to be much better established than those that involve CLEMs.

FURTHER READING

BRYDEN, M. P. Strategies in the assessment of hemispheric asymmetry. In G. Underwood (Ed.), *Strategies of information processing*. New York: Academic Press, 1978.

HELLIGE, J. B. Visual laterality and cerebral hemisphere specialization: Methodological and theoretical considerations. In J. B. Sidowski (Ed.), *Conditioning, cognition and methodology*. New York: Lawrence Erlbaum, in press.

KIMURA, D. The asymmetry of the human brain. *Scientific American*, 1973, *228*, 70–78.

KRASHEN, S. Cerebral asymmetry. In H. Whitaker & H. A. Whitaker (Eds.), *Studies in neurolinguistics* (Vol. 1). New York: Academic Press, 1976.

MOSCOVITCH, M. Information processing and the cerebral hemispheres. In M. S. Gazzaniga (Ed.), *Handbook of behavioral neurobiology, Vol. 2: Neuropsychology.* New York: Plenum, 1979.

PROHOVNIK, I. Cerebral lateralization of psychological processes: A literature review. *Archiv für Psychologie,* 1978, *130,* 161–211.

SPRINGER, S. P. Tachistoscopic and dichotic listening investigations of laterality in human subjects. In S. Harnad, R. W. Doty, L. Goldstein, J. Jaynes, & G. Krauthamer (Eds.), *Lateralization in the nervous system.* New York: Academic Press, 1977.

WITTROCK, M. C. *The human brain.* Englewood Cliffs, N.J.: Prentice-Hall, 1977.

CHAPTER SEVEN
Load, Novelty, Practice, Arousal, and Attention

In reviewing the evidence for cerebral asymmetry, we have assumed up to this point that the hemispheres are specialized, relatively if not absolutely, for the processing of different types of material. We shall discuss the ultimate nature of this specialization (verbal versus visuospatial, or analytic versus holistic) in Chapter Nine; in this chapter we shall examine the pattern of interhemispheric interaction. Kimura (1966, 1973a) proposed a structural account of hemispheric asymmetry when she argued that ear and visual field superiorities reflect privileged access, via superior contralateral pathways, to hemispheres uniquely able to process a given type of information; information that cannot be processed in a certain hemisphere is transmitted across the commissures to the hemisphere that is competent to do so, and ear and visual field differences (in terms of reaction time or accuracy) reflect either transmission delays or signal degradation during such transfer. It was later suggested (e.g., Geffen, Bradshaw, & Wallace, 1971) that the hemispheres may merely differ in their relative capacities for performing a particular function, and laterality differences reflect these differential processing capacities. Kimura's original structural account was supported by such findings as the observation that, although commissurotomy patients could comprehend speech well through either ear with monaural stimulation, with dichotic listening there appeared to be complete left-ear suppression (B. Milner, Taylor, & Sperry, 1968; Sparks & Geschwind, 1968; Springer & Gazzaniga, 1975). It was proposed that during dichotic listening a left-ear input can normally arrive at the ipsilateral (left) hemisphere only via the contralateral hemisphere and the commissures. This route, of course, is lost after commissurotomy.

However, in time the performance of the left ear of commissurotomy patients improved, and Gordon (1980a) showed that when the stimulus in the left ear (ipsilateral pathway) is necessary or important to the left hemisphere for completing a task, words from *both* pathways are reported, suggesting that any gating of the ipsilateral pathway may be *central* rather than *peripheral*. Kimura's structural model also has difficulty in coping with the dynamic aspects of laterality, whereby effects often shift as a function of load, expectancy, practice, adopted strategies, and so on. We shall discuss alternatives to Kimura's structural model in a later section of this chapter but first shall discuss certain circumstances where information may actually require transmission between the hemispheres and other circumstances where such transmission may even be disadvantageous.

Double Tasks

In Chapter Five we saw that there is dispute whether commissural section augments or decreases the overall capacity of the brain to carry out more than one task simultaneously. According to one viewpoint, that of Sperry and his coworkers, commissurotomy effectively increases the brain's capacity to deal independently with two parallel streams of information, as long as the two tasks are relatively simple and can be performed from a common posture and set. According to another viewpoint, that of Trevarthen and of Kinsbourne, for example, commissural section can lead to problems in the unilateral allocation of attention and to an overall decrease in processing capacity. These authors suggest that interference, and performance deficit, will be maximal when the two tasks are very similar, the opposite position to that of Sperry and colleagues. Obviously, the issue is not yet fully resolved, but we concluded that the observed effects are likely to depend on the complexity and the degree of mutual similarity of the two tasks, on the subject's level of expertise, and on whether stimulus identification or response selection is the more important component in the task. Thus even *normal* subjects with undivided commissures are quite capable of simultaneously processing several stimulus streams in parallel, as long as separate overt responses are not required.

Turning now to normal performance, we discussed in Chapter Six the use of the concurrent task technique as an index of cerebral asymmetry; right-hand performance in dowel balancing or simple tapping was decremented more than left-hand performance when subjects simultaneously engaged in a verbal task, presumably because both tasks were vying for limited processing space in the left hemisphere. We saw that under certain circumstances the opposite effects occurred with nonverbal concurrent tasks. A related phenomenon occurs when the concurrent task is so difficult as to fully occupy the processing capacity of its mediating hemisphere: Then the primary task, normally mediated by the same hemisphere as the concurrent task, may be mediated by the other, normally inferior, hemisphere, which now has the spare capacity. Thus, the normal field or ear asymmetries for a primary task may reverse when there is a demanding concurrent task of the same (i.e., verbal or nonverbal) nature (Geffen, Bradshaw, & Nettleton, 1973; Moscovitch & Klein, 1980; M. O. Smith, Chu, & Edmonston, 1977).

There is, however, another simultaneous-task paradigm with normal subjects that we have not yet discussed. Two signals are simultaneously sent either one to each or both to the same hemisphere, each requires a separate response, and the signals chosen are kept sufficiently simple and neutral as to be likely to be processed equally readily by either hemisphere. Elithorn and Barnett (1967) presented their subjects with a signal in either or both visual fields and required them to respond with the hand or hands so indicated. They found that subjects were able to respond in a partly independent manner to signals presented to opposite hemispheres. Dimond (1970) likewise found that when a double, two-handed response was required, performance was faster when the two signals for these responses went to opposite visual fields and hemispheres than when both went to the same visual field and hemisphere. In both cases, however, performance was slower than where only a single signal was presented and only one response was required, suggesting that the two hemispheres are not operating with complete independence. Dimond and Beaumont (1971) subsequently found that when the subject was simultaneously occupied with another demanding concurrent task, he or she could report more digits when two sets of numbers were presented to opposite fields than when both sets went to the same visual field. Dimond and Beaumont (1974) review a number of their other studies, which also indicate superior performance when information is divided between hemispheres rather than sent to one, though it should also be noted that some of their own studies give the opposite results (Dimond, 1969; Dimond & Beaumont, 1972a).

Yet another closely related paradigm returns us to one of the main considerations of this chapter, interhemispheric communication rather than hemispheric independence. In this paradigm a number of experiments apparently demonstrate a substantial advantage for distributed input (two signals divided between the hemispheres, rather than both going to a single hemisphere) when the task itself requires integration of the information, since the two signals must be compared or crossmatched. Obviously, where such an advantage *is* demonstrated for distributed input, it must reflect the fact that it more than outweighs any disadvantage (in terms of delay in interhemispheric transmission time or signal degradation during transfer) associated with the need for subsequent interhemispheric communication. (In a subsequent section of this chapter we shall see that interhemispheric transmission time, contrary to widespread belief, is only a few milliseconds). Dimond and Beaumont (1972b) required two simultaneously presented figures to be crossmatched when the figures were projected either both to the same hemisphere or one to each. The latter condition proved superior. Similar findings were reported by R. Davis and Schmit (1971, 1973) with digit and letter stimuli, and by Annett and Annett (1979). We can therefore conclude that any limitations imposed by interhemispheric intercommunication (e.g., signal delay or degradation) cannot be very substantial.

Interhemispheric Transmission Time
and Other Explanations

With normal subjects tachistoscopic and dichotic techniques do not allow the functioning of each hemisphere to be examined in isolation, so it is not immediately apparent whether stimuli are processed within the hemisphere to which they are immediately projected or whether the input has been transmitted across the commissures for processing in the other hemisphere. Studies of clinical patients often seem to suggest the absolute superiority of one or the other hemisphere for processing in a particular mode and the complete inability of its fellow to mediate such a function; however, it must be remembered that persisting inhibitory influences from the damaged hemisphere may be partially responsible. Such influences are of course largely absent with commissurotomized subjects, and workers in this area are far more inclined to the view that interhemispheric differences are relative and quantitative rather than absolute and qualitative. However, in the case of split-brain patients, long-standing preoperative morbidity may well have led to functional reorganization and the development of some degree of bilaterality. What then can we learn from studies with normal subjects? Do ear and visual field superiorities reflect relatively more or less efficient processing by one or the other hemisphere? Or are the hemispheres uniquely and absolutely specialized, with speed and accuracy differences between the hemispheres reflecting either interhemispheric transmission time or signal degradation during interhemispheric transfer or both? As we shall see, the considerable intersubject, intertask and even intertrial variability in such reaction-time differences tends to argue against the long-accepted interhemispheric transmission-time explanation. With respect to the signal-degradation account, one might expect more complex information to experience more degradation and to be associated with greater field and ear differences. While there is indeed evidence, which we shall review below, of asymmetries being stronger at "deeper" or "higher" levels of required (or achieved) processing, there is no actual evidence of the magnitude of such asymmetries correlating with the *complexity* of stimulus information *per se*. We are ourselves inclined to the view that laterality differences reflect relative (rather than absolute) differences between the hemispheres in their processing capacities for the types of materials under test. There are, however, other possible explanations, including a number invoking aspects of attention, which we shall consider later in this chapter. At the moment we wish to review the studies that have specifically sought to measure empirically interhemispheric (transcallosal) transmission times.

A number of studies (recently reviewed by Anzola, Bertoloni, Buchtel, & Rizzolatti, 1977; Di Stefano, Morelli, Marzi, & Berlucchi, 1980; Rizzolatti, 1979) have compared reaction-time performance when subjects detect the presence of a light flash in one or the other visual field and respond by pressing a button with the hand that happens to be placed on the same or the opposite side as the stimulus event. Response times are typically faster in the ipsilateral, or "uncrossed," condition (light flash and hand on the same side) than when the relationship is contralateral. An explanation in terms of the longer interhemispheric pathway required in the latter instance has usually been offered (see, e.g., Poffenberger, 1912; J. L. Bradshaw & Perriment, 1970; Jeeves, 1969, 1972; Jeeves & Dixon, 1970). One problem, however, is that one group of studies reports differences of about two or three milliseconds; another finds the difference to be in the order of tens of milliseconds. A second problem is that when subjects are made to respond with their arms crossing the body midline, the right hand now on the left side and the left hand on the right, again one group finds that faster responses occur not with ipsilateral *hand*-visual field relationships but with ipsilateral *body side*-visual field relationships; that is, the *right* hand in the *left* body space now responds faster to stimuli in the *left* visual field (see, e.g., Wallace, 1971). On the other hand, other groups (see, e.g., Anzola et al., 1977; Rizzolatti, 1979) obtained faster right-hand responses to RVF stimuli and faster left-hand responses to LVF stimuli *regardless* of whether the hands were crossed or not. Moreover, the two groups of studies completely segregate with respect to the above two variables and to a third variable, which in fact may completely account for the various findings. All studies finding the small (2-3 msec) interhemispheric transmission time used a *simple* reaction-time procedure; that is, subjects responded with a single hand or a single finger, regardless of the visual field of presentation. All studies obtaining the larger value (10-40 msec) employed a *choice* reaction-time paradigm; either subjects were ready and able to respond with either hand, depending on whether the signal occurred in the LVF or RVF, or subjects were ready and able to respond with one of two fingers on a single hand, again as a function of field of stimulation. Moreover, when the crossed-arms condition was run under simple or choice reaction-time conditions (see, e.g., Berlucchi, 1978; Berlucchi, Crea, Di Stefano, & Tassinari, 1977), ipsilateral responses proved faster (by a few milliseconds) than contralateral responses *regardless* of hand position with the *simple* reaction-time paradigm. Thus the right hand, though in the left body space, still responded faster to stimuli in the RVF, and the left hand still responded faster to stimuli in the LVF, even when located in the right body space. Conversely, with the *choice* reaction-time paradigm, the responding hand on the side of the stimulus event proved faster (by about 30 msec). Compatible findings are also reported by Harvey (1978) and Swanson, Ledlow, and Kinsbourne (1978). We may conclude that the simple reaction-time paradigm probably measures the true, anatomic, interhemispheric transmission time; it certainly accords with our knowledge of axon length and number of synapses and with recent evoked potential measurements of latency differences of arrival times in the two hemispheres (see, e.g., Swadlow, Geschwind, & Waxman, 1979). The choice reaction-time paradigm, on the other hand, may well be contaminated by attentional effects, with attention divided between two sides of body space or of sensory and motor space, not just in terms of detecting a sensory event, but also of deciding where it occurred and which *limb* should respond. (For similar ideas on hemispace and their development, see Bowers & Heilman, 1980; Cotton, Tzeng, & Wang, 1980; Heilman, 1979b). If this conclusion is correct, and we believe it is, it will account for the finding (Provine & Westerman, 1979; Schofield, 1976) that infants are unable to make hand or arm movements across the body midline, whether or not visually guided. Our conclusion also has two further consequences:

1. "Cognitive" laterality effects (e.g., for verbal or visuospatial processing) reflect the much longer (and more variable) differences in hemispheric capacity for processing that particular mode of stimulus, rather than interhemispheric transmission times.

2. It makes little difference, in terms of interhemispheric transmission times, whether a left- or right-hand response is used in cognitive studies since the interhemispheric transmission-time effect is only of the order of a few milliseconds, while the cognitive laterality effect is typically measured in tens of milliseconds. However, this does *not* mean that *unimanual* responding should be employed, since this procedure may well lead to directional attentional biases, and/or "priming" of the contralateral hemisphere, with artifactual results. It *does* mean, though, that *bimanual* responding (e.g., use of the two forefingers for "target" responses and the two middle fingers for "nontarget responses," or vice versa) can safely be employed, since any interhemispheric difference will again be only one or two milliseconds. Indeed, organization of a bimanual response (probably within a single hemisphere) will itself tend to obliterate any consistent hand differences. In an unpublished series of experiments, we found that laterality effects were the same whether measurements were made of left or right hand, ipsilateral or contralateral hand (in terms either of field of presentation or of presumed hemisphere of stimulus processing), or *faster* hand. Other independent evidence (see, e.g., Babkoff, Ben-Uriah, & Eliasher, 1980; Isseroff, Carmon, & Nachshon, 1974; Moscovitch, 1976; Reynolds & Jeeves, 1978; Shefsky, Stenson, & Miller, 1980) indicates that field differences in cognitive laterality tasks are not a function of the hand making the (reaction-time) responses. Any effect contributed by the responding hand is only a few milliseconds, a value that is normally nonsignificant unless a very large number of trials are measured.

We conclude, therefore, that transcallosal transmission times are very small and do not determine the often considerable, and usually variable, laterality differences found with cognitive tasks. Such differences reflect either differential processing capacities in the two hemispheres for different kinds of material or differential attentional tendencies to one or other side of body space. These attentional biases may be a function of the location of the stimulus and the responding limb or of the nature of the required processing (leading to a differential activation of the hemispheres), or of both. In the subsequent sections of this chapter we shall examine in detail the various versions of the attentional and activational accounts.

Kinsbourne's Attentional Model

Kinsbourne (1970, 1973, 1975) contends that the levels of activation in hemispheres are normally in a reciprocal balance and that this balanced state is associated with a straight-ahead orientation of receptors and attentional tendencies.

Eccentric stimulation or, conversely, endogenously generated activation in the contralateral hemisphere, both of which disturb this balanced equilibrium, will lead to an orientational response in that direction, to inhibition of orienting responses in the other hemisphere, and to a biased readiness to accept stimulation and emit responses in a direction contralateral to the activated hemisphere. Thus readiness to process stimuli appearing in either visual field is determined by the relative levels of activation of the two hemispheres. Verbal processes activate the left hemisphere and thus bias attention toward the RVF and/or the right ear; visuospatial processes activate the right hemisphere and bias attention in the opposite direction. This account consequently sees visual field and ear superiorities not as due to structural determinants, privileged access of stimuli from one side of the body to specialized neural processing centers, but as a consequence of attentional and activational biases. Moreover, an orientational movement (overt or covert) to one side will momentarily render the brain more ready for the mode or form of processing (verbal or nonverbal) in which the hemisphere contralateral to that side specializes. Lateral shifts in the direction of attention will affect the momentary balance of activation between the hemispheres. Conversely, activation in one hemisphere, apart from rendering the subject better able to process those stimuli for which the activated hemisphere is specialized and which arrive in the contralateral side of attentional space, will also overflow to adjacent motor structures for hand, arm, head, and eye movements and will produce measurable deflections of the receptors. The subject will orient head or eyes in a direction contralateral to the activated hemisphere (Kinsbourne, 1972), thus providing the researcher with a ready index of lateralized cerebral activation, such as conjugate lateral eye movements, CLEMs (see Chapter Six). The model also nicely accounts for EEG asymmetries. The source of this hemispheric activation or priming is never made explicit; however, it appears to be regarded as originating in the thalamus or brainstem, with feedback control via the corpus callosum.

A number of studies have supported Kinsbourne's attentional model. Kinsbourne (1970) found that in a task requiring the subject to detect a threshold-sized gap on the side of a square, a RVF superiority appeared only if the subject was concurrently engaged with a verbal memory load, which presumably activated the left hemisphere and biased it for the detection of events to the right. Spellacy and Blumstein (1970) obtained a REA in a dichotic task employing vowels only when the subjects were expecting speech, otherwise a LEA (in a nonspeech context) appeared. Morais and Landercy (1977) reported that a REA for dichotically presented nonsense syllables decreased when subjects concurrently stored short musical passages. Kershner, Thomae, and Callaway (1977) found that a nonverbal fixation control stimulus induced a (nonsignificant) LVF superiority in digit recall, and a verbal fixation stimulus produced (nonsignificant) RVF superiorities, though others have failed to replicate this effect (see Chapter Six). G. Cohen (1975b) presented such stimuli as FOUR, FIVE; 4, 5, and °°, °°° and required her subjects to decide whether or not the cardinal numbers *four* or *five* had been presented. Significant differences only appeared when subjects were precued as to the type of stimulus immediately to follow; then a significant RVF superiority appeared for such stimuli as FOUR and FIVE, and a (nonsignificant) LVF superiority for the dot configurations. Klein, Moscovitch, and Vigna (1976) found that a LVF superiority in a face-processing task only appeared when it was not immediately preceded by a word-processing task or by the subject's reporting a verbal stimulus. Honda (1978) reported that a LVF superiority in recognizing line orientations increased with nonverbal loads and disappeared with verbal loads, and RVF superiorities in recognizing letters increased with a verbal load and disappeared with a nonverbal load. Heilman and Van Den Abell (1979) showed that a warning signal directed to one or the other visual field effected a significant reduction in simple reaction time to a stimulus subsequently presented to the same visual field. Bowers and Heilman (1980) extended these findings by using verbal and nonverbal warning signals and found further support for the notion of differential hemispheric activation.

However, a very considerable number of studies have failed to support Kinsbourne's account; some have even failed to replicate his original findings (Boles, 1979; E. B. Gardner & Branski, 1976). Those who have failed to support the predictions of his model include, among others, Allard and Bryden (1979), Berlucchi, Brizzolara, Marzi, Rizzolatti, and Umiltà (1979), Guiard (1980), Hansch and Pirozzolo (1980), Haun (1978), Kallman (1978), Kirsner (1980), Pirozzolo (1977), Pirozzolo and Rayner (1977), and Wexler and Heninger (1980). One of the best and easiest tests of Kinsbourne's account is to compare the effects of blocking and randomizing visual field (or ear) of presentation, on the one hand, and on the other, of blocking and randomizing the type of stimulus, verbal or nonverbal, when both are present in a single experiment. If visual field or ear asymmetries still occur when the stimuli are scrambled as to type (verbal or nonverbal processing modes), this counts against Kinsbourne's account, since subjects cannot establish the appropriate processing sets, which Kinsbourne claims underpin his attentional account. While G. Cohen (1975a) did find that appropriate asymmetries only appeared when subjects knew in advance the nature of each stimulus, Geffen, Bradshaw, and Nettleton (1972) found in a physical and nominal letter-matching task that directional asymmetries were equally strong whether the verbal and visuospatial comparisons were blocked or scrambled. This finding was confirmed by Ledlow, Swanson, and Kinsbourne (1978). Berlucchi et al. (1974) found the same: a LVF superiority for faces and a RVF superiority for letters, whether blocked or scrambled. Kallman (1978) obtained a REA to monaurally presented syllables and a LEA to musical notes whether or not subjects knew in advance the nature of each stimulus before a trial. Goodglass and Calderon (1977) simultaneously presented verbal and tonal materials for parallel processing under dichotic conditions and obtained independent REAs for the verbal and LEAs for the tonal components. The fact that the two hemispheres could concurrently and independently process that component of a complex stimulus for which each is dominant is contrary to the predictions of the Kinsbourne model.

We have just seen that according to Kinsbourne, visual field or ear asymmetries should be lost when subjects cannot predict the verbal or visuospatial *nature* of the immediately subsequent stimulus. According to him these asymmetries should also be lost when the subject *can* predict the visual field (or ear) of the oncoming stimulus, since such foreknowledge should overcome the effects of any preexisting lateral biases in attention arising from unilateral hemispheric activation, when the latter is a consequence of verbal or nonverbal processing. Indeed, Geffen et al. (1972) and J. L. Bradshaw, Farrelly, and Taylor (1981) found very strong visual field and ear asymmetries, respectively, when stimuli were blocked as to side of presentation—as strong as when they were randomized in the former study and even stronger in the latter. Moreover, the demonstration of *monaural* ear asymmetries, since a blocked mode of presentation has usually been employed, is itself evidence against the Kinsbourne model. We are only aware of one study, that of Ledlow et al. (1978), which lost the expected verbal RVF superiority when stimuli were blocked as to side of presentation.

In conclusion, we believe that attentional and activational influences of the sort envisaged by Kinsbourne are very probably present, but do not wholly account for the laterality findings. They show their greatest effect with material that does not strongly engage laterally specialized processors. Aspects of both the structural and the activational-attentional models probably need to be combined (Klein, Moscovitch, & Vigna, 1976), together with the concept of lateralized and overall processing load (Hellige, Cox, & Litvac, 1979, and see the section that follows). Moreover, we shall in a later section argue for further modifications in the actual concept of attention itself.

The Attentional Account of Morais and Bertelson

Morais and Bertelson (1973) used loudspeakers rather than headphones in an analogue of the dichotic listening paradigm, positioning a loudspeaker on each side of the subject's head. In this way both messages, one via each speaker, ultimately reached both ears. In a nonsense syllable recall task they found a right-side advantage equal in magnitude to the true REA from a dichotic condition. In a subsequent study (1975) they contrasted the effects of intensity differences and stimulus asynchrony independently of each other in this loudspeaker paradigm, employing stereophonic techniques. A message was subjectively lateralized to one or the other side of the subject's head either by leading one message or by increasing its intensity. They obtained a right-side advantage with time delay but not with intensity differences, showing that apparent spatial origin was a more important determinant than either ear of entry or spatial direction. Hublet, Morais, and Bertelson (1977) later found that competition between messages from a single direction was as effective in determining auditory spatial effects as competition between spatially distinct sources. Finally, Morais (1978) found that the *apparent* spatial origin of these auditory signals (as a result of the employment of dummy loudspeakers) was sufficient to eliminate (but not to create) an asymmetry in performance. He asks whether sounds from particular directions in perceived auditory space have a stronger representation in the primary auditory cortex of the left hemisphere than sounds apparently coming from other directions.

So far we appear to be describing a model that is fairly similar to that offered by Kinsbourne, and indeed the effects so far described are compatible with and support his position. However, the activational aspect, which is an essential component of Kinsbourne's account, is not needed by Morais and Bertelson. Moreover, as Morais and Landercy (1977) observe, the fact that placing real loudspeakers at 45° and fictitious ones at 90° rather than 45° is not sufficient to create a right-side advantage, is inconsistent with Kinsbourne's assumption that focusing attention 90° to the right favors left hemisphere processing while focusing it 90° to the left has a detrimental effect on these processes. Furthermore, Tweedy, Rinn, and Springer (1980) compared the magnitude of the right-side advantage with headphones (normal dichotic listening) and loudspeakers (in the Morais and Bertelson paradigm) for both normal and commissurotomized subjects. They found that the right-side advantage was in fact greater with headphones (which is contrary to the predictions of Kinsbourne's model) and for commissurotomy subjects. The fact that the latter group of subjects was more sensitive to a change between headphones and speakers is also incompatible with (Kinsbourne's) viewpoint that the major or only role of the corpus callosum is in the balanced distribution of attention across the two halves of auditory space and would suggest instead that it does serve (when present) to convey some information from the left ear (and right hemisphere) to the left hemisphere. Tweedy et al. conclude that the fact that a right-side advantage does occur even with loudspeakers suggests that attentional processes *in some form* must be included *along with* a structural account (such as Kimura's) of cerebral asymmetry.

Some such compromise between the two theories, the structural and the attentional, is implied by Heilman (1979b). He argues that each hemisphere is responsible not only for mediating the distal movements of the contralateral extremities and for processing the contralateral sensory input but *also* for mediating behavior in the contralateral spatial field *independently* of whichever extremity (or visual field) is actually used. This account explains the findings from the reaction-time experiments with crossed arms, which we discussed in a previous section: The crossed arm enters the other hemisphere's field and interhemispheric communication is needed. It also explains why, with right hemisphere damage and hemineglect, patients tend to ignore whatever is to the left of their *body* midlines (whether it is the left side of their plates or of a sheet of paper or even of their clothing while dressing) despite being able to move head, eyes, and trunk so as to be able to put the unattended section in foveal vision. Finally, such an account satisfactorily explains why a normal person, with arms out from the body, is superior with the left hand (right hemisphere) in halving a rod (with tactile information alone), and why, with arms crossing the body midline, the person is better with the right hand and better with *either* hand in left hemispace than in right hemispace (Bowers & Heilman, 1980). This is of course a demonstration of something akin to visual hemineglect in normals and again would suggest that Kimura's structural model is incomplete; field, ear, and hand superiorities perhaps depend as much on the side of *hemispace* in which a stimulus is presented (the external space to one or the other side of the body midline) as on direct anatomical access to lateralized processing centers. A further test of such an account would be to determine whether the blind reading of Braille is better accomplished not so much by the left hand but by either hand in the left hemispace.

We would ourselves argue that it is not just ears, visual fields, or proximal receptor surfaces that map on the cortex but also auditory, tactile, or visual hemispace—all of which of course are normally confounded unless artificial conditions such as crossing the limbs are employed. If both Kimura's structural model and Kinsbourne's attentional account are seen as incomplete on their own, we can perhaps conclude that behavioral asymmetries also reflect the cortical mapping of perceived visual or auditory space as well as perhaps biased attentional tendencies toward that space and the neural representation of the proximal locus of stimulation in one or the other ear or hemiretina. This would account for the otherwise ignored and inexplicable findings of Corballis, Anuza, and Blake (1978) that lateral asymmetries depend more on a *perceptual* than on a *retinal* interpretation of visual fields. They found that accuracy of single-letter recognition was partly a function of *gravitational* coordinates, sometimes overriding hemiretinal location when subjects' heads were tilted.

Levels of Coding:
Memory Versus Perceptual Factors in Cerebral Asymmetry

It is a common observation that laterality effects tend to be larger when a comparison to memory rather than purely perceptual matching is required (Dee & Fontenot, 1973; Hannay & Malone, 1976; Hines, Satz, & Clementino, 1973; Moscovitch, Scullion, & Christie, 1976). In a dichaptic tactile task Oscar-Berman, Rehbein, Porfert, and Goodglass (1978) obtained right-hand superiorities for letter recognition and left-hand superiorities for the recognition of line orientations, but only for the hands reported second—that is, after a storage interval while the reports were being completed for the first hands. Thus, tactile storage was more sensitive to laterality differences than measures closer in time to the actual stimulus events. Hardyck, Tzeng, and Wang (1978) in fact proposed that lateralization effects are not a function of immediate cognitive processing in specialized cortical areas but instead reflect differences in storage locations. If subjects are required to evaluate new material on every trial, reaction times will not show the asymmetry that is reported in experiments employing a small set of stimuli and a large number of trials. Hardyck et al. claimed to have demonstrated this when visual field superiorities only emerged in their fourth experiment, which employed a small stimulus set repeatedly encountered. In their preceding experiments new stimuli were employed on every trial and no asymmetries emerged. Thus, they argued that laterality effects only appear with a restricted number of stimuli and a large number of trials, where memory rather than perceptual effects are being tested. As we have ourselves found (J. L. Bradshaw & Gates, 1978) and as we shall discuss further in a later section, practice certainly is important in determining the extent and direction of laterality effects, but it must also be noted that with words large laterality effects may be demonstrated when many words are presented each time only once (J. L. Bradshaw & Gates, 1978; J. L. Bradshaw & Taylor, 1979; J. L. Bradshaw, Nettleton, & Taylor, 1981a). However, words of course are familiar long-term memory items, so this objection may not be entirely valid. We have tended to find weaker field effects for nonwords, which are *not* in long-term memory. Another study that has reported enhanced (LVF) effects for more frequently occurring stimuli (polygons) is that of Hellige (1980a). He found field effects were enhanced when a small number of stimuli were used repeatedly, as compared with when a large number were each infrequently presented, just as Hardyck et al. reported.

As we have seen, before asymmetries emerge retention intervals must often exceed a certain lower limit (for review of the very considerable body of research that demonstrates this, see Moscovitch, 1979), or stimuli must be subjected to some form of masking degradation (Hellige, 1980a; Moscovitch et al., 1976) or abstraction (e.g. caricaturing, Moscovitch et al., 1976) or the subject must identify a test face that appears with changes in viewing angle (and possibly also in expression, age, and health) as compared with the target (Bertelson, Vanhaelen, & Morais, 1979). This has led Moscovitch (1979) to propose that functions of the two hemispheres diverge more clearly at the later, higher, postcategorical stages of information processing. During the earlier stages he believes that the hemispheres process information in a largely similar manner. He claims that visual field and ear differences for intensity, brightness, color, hue, pitch, pressure, and touch are small and weak (though we would dispute whether they are nonsignificant) and are basic to the later, stronger asymmetries that arise at deeper or high levels of cognitive processing.

Hellige and his coworkers (e.g., Hellige, Cox, & Litvac, 1979) have taken these ideas one stage further and attempted to marry them to Kinsbourne's attention-activation account. It will be remembered that according to Kinsbourne, functional specialization of the hemispheres accounts for, at most, only a very small part of the asymmetry effect. The latter is largely due to differential allocation of attention, itself a consequence both of cognitive set or expectancy and of concurrent processing load. It is this aspect that interests Hellige. Kinsbourne's model holds that concurrent work loads can prime or activate either the hemisphere appropriate for that type of processing or an inappropriate one, in each case leading to a bias towards the contralateral side of space and superior processing of stimuli arriving in that space. Small loads may prime a particular hemisphere, enhancing its superiority; larger loads may overload it, depressing its performance. Hellige attempted to quantify these loads and to determine the direction of their effects at various levels, to avoid the problem of Kinsbourne's version's having too much explanatory and too little predictive power. It had been known for some time (e.g., Geffen et al., 1973) that a heavy concurrent load, far from enhancing the RVF superiority

of a primary verbal task, can overload the left hemisphere so that the field superiorities (and presumably the mediating hemispheres) reverse, generating a LVF superiority as the spare capacity of the right hemisphere takes over. Hellige and Cox
(1976) and Hellige et al. (1979) confirmed these findings, showing that whether
primary-task field asymmetries are enhanced or reversed by adding a secondary
task depends on the magnitude of the processing demands imposed by the added
task. However, as G. Cohen (1979) observes, there is still an *ad hoc* quality about
the way Hellige is forced to quantify and manipulate his measures of load, and so
far from invoking activation levels or attentional shifts, one could perhaps simply
appeal to changes in strategy that subjects adopt when single, multiple, or composite tasks become too difficult (or too easy) for them to continue as before.

Obviously, the issue is as yet unresolved. Kimura's structural account, though
needing modification to take into account the dynamic aspects of cerebral asymmetry, such as changes due to practice and familiarity or difficulty of task or stimuli,
cannot be abandoned *in toto*. It will eventually have to be incorporated into a more
dynamic model that recognizes the roles played by activation, attention, practice,
and processing loads, as well as the possibility that the cortex codes body space in
addition to its classic role of mapping the proximal receptor surfaces. Further
progress in laterality research will probably depend on programs of study of the
sort we discussed in preceding sections, but there is still a long way to go. Any
grand, all-encompassing resolution will eventually have to accommodate the issues
discussed above together with the question of more fundamental asymmetries (e.g.,
analytic–holistic) underlying the traditional verbal–visuospatial dichotomy (see
Chapter Nine) and the possible auxiliary role of the right hemisphere in mediating
the emotions, awareness of body space, arousal, vigilance, and novelty. It is with
these last issues that the rest of this chapter is concerned.

Auxiliary Functions of the Right Hemisphere: Emotionality, Hemineglect, Arousal, Vigilance, and Novelty

In the last section of this chapter we wish to review a number of interrelated issues,
all of which involve right hemisphere activation, and from the conclusions derived
from such a review return to a general theory of cerebral asymmetry to account for
the effects of novelty, practice, and experience.

The right hemisphere and emotions. Detailed reviews of laterality differences in emotional affect have recently been provided by Cacioppo, Petty, and
Snyder (1979), Gainotti (1979) and Ley and Bryden (1981). The right hemisphere
seems, relative to the left, to be more specialized for emotional reactivity, possibly
due to its mediation of synthetic, holistic, and integrative functions (see Chapter
Nine). With hysterical illnesses of the conversion type, where symptoms of physical
illness appear without underlying organic pathology, perhaps permitting the indi-

vidual to avoid stressful experiences, disorders such as hysterical blindness and deafness, motor paralyses, and visceral disorders tend to predominate on the left. Psychogenic pain is also more common on the left, suggesting that the right hemisphere may play a role in mediating affectively determined conversion reactions. Conversely, anosognosia (unawareness of or indifference towards or denial of a *real* neurological deficit) is also more common for problems manifesting on the left side of the body. Other asymmetries of psychiatric symptoms are apparent with the temporal lobe epilepsies: Those on the left side of the brain are more often associated with aggressiveness and those on the right with neurotic depression and manic-depressive psychoses. Similar asymmetries are reported with unilateral brain trauma: Damage on the left side of the brain is more often associated with the so-called catastrophic reaction (crying, swearing, refusals, anxiety, and depression); those on the right with indifference (joking, minimization, anosognosia). In addition, right hemisphere lesions may impair the ability to recall emotional stories, discriminate emotionally intoned speech, or generate the appropriate emotional reaction to humorous cartoons. Such asymmetries can also be temporarily induced by the Wada (amytal) technique, depression of the left hemisphere being associated with a depressive catastrophic reaction, that of the right frequently with a euphoric or maniacal response.

One can obviously ask whether, under these circumstances, the effects are partly determined by the traumatic loss of speech associated with left hemisphere inactivation, and also whether the effects are due to the affected side being interfered with, or alternatively the *unaffected* side being released from inhibition. Unilateral electroconvulsive therapy (ECT) simulates many of the effects of unilateral sodium amytal; nondominant (right hemisphere) ECT is possibly more beneficial, therapeutically, than bilateral or left hemisphere ECT and also minimizes sensory or language disruptions. With normal subjects, a LEA is found for the identification of nonverbal human vocalizations, such as laughing, crying, or sighing, and for the identification of emotional intonation. There is a greater LVF advantage in matching faces to stored memory targets when the faces are emotional rather than neutral, though LVF superiorities for the recognition of faces and the processing of emotions appear to be distinct and dissociable. When a contact lens system is used (with normal subjects) to permit the subject to view the world through one or the other visual field, emotionally charged films are seen as more horrifying when viewed through the LVF, and autonomic indices such as heart rate tend to bear out these conclusions. Such findings and their associated references are tabulated in detail in the three review articles listed at the beginning of this section.

Unilateral hemineglect, alerting, and the right hemisphere. In Chapter Four we discussed the phenomenon accompanying unilateral brain trauma in which the left side of the body is far more likely to be ignored, disowned, or neglected after right hemisphere injury than is the right side of the body after damage to the left. Heilman (1979b) reviews these findings in detail, together with the observations that right hemisphere injury is likely to be associated with a generalized lowering of affect, defects in alerting responses, poorer arousal, and reaction-time decrements (with either hand), all suggesting that the right hemisphere may be concerned with *bilateral* manifestations of arousal as well as unilateral aspects. Abnormal galvanic skin responses and evoked potentials are more likely to follow right than left hemisphere lesions. Heilman suggests that in health the right hemisphere may be alerted by any of a range of possible stimuli, but the left is more specific in the nature of stimuli (e.g., verbal) to which it is responsive. Van Den Abell and Heilman (1978) studied reaction times in normal subjects and found that warning signals in the LVF (right hemisphere) reduced subsequent reaction times of the right hand (i.e., increased left hemisphere arousal) more than did warning signals to the RVF (left hemisphere).

A considerable number of studies have independently, and usually in the context of some unrelated investigation, observed that with simple reaction times (without warning signals), stimuli in the LVF or left ear are responded to faster than those in the RVF or right ear (see, e.g., Annett & Annett, 1979; Anzola, Bertoloni, Buchtel, & Rizzolatti, 1977; Berlucchi, Crea, Di Stefano, & Tassinari, 1977; J. L. Bradshaw & Perriment, 1970; Jeeves & Dixon, 1970; Rizzolatti, Bertoloni, & Buchtel, 1979).

The right hemisphere and vigilance. Dimond (1979a, b) with commissurotomy patients and Dimond and Beaumont (1973) with normal subjects reported that in lateralized vigilance tasks where the subject is required to detect the occurrence of prespecified signals that occur randomly and infrequently, in the LVF or RVF or the left or right ear, performance by the left hemisphere declines in a way that is not evident with signals presented to the right hemisphere. The right hemisphere seemed to be better at sustained attention, with attentional gaps appearing in the left hemisphere performance. These findings with commissurotomy patients were disputed and not replicated by Ellenberg and Sperry (1979), and Salmaso (1980), working with normals, found that the RVF (left hemisphere) had the higher sensitivity and was more accurate in detecting novel stimuli. He suggested that the left hemisphere may be concerned with the categorization of environmental changes. Warm, Richter, Sprague, Porter, and Schumsky (1980), however, confirmed Dimond's findings, observing that in an auditory vigilance task right-ear responses were sluggish early in the vigil (thus perhaps accounting for Salmaso's findings) but remained stable over time, while those for the left ear increased in a negatively accelerated fashion over time. They concluded that during sustained attention the right hemisphere may dominate.

The right hemisphere and the preprocessing of degraded stimuli. We briefly mentioned findings in Chapter Six that when letter stimuli are unusual, unfamiliar, "florid" in design, or perceptually degraded, LVF rather than the "expected" RVF superiorities may eventuate (see, e.g., Bryden & Allard, 1976; Hellige, 1976; Hellige & Webster, 1979; Polich, 1978). We shall discuss related aspects of this phenomenon in more detail in Chapter Eight in the context of right hemisphere language mechanisms. Silverberg, Gordon, Pollack, and Bentin (1980) noted that when individuals first learn to read a script, a LVF superiority appears for the (presumably unfamiliar) script, which gives way with increasing experience to the "normal" RVF superiority. Such observations, apart from underlining the point that the right hemisphere may be called in to deal with novel, unfamiliar stimuli that require some level of preprocessing (see also J. L. Bradshaw & Gates, 1978; Hellige, 1980b), also suggest that tachistoscopic studies may be intrinsically artifactual. They employ abnormally brief and unnaturally nonfoveal exposures, which in themselves may tend to call in right hemisphere functions of the sort just discussed, and they do not engage the full perceptual capacities of the brain. It may well be that many of the findings in the literature are partly or wholly a consequence of the nature of stimulus presentation and of the choice of stimuli. Such considerations bring us to the topic of consideration for the next section, practice effects.

Practice Effects

While asymmetries may still occur when the subject is unable to inhibit automatic processing, as in the delayed auditory feedback (DAF) studies (J. L. Bradshaw, Nettleton, & Geffen, 1971, 1972) and the visual and auditory Stroop studies (G. Cohen & Martin, 1975; Schmit & Davis, 1974) reviewed in Chapter Six, practice and increasing automaticity may nevertheless lead to reduction or reversals in the "normal" asymmetry patterns. This may occur if the "inferior" hemisphere develops enough skill, with practice, to handle the stimuli or if the stimuli no longer need to be processed at as deep a level as was required earlier (Moscovitch, 1979). Thus, in addition to possible reductions in the right hemisphere "novelty" effect reviewed in the immediately previous sections, laterality effects may decrease with practice (see, e.g., Kallman & Corballis, 1975; Murray & Richards, 1978; Ward & Ross, 1977); they may also *increase* (J. L. Bradshaw & Gates, 1978; Gordon & Carmon, 1976; Miller & Butler, 1980; Perl & Haggard, 1975; Yeni-Komshian & Gordon, 1974) as appropriate processing mechanisms are switched in (see Hardyck et al., 1978, and earlier sections of this chapter) or as right hemisphere "novelty" or preprocessing mechanisms are switched out, or simply as variability in response times is reduced as the subjects become more comfortable with the task. A problem in comparing the effects of practice across tasks is that studies differ widely in the number of trials used and in block size as well as task difficulty and competence of the subjects. In some laboratories the same subjects take part in several different experiments and so become familiar with the general routine.

Goldberg and Costa (1981) have recently proposed a model to account for both the effects of practice and the sundry right hemisphere involvements in emotionality, novelty, and arousal just reviewed. One of the principles of this model is that left hemisphere processing, which is contingent on stimulus encodability in terms of some kind of established descriptive system, follows at a later stage from an initial right hemisphere involvement. Because of the rather diffuse patterning of motor and sensory representation in the right hemisphere (Goldberg & Costa review anatomical and physiological findings in support of this position), these authors argue that the right hemisphere is better equipped to deal with novel stimuli. Right hemisphere processing is more likely to be present when the stimuli do not lend themselves to encoding according to a preordained descriptive system or when no task-relevant descriptive system is immediately available in the subject's repertoire. The left hemisphere, on the other hand, can accept any class of stimuli that can be fitted into a routine descriptive system. This model has sufficient flexibility to enable it to account for individual differences and for the effects of development, experience, and practice that may be associated with right-to-left hemisphere shifts.

Evidence in favor of the Goldberg and Costa hypothesis comes from the findings (reviewed by Umiltà, Brizzolara, Tabossi, & Fairweather, 1978) of a RVF superiority in the recognition of well-known, famous, or familiar faces, instead of the LVF superiority usually associated with face processing. (It should, however, be noted that at least two other studies, S. C. Leehey & Cahn, 1979, and A. W. Young & Bion, 1980b, found LVF superiorities even with familiar faces.) Bever (1980) also reviews the evidence of an initial tendency for nonmusicians to process musical tasks holistically in the right hemisphere, but notes that this effect gives way to a left hemisphere analytic mode of processing among musicians. However, in Chapter Nine we shall review evidence that is not always compatible with this position. Spellacy (1970) and Kallman and Corballis (1975) obtained a LEA for tonal or musical stimuli only in the early stages of practice, losing it later in practice. Sidtis and Bryden (1978) found that an initial LEA in a verbal task gave way to a REA with practice; however, contrary to the Goldberg and Costa model, an inital REA in a tonal task later gave way to a LEA. Also incompatible are the findings of Murray and Richards (1978) and Ward and Ross (1977). In the former study a REA (monaural) for naming words only occurred early in practice and was later lost. Analogous effects in a visual matching paradigm also occurred in the second study. We ourselves (J. L. Bradshaw & Sherlock, 1982) have found that in tasks involving the discrimination of schematic faces and bugs, the predicted visual effects are stronger in the second of two consecutive tasks and with subjects given previous practice, whether left hemisphere analytic or right hemisphere holistic processes are being investigated.

Despite the obvious appeal of Goldberg and Costa's model, and the neat way in which it follows from the predictions made and the points raised in the earlier sections of this chapter, we regretfully have to conclude that at this moment there is insufficient evidence to support it. The best general statement that can be made so far is that practice is likely to result in the normal or "predicted" pattern of field asymmetries, unless it is such as either to so increase the capability of the "inferior" hemisphere as to reduce its inferiority, or to bring about changes in processing strategies that themselves reverse the patterns of asymmetry. Although the right hemisphere does seem to be more readily aroused than the left, perhaps to be more responsive to novel stimuli, and certainly to be better able to preprocess degraded or unfamiliar patterns, we believe that the best characterization of hemispheric asymmetry is some version of the analytic–holistic processing dichotomy. This will be the subject of Chapter Nine.

Summary and Conclusions

According to Kimura's structural account of hemispheric asymmetry, laterality differences reflect privileged access, via superior contralateral pathways, to hemispheres uniquely specialized for processing a given type of information. Material received in the nonspecialized hemisphere is sent across the commissures to the competent hemisphere. Laterality differences thus reflect either transmission times or signal degradation during transmission. However, not everyone agrees that the hemispheres are absolutely and qualitatively rather than relatively and quantitatively specialized, and the inflexibility of Kimura's model as it stands renders it unable to account for the dynamic, changing aspects of lateral superiorities.

There is some evidence that commissurotomy patients and even normal subjects may process simultaneous stimuli better when each stream of information goes to a separate hemisphere than when both are presented to the same hemisphere. While this may be more evident in commissurotomy patients, even here the two parallel functions must be relatively simple and capable of being performed from a common posture and mental set. Superior processing of simultaneously presented streams of information directed to different hemispheres extends even to the situation where the two streams must be integrated, compared, and cross-matched, *despite* any delay or signal degradation that might result from such interhemispheric communication, suggesting that the latter does not impose any substantial limitations.

Further evidence against the idea of unique, absolute hemispheric superiorities is the magnitude of the intersubject, intertask, and intertrial variability in laterality effects as measured by reaction time. Reaction times may be compared when subjects respond to the presence of a light flash in one or the other visual field by pressing a button with a hand on the same or opposite side as the light. Responses are typically faster when hand and the visual field are on the same side (uncrossed or ipsilateral sensory-motor relationships) than when they are on opposite sides (crossed or contralateral sensory-motor relationships). There is evidence, however, that this effect occurs not simply because sensory or motor information has to cross the commissures in the contralateral situation. The relevant studies all appear to segregate themselves in terms of whether the reaction-time differences are two or three milliseconds or tens of milliseconds; whether it makes a difference if the arms cross the body midline or instead extend out from it (i.e., some studies find that side of body space is a more important determinant than anatomical relationships between visual field and limb); and finally whether a simple or a choice reaction-time paradigm is used. These three groupings of the relevant studies completely segregate, indicating that true transcallosal transmission time (two or three milliseconds) is demonstrable by the simple reaction-time paradigm. The longer values, which can be obtained with the choice reaction-time design and which are subject to how the limbs are positioned with reference to the body midline, reflect the effects of a division of attention between the two sides of sensory and motor hemispace. Since most cognitive laterality studies find differences of the order of tens of milliseconds, we conclude that such differences do *not* reflect transcommissural transmission time (which is only a few milliseconds).

An alternative to Kimura's structural model is Kinsbourne's attentional account, in which laterality differences reflect activation of one or the other hemisphere as a function of expectancies as to the likely nature (verbal or nonverbal) of the processing that a particular stimulus may require. Many studies have wholly or partially supported Kinsbourne's model, but many have failed to do so, and often have been unable even to replicate his original findings. In particular, laterality effects have often been shown to occur even when the subject cannot predict the verbal or nonverbal nature of each stimulus, thus preventing the hemispheric activation that Kinsbourne believes to be necessary, or when stimuli that require *both* modes of processing are simultaneously presented. Laterality effects also occur when the subject knows in advance which visual field or ear will be stimulated; this knowledge should tend to offset the development of hemispheric-specific activation for processing in a particular mode. At the very least aspects of both Kinsbourne's and Kimura's accounts may need combining, as Hellige has tried to do.

Morais and Bertelson propose another attentional account. They showed that left or right ear advantages could be obtained with loudspeakers as well as earphones, and that *apparent* spatial origin is an important determinant of laterality. Thus the auditory cortex may map perceived auditory space as well as or maybe instead of simply mapping the proximal receptor surfaces. This account does not invoke the *activational* aspects of Kinsbourne's model. Kinsbourne's model would, in any case, predict equal laterality effects for both loudspeakers and earphones, while earphones provided the stronger effects. Kimura's account is still required in some form, together with components involving the ideas of attention and the cortical mapping of hemispace. The hemispace account is given further support by the results of tactile laterality experiments conducted with crossed arms, and of visual studies conducted with tilted subjects, and by the phenomenon of unilateral hemineglect.

Laterality effects tend to be larger when *memory* rather than purely *perceptual* processes are tapped, when subjects become thoroughly familiar with the nature of the actual stimuli and of the task, or when deep (postcategorical) levels of stimulus processing are required. The nature and extent of concurrent tasks may also be important in priming or overloading a given hemisphere, so that at relatively low activation and/or load levels, hemispheric superiority may be increased, and at high levels, when a processing hemisphere is overloaded, laterality effects may reverse.

The right hemisphere seems to play its own role in activation, arousal, and attention. The right hemisphere may be more specialized than the left for emotional reactivity, perhaps especially so for the more negative emotions. It also appears to be particularly involved in the phenomenon of unilateral hemineglect, in activation in response to warning signals, response signals, and vigilance tasks, in mediating sustained attention, and in detecting novel stimuli. It is also involved in preprocessing degraded stimuli.

Practice and increasing automaticity may alter the magnitude of laterality effects, reducing them if the normally inferior hemisphere is given enough practice, or increasing them as appropriate processing mechanisms are switched in or as right hemisphere novelty or preprocessing mechanisms are switched out. There are, however, many empirical and methodological problems in interpreting the effects of practice on laterality measures. A recent model suggests that right hemisphere processing is more likely to occur when stimuli do not lend themselves to encoding according to a preordained descriptive system, or when such a task-relevant descriptive system is not immediately available. Otherwise, a left hemisphere superiority should occur. While there is considerable independent support for such an account, there is also contrary evidence. We conclude that practice is likely to result in the "normal" or "predicted" pattern of asymmetries unless either the capacity of the "inferior" hemisphere is so increased as to eliminate its inferiority, or changes in processing strategies eventuate that themselves reverse the patterns of asymmetry.

FURTHER READING

BERLUCCHI, G. Interhemispheric integration of simple visuomotor responses. In P. A. Buser & A. Rougeul-Buser (Eds.), *Cerebral correlates of conscious experience*. Amsterdam: Elsevier, North-Holland, 1978.

COHEN, G. Comment on "Information processing in the cerebral hemispheres: Selective activation and capacity limitations" by Hellige, Cox, & Litvac. *Journal of Experimental Psychology: General*, 1979, *108*, 309–315.

GAINOTTI, G. Affectivity and brain dominance: A survey. In J. Obiols, C. Ballús, E. González Monclús, & J. Pujol (Eds.), *Biological psychiatry today*. Amsterdam: Elsevier, North-Holland, 1979.

GOLDBERG, E., & COSTA, L. Hemisphere differences in the acquisition and use of descriptive systems. *Brain and Language*, 1981, *14*, 144–173.

HEILMAN, K. M. Neglect and related disorders. In K. M. Heilman & E. Valenstein (Eds.), *Clinical neuropsychology*. Oxford: Oxford University Press, 1979.

HELLIGE, J. B. Visual laterality and cerebral hemisphere specialization: Methodological and theoretical considerations. In J. B. Sidowski (Ed.), *Conditioning, cognition and methodology: Contemporary issues in experimental psychology*. Hillsdale, N.J.: Lawrence Erlbaum, (in press).

HELLIGE, J. B., COX, P. J., & LITVAC, L. Information processing in the cerebral hemispheres: Selective hemispheric activation and capacity limitations. *Journal of Experimental Psychology: General*, 1979, *108*, 251–279.

LEY, R. G., & BRYDEN, M. P. The right hemisphere and emotion. In G. Underwood & R. Stevens (Eds.), *Aspects of consciousness* (Vol. 2). New York: Academic Press, 1980.

MORAIS, J. Spatial constraints on attention to speech. In J. Requin (Ed.), *Attention and performance VII*. Hillsdale, N.J.: Lawrence Erlbaum, 1978.

MOSCOVITCH, M. Information processing and the cerebral hemispheres. In M. S. Gazzaniga (Ed.), *Handbook of behavioral neurobiology, Vol. 2: Neuropsychology*. New York: Plenum, 1979.

RIZZOLATTI, G. Interfield differences in reaction times to lateralized visual stimuli in normal subjects. In I. Steele-Russel, M. W. Hof, & G. Berlucchi (Eds.), *Structure and function of cerebral commissures*. London: Macmillan, 1979.

CHAPTER EIGHT
Language and the Nondominant Hemisphere

The evidence reviewed so far points to a generally superior capability of the left hemisphere to mediate language functions in humans. This superiority is perhaps more pronounced in right-handed people, and perhaps particularly so in those whose parents are also dextral (see Chapter Ten), in males (see Chapter Eleven), and in adults (see Chapter Twelve). Possible reasons for the left hemisphere's assumption of language functions will be discussed in the next chapter. However, at this stage we must consider the extent to which the right hemisphere can participate in speech and language (regardless of sex, age, and handedness differences), both in normal healthy adults and in those with various clinical syndromes, either long-standing or of an acute, rapid onset in adulthood.

A number of sources give evidence of participation by the right hemisphere in certain language functions. The major pieces of evidence, with which we shall deal in turn, are: the effect of temporary anaesthesia of the major hemisphere by barbiturate (e.g., sodium amytal) injection to the (usually right) carotid artery; the performance of commissurotomized subjects on verbal materials routed to the minor hemisphere; the effects of lesions to the minor hemisphere on language functions; tests of language functions in adults who have undergone partial or complete hemispherectomy; preserved reading functions in those who acquired deep dyslexia in adulthood; the study of Japanese *kana* and *kanji* in both normal subjects and patients with left or right hemisphere lesions; possible performance differences in normal subjects with different classes of lateralized verbal stimuli.

None of these sources of information is entirely satisfactory. Unilateral anaesthesia is short-lived, sometimes incomplete, and often disturbing to the patient. It is also a hazardous procedure and is only administered to patients who have gross pre-existing disturbances of normal function. Adults who had hemispherectomies as infants will have had a long period of development and reorganization, which would probably permit unusual levels of language ability to be acquired by the minor hemisphere; in consequence, such minor hemisphere capacities may be regarded as the upper limit possible after maximum potential for plastic reorganization. The recovery of language in an aphasic patient who has sustained left hemisphere damage may be due either to the transitory nature of the injury, to compensatory functioning of undamaged neighboring left hemisphere tissue, or to the right hemisphere's taking over language functions. Conversely, continuing aphasia after left hemisphere trauma may reflect the limits of right hemisphere language functions, inhibition of right hemisphere capacities by existing portions of the damaged left hemisphere, or even facilitation by the damaged left hemisphere of still more elementary linguistic capacities in the right. Language deficits after right hemisphere injury could conceivably even be due to the damaged right hemisphere's sending over "neural noise" to the dominant, verbal left hemisphere.

Although such facilitatory or inhibitory influences cannot occur with commissurotomy patients, these patients will generally have had more or less long-standing epilepsy. This, coupled with concomitant likelihood of massive cerebral reorganization and the probability of at least some degree of cortical trauma resulting from the operation itself, will mean that the minor hemispheres of commissurotomy patients are hardly representative of those of the general population. In addition these subjects, like normal subjects, can be tested only with certain restricted types of stimuli that can be presented, usually under highly artificial and limiting conditions, to one or the other hemisphere. The deep dyslexic patients who were clinically normal until their injury in adulthood usually have naturally occurring lesions whose extent and limits are either unknown or unclear (until autopsy); in any case they rarely correspond exactly to structures known to be important for certain specific language functions.

Clinical patients, including commissurotomies, are generally grossly disparate in such relevant variables as age, intelligence, motivation, and education, and should not be grouped together and treated statistically as a homogeneous sample simply because they all underwent similar treatment. The studies of *kana* and *kanji,* two different types of script in Japanese thought to involve respectively phonological and ideographic processing mechanisms to a greater or lesser extent, are subject to all the limitations already discussed for normal subjects and clinical patients, and in any case by their very nature relate to a unique language. Perhaps technically the cleanest source of evidence for the extent and nature of right hemisphere language mediation would come from adult dextral males who have recently undergone dominant hemisperectomy for a recent condition of very rapid onset. Such cases are of course extremely rare.

Notwithstanding these limitations, a general picture does emerge. This picture shows that the minor hemisphere has very considerable but probably not complete ability to assume language functions when the major hemisphere is damaged or removed in infancy. Among adults, the minor hemisphere's capacities seem largely limited to comprehension; this hemisphere has little or no expressive ability and is mute. While it is by no means uncomprehending, its power of comprehension seems considerably less than that of the major hemisphere. Indeed, as early as 1874 Hughlings Jackson believed that the right hemisphere could produce automatic speech, expletives, and well-known phrases (Joynt & Goldstein, 1975) but was even more actively engaged in lexical decoding and speech comprehension. Despite the advance of knowledge, the picture is still much the same today. The "minor hemisphere is much like a patient with nominal aphasia, who, while knowing an object's use and the things and qualities with which it is associated, cannot produce its name" (Nebes, 1974, p. 5).

Studies Involving Major Hemisphere Suppression by Unilateral Barbiturate Anaesthesia

In Chapter Four we described the Wada test, a form of reversible hemispherectomy in which a barbiturate anaesthetic, sodium amytal, is unilaterally injected into the carotid artery to suppress activity for a brief period in one or the other hemisphere. As we mentioned then, the technique is not entirely without hazard, the effect usually lasts only a few minutes, and it tells us more about the locus of speech production than speech perception. We do not know whether the described effects would persist unchanged were it in fact possible to maintain the condition for lengthy periods, or whether, for example, the initial total muteness would gradually give way to some form of aphasic utterance, either propositional or consisting merely of overlearned phrases. Nor has anyone seen fit, for the reasons outlined above, to determine systematically the nature and extent of possible deficits in comprehension when only the minor hemisphere is active. Within the limits of obeying simple instructions (e.g., "lift your hand, clench your fist"), the active minor hemisphere is obviously not uncomprehending, but we do not know whether the minor hemisphere would be able to cope with syntactically complex sentences or with unfamiliar, abstract words. The evidence from the other types of study, which we shall review, suggests that such complex material would not be readily comprehended, but confirmation is urgently needed.

The Wada test has demonstrated that the right hemisphere can sometimes become the source of aphasic speech after left hemisphere injury. A left-sided Wada test was administered to three dextrals who had become aphasic, though not entirely speechless, after left hemisphere damage (Kinsbourne, 1971). This left-sided injection did not interrupt their residual speech capabilities. Two of the patients then had to undergo right-sided testing, whereupon they became totally aphasic. Since, as Kinsbourne pointed out, other aphasic patients similarly tested did not demonstrate evidence of right hemisphere (aphasic) speech, it would be beneficial both clinically and theoretically to determine why the right hemisphere can sometimes take over (Searleman, 1977). Similar findings (loss of aphasic speech in left-lesioned patients after right-sided administration of the Wada test) are also reported by Czopf (1972, cited by Hécaen, 1978).

Studies Involving Commissurotomized Patients

In Chapter Five we discussed how section of the interhemispheric tracts to control epilepsy eliminates much of the normal integration of sensory information between the two sides of the brain, leaving each hemisphere cognizant only of contralateral sensory input. The left hemisphere thus receives detailed visual information only via the RVF and detailed somesthetic information only from stimuli presented to the right side of the body (see, e.g., Sperry, Gazzaniga, & Bogen, 1969). This division of the subject's peripheral sensory world makes it possible for us to test one or the other hemisphere more or less exclusively by appropriately lateralizing the test stimuli. Relatively few subjects are available for testing and special tachistoscopic techniques must be employed. Moreover, the patients' previous history of epilepsy may well have resulted in organizational changes, prior to surgery, in the hemispheres, making them perhaps not wholly representative of the general population. Nevertheless, both hemispheres are available as matched controls for each other, a great research advantage.

As might be expected, the left hemisphere in commissurotomized patients is proficient in all language skills (Gazzaniga & Sperry, 1967; Sperry & Gazzaniga, 1967). When stimuli such as words or objects are presented to the left hemisphere either visually through the RVF or haptically in the right hand, they are readily identified both verbally and in writing by the right hand. In time the major hemisphere may gain some motor control over the left hand also, allowing the left hand to respond in writing to stimuli received in the left hemisphere. The major hemisphere's comprehension of language can be demonstrated by the correct tactile retrieval with the right hand of items named, described, or defined by the examiner, and by the correct performance of printed commands flashed to the RVF (Nebes, 1978).

With respect to minor hemisphere language, early reports all emphasized the lack of any evidence of expressive capacity (Gazzaniga, Bogen, & Sperry, 1962; Gazzaniga & Sperry, 1967). The subjects were unable to name, verbally or in writing, words or objects seen in the LVF or felt in the left hand, although the results of nonverbal testing clearly showed that the minor hemisphere had perceived and comprehended the nature of these items. It could often use the left hand to correctly select an object named by the examiner, spelled tactually, or flashed to the LVF. It could even correctly pick out verbally described objects, selecting, for example, a magnifying glass for "something that makes things look bigger" (Nebes & Sperry, 1971). Expressive language, however, seemed to be purely a left hemisphere function.

As new subjects were tested and old ones were retested over the years, instances of limited right hemisphere expression were reported, particularly if the subject was allowed sufficient time, if the number of possible stimuli was limited, and if the identity of the stimuli was known to the subject ahead of time. Nebes (1978) in this context discusses a possible cross-cueing mechanism whereby, for example, the left hemisphere silently listed the possible choices and the right monitored this either through the peripheral mouth and throat movements or the covert internal speech, signaling the left hemisphere when it came to the proper name.

Although the earlier reports had indicated that the right hemisphere could recognize only a few nonmorphemic nouns and adjectives and had little or no syntactic capacity (Gazzaniga, 1970; Gazzaniga & Hillyard, 1971), it soon became apparent that the right hemisphere could comprehend verbs, carry out spoken commands, and link an appropriate noun to a verb by, for example, picking out a toy chair in response to the spoken command "sit"—but only if the response was not verbal and did not require the subject to actually *perform* the named act (J. Levy, 1970); otherwise, interference from the major hemisphere seemed to block the response of the minor. Thus with appropriate testing, the minor hemisphere was shown to make reasonably complex verbal associations between nouns and verbs. In similar vein, Gordon (1973) and Milner, Taylor, and Sperry (1968) showed that in response to dichotically presented commands (different commands simultaneously presented to each ear), commissurotomy patients could carry out an order to the left ear but still were unable to *say* what the command had been. This showed that the act must have been initiated by the minor hemisphere.

Evidence for minor hemisphere writing abilities appeared with two *young* commissurotomized patients. Both could produce words blindly with the left hand, but they could not then say what they had written (Nebes & Sperry, 1971), again indicating lack of major hemisphere involvement. Apart from copying words, however, anything else, such as writing the name of an object flashed to the LVF, was achieved only with great difficulty if at all and often with considerable blocking interference from the left hemisphere. In general, at least in these young patients who had cerebral birth injuries and had undergone the commissurotomy operation by age thirteen, the minor hemisphere did appear to have access to the motor patterning necessary to write words, but as in patients with nominal aphasia, it could not generate the name itself.

J. Levy and Trevarthen (1977) and J. Levy, Trevarthen, and Sperry (1972) pioneered a new technique, chimeric stimulation, for testing commissurotomized patients (see Chapter Five). Each stimulus was made up of two different half-pictures or half-words joined down the vertical midline. The midline was accurately placed to coincide with the fixation point and the subject's vertical retinal meridian. Under these conditions each half of the chimera is perceived as complete by one cerebral hemisphere, although each hemisphere receives detailed perceptual information about only one half of the stimulus. J. Levy and Trevarthen found that the right hemisphere, while comprehending verbal stimuli (e.g., the meaning of words such as *ache* and *lake*), could not make phonological transformations (i.e., recognize that the name of a picture rhymed with a previously spoken word). The right hemisphere was dominant for the visual recognition of words when no semantic or phonetic decoding was required; the left assumed control of behavior when written words had to be matched semantically to pictures, though the right hemisphere was also competent at this task. E. Zaidel (1978a) confirmed that commissurotomized patients cannot match pictures to words by rhyme with their right hemispheres, though they can match them by meaning. Interestingly, they *can* match *pictures* by rhyme, suggesting that the isolated right hemisphere can derive phonology from *pictures* but not from *print.*

E. Zaidel has extensively employed his scleral contact lens system (see Chapter Five) to investigate the limits of right hemisphere language. Typically, the experimenter speaks the stimulus message aloud while the subject views an array of pictures presented to one hemisphere. The subject then points with the hand controlled by the viewing hemisphere to the picture that best corresponds to the auditory stimulus. The remaining decoy pictures are chosen to make precisely the phonological, semantic, or syntactic distinctions at issue. E. Zaidel (1978a, b) found that the right hemisphere, although never doing as well as the left and lacking the left's phonological and syntactic capacities, did attain the vocabulary level of a child around puberty. Both hemispheres did better on nouns than on verbs and better on verbs than on adjectives, and both showed a similar effect from word frequency. The right hemisphere could understand orally presented abstract words and verbs when asked to select pictures depicting actions. With respect to syntax, the right hemisphere did significantly better than chance in understanding almost all types of syntactic constructions but still performed at a rudimentary level compared to the left; the most important limitations were the length of the construction and the word order. The right hemisphere's greatest limitation may be a highly restricted (perhaps as small as three-item) short-term verbal memory. The right hemisphere was consistently poorer at reading than at auditory comprehension and had a smaller visual than auditory vocabulary. It seemed to read by "direct access" rather than by applying grapheme-to-phoneme translation rules. E. Zaidel concluded that Gazzaniga's earlier findings of grossly deficient syntactic competence in the right hemisphere may have stemmed from limitations of the tachistoscopic technique he used. The right hemisphere, E. Zaidel claimed, still possesses a richly endowed lexicon, though it is perhaps connotative, associative, and imaginal rather than precise, denotative, and phonological. It may normally act in a supportive role, identifying input by visual and auditory gestalts and attending to extralinguistic contexts.

Lesion Studies

Lesions in the left hemisphere invariably cause massive disruption of language processes. This well-worn observation in itself tells us little about right hemisphere involvement in such processes, though a lot about the extent of the involvement of the left. Perhaps the most careful and systematic study was that reported by Rasmussen and Milner (1977). They employed the Wada (amytal) test to study the hemispheric representation of speech *production* in 134 patients with left hemisphere lesions incurred before the age of six and in most cases perinatally. They found that an early lesion that does not modify hand preference is unlikely to change the side of speech representation. There was a strong tendency in most subjects, especially dextrals, for the left hemisphere to become and remain dominant for speech, even though it had sustained gross injuries at the time of birth. Childhood injuries to the left hemisphere that occurred after the age of five rarely changed the adult pattern of speech representation, and while such patients generally recovered better than adults would after comparable injury, the recovery was apparently achieved by *intra*hemispheric reorganization (recruitment of neighboring cortex, which normally does not participate in speech) rather than by the development of speech functions in the right hemisphere. Only if the parietal and frontal speech areas were very extensively damaged was there apparently any likelihood of right hemisphere involvement. However, we must emphasize that since these studies employed the Wada test, they were necessarily of short duration and measured *expressive* speech.

Turning to *speech comprehension,* a number of studies have measured the extent and direction of ear and visual field superiorities after left hemisphere trauma (see Searleman, 1977, for review). Unfortunately, for obvious reasons, data are not available on premorbid values, which make the findings less than conclusive. A further problem is that the effects could also be due, in part, to sensory or other decrements, rather than being purely cognitive or linguistic. Generally, dextral aphasics with left hemisphere lesions tend to show (reversed) LVF superiorities or LEAs, which indicate a shift in language lateralization; those with right hemisphere damage show equal or greater REAs or RVF superiorities than normal subjects (Berlin, Cullen, Lowe-Bell, & Berlin, 1974; Oscar-Berman, Zurif, & Blumstein, 1975; Castro-Caldas & Botelho, 1980; Moore & Weidner, 1974; Pettit & Noll, 1979; Pohl, 1979; Schulhoff & Goodglass, 1969). Left temporal lobectomies show gradually improving left ear scores, with no improvement in scores for the right ear (Berlin, Hughes, Lowe-Bell, & Berlin, 1973), indicating that there is a true, if gradually developing, language shift to the right hemisphere after left hemisphere trauma. If such a shift does take place, we may ask why *some* patients with intact right hemispheres and damage to the left are quite unable to process *any* linguistic information. Possibly in these patients areas of the left hemisphere that are still intact may send over inhibitory signals to prevent the right from taking over. This hypothesis would explain why such patients perform at a far lower level verbally than commissurotomy patients tested via the right hemisphere, which, being disconnected, is free from inhibition by the left hemisphere. It also accounts for the finding that if the damaged left hemisphere is removed, there may be an *improvement* in speech (A. Smith, 1969). Again, for theoretical and therapeutic reasons one would like to know under what circumstances a damaged left hemisphere is more of a hindrance than a help.

When we turn to the effects of right hemisphere damage on language, we find that there are usually no very obvious signs of aphasia. Nielsen (1946) reported that some of his left hemisphere patients who had partly recovered became aphasic again after sustaining additional damage to their right hemispheres. This further confirms the point we made immediately above: The right hemisphere can sometimes partly take over from the damaged left. Careful testing by some earlier workers did sometimes uncover subtle deficits among patients who had experienced only right hemisphere damage. Thus Eisenson (1962) found some evidence of slight impairment on vocabulary and sentence completion tests, especially when the tasks involved the use of abstract concepts and abstract words to complete sentences. Critchley (1962) noted some problems in articulation, verbal creativity, finding words, and learning novel linguistic material. Simernitskaya (1974) reported impairment in writing well-known automatic phrases. Marcie, Hécaen, Dubois, and Angelergues (1965) found a tendency towards vocal perseveration, repetition of syllables, disorders of articulation and dysprosody in spontaneous expression, and disorders of syntactic transformation and vocabulary selection, with lengthening of sentences. Hécaen and Marcie (1974) reported perseveration in writing and iteration of strokes and letters. Kimura (1963), B. Milner (1968), E. A. Weinstein (1964), and E. A. Weinstein and Keller (1963) all reported a variety of naming difficulties.

Some very recent studies on the effects of right hemisphere trauma on language processes have confirmed and extended the above findings. Rivers and Love (1980) found minor changes in language performance. Cooper (1981) comments that the speech of patients with right hemisphere damage seems to exhibit prosodic abnormalities that involve fundamental frequency (e.g., speaking in a monotone) more than the temporal control of speech flow, word and pause durations, and so on. However, as he points out and as we ourselves must also conclude, the effects of various subtypes of right hemisphere damage on speech have not been studied nearly as systematically as has the speech of aphasics.

Effects of Hemispherectomies:
Evidence for Right Hemisphere Language

The term *hemispherectomy* is very often a misnomer. The more appropriate one is probably *hemidecortication,* since parts of the thalamus and the basal ganglia are normally left intact (Nebes, 1978; Searleman, 1977), though some subcortical tissue may be removed. The operation is performed either to remove a large and invasive tumor or to help alleviate the crippling effects of infantile hemiplegia or epileptic seizures, the results of extensive unilateral damage at birth. Hemispherectomy for tumor in adults, and especially removal of the left hemisphere, is rare, and extensive neuropsychological testing of such patients is even rarer. Control or baseline testing prior to morbidity in such cases is of course nonexistent. These individuals, however, are very important, as with them there is no doubt about which hemisphere is performing the task, nor can one hemisphere be suppressing, inhibiting, or facilitating abilities present in the other, a possibility with brain-damaged patients. One can also follow recovery processes in a relatively uncontaminated form. Ideally, one would seek patients with a short-onset, rapidly growing tumor and be able to assess (lateralized) language performance both before and after surgery. These conditions have not yet been met.

Just as with the studies of right hemisphere lesions, in the few cases of right hemispherectomy that have been studied, no obvious aphasia or gross deficit in language abilities, as measured on standardized tests, has been reported. Vocabulary is generally normal, though Dennis (1980a) does claim there may be some alterations in syntactic comprehension after right hemidecortication.

Left hemispherectomy in adults. Very few cases of left hemispherectomy in adults have been reported, as the effects are very debilitating, and postoperative survival times have generally been short (Hécaen, 1978; Nebes, 1978; Searleman, 1977). A patient studied by A. Smith (1966) showed markedly restricted language behavior, but later demonstrated a significant return of certain functions. He could produce short, well-constructed sentences and showed fair levels of comprehension but poor writing ability. Similar recovery effects were reported by Burklund and Smith (1977) and Rossing (1975, cited by Hécaen, 1978). These and other cases are also reviewed by Searleman (1977).

Generally, despite wide differences in intelligence, age of onset of illness, sex, associated physiological and psychological disorders, degree of damage to the remaining hemisphere, and methods of testing, all patients were found to be severely impaired in their ability to produce voluntary propositional speech, though their comprehension remained comparatively intact, just as in the sodium amytal studies. Patients were generally able to utter expletives and phrase automatisms, often they remained able to sing (Gott, 1973; A. Smith, 1966; A. Smith & Burklund, 1966). Some, after a recovery period, could even produce some very limited propositional speech (Gott, 1973; A. Smith, 1966; A. Smith & Burklund, 1966; E. Zaidel, 1973; Zangwill, 1967), but they usually showed very little improvement in communication. A similar picture emerges when writing is examined; in a case not involving hemispherectomy but rather left occipital lobectomy, Hécaen, Ajuriaguerra, and David (1952, cited in Hécaen, 1978) found that initial total alexia was followed by a very marked recovery after six weeks. E. Zaidel (1973), in a thorough investigation of a left hemispherectomy patient, found no deficit in phonemic discrimination. The patient was adept at picking out pictures of objects and actions named by the examiner and in understanding prepositions of place (except, interestingly, for left and right) and various syntactic constructions, including the passive. The patient's ability, however, rapidly deteriorated when she was given long sentences, several elements to be related within a sentence, or complex syntax. Much of her difficulty may have stemmed from a poor verbal short-term memory. Finally, she was almost completely alexic.

Left hemispherectomy performed in infancy. A left hemispherectomy performed in infancy never seems to lead to permanent dysphasia if performed *before* language is acquired. Recovery of *nearly* all language functions by the right hemisphere is often dramatic (Searleman, 1977). Thus, people have long viewed the two hemispheres as equipotential (for language development) at birth (Lenneberg, 1967; Zangwill, 1964; but see Chapter Twelve). Only recently have subtle deficiencies begun to emerge, mainly of abstract linguistic functioning in language development. These findings have been reported in a series of studies on infantile hemispherectomies tested as adults or near-adults, by Dennis and her colleagues (Dennis & Kohn, 1975; Dennis & Whitaker, 1976; Dennis, 1980a, b). She found that syntactic competence was generally inferior in the isolated right hemisphere compared to the left. The right half-brain was deficient in coping with syntactic diversity, detecting and correcting errors of surface syntactic structure, repeating stylistically permuted sentences, producing tag questions to match the grammatical features of a heard statement, determining sentence implication, and performing judgments of word interrelationships in sentences. The left hemidecorticates in her study (1980b) also had considerable difficulty with rhyming cues and appeared to have limited access to a phonological retrieval system for common words. Finally, she found that semantic space is both more lawful and tightly organized in the right hemidecorticate. She concludes that language development in an isolated right hemisphere, even under seizure-free conditions, results in incomplete language acquisition.

In opposition to this position is a study by A. Smith and Sugar (1975), who examined the language development of a patient twenty-one years after left hemispherectomy for seizures at age five and a half. He developed superior language ability (Verbal IQ of 126), though at the expense of an (average) Performance IQ of 102. Two points should be made: first, in this instance the right hemisphere was able to subserve *superior* language skills (though it is just possible that the tests were not sensitive to hidden phonological and syntactic deficiencies); second, the language "invasion" was apparently at the expense of the right hemisphere's *nonverbal* capacities. We shall meet this situation again in the context of female verbal superiority and nonverbal inferiority and of normal verbal and deficient visuospatial functioning in congenital acallosal cases.

Finally, in a recent study on infantile hemidecorticates tested as adults, Dennis, Lovett, and Wiegel-Crump (1981) found that while right hemidecorticates were superior to left hemidecorticates on morphophonemic processing, they were inferior on logographic processing, neatly demonstrating the complementary role of the two hemispheres in the phonological and ideographic aspects of speech and writing.

Deep Dyslexia and Right Hemisphere Reading

One dispute currently engaging psycholinguists is whether words are recognized as wholes, in terms of the gross features of the word itself, or in terms of the constituent letters (for reviews, see Henderson & Chard, 1980; Massaro, 1975). Another dispute, also occurring largely apart from laterality research, is whether words are "directly" recognized or must first undergo letter-to-sound (grapheme-to-phoneme) conversion, by rule, before their meaning can be "accessed" in the "internal lexicon" (see, e.g., Coltheart, 1980b). The first approach will obviously not work for novel nonwords, such as *gope,* that do not have existing "lexical entries." The second will not work well for irregularly spelled or pronounced words like *yacht, bread,* or *sword* that do not conform to conventional grapheme-to-phoneme rules. How these psycholinguistic disputes are ultimately resolved will have important implications for neuropsychological theories of reading disorders.

In the meantime, amidst the historical welter of typologies that have been proposed for the different kinds of alexia or reading difficulty (see Chapter Four), one particular syndrome is of special interest in the study of right-hemisphere language processes. This syndrome has only recently been described in any detail, though Hughlings Jackson is said in 1878 to have reported a patient in whom left hemisphere damage in adulthood had produced a reading disorder (Coltheart, 1979). This patient, when asked, for example, to read aloud the printed word *table* had responded with *chair.* A semantic error of this type is known as a paralexic error; although the response is visually and phonologically "wrong," it is *semantically* related to the stimulus. The patient must have understood at least to some extent the meaning of the word he was shown. Such paralexic errors typify the syndrome known as deep dyslexia. The ability of such patients to read a single printed word aloud depends on the part of speech the word represents. They read nouns best, followed by adjectives, then verbs; function words (articles, prepositions, conjunctions, etc.) are read least well, despite their great frequency in English. Thus a patient who could not read *be* could do so when an extra *e* was added *(bee).* A French patient could not read the second *car* in the printed sentence *Le car ralentit car le moteur chauffe* ("The bus slows because the motor overheats") (Andreewsky, Deloche, & Kossanyi, 1980). The first *car,* meaning "vehicle," is a noun and posed no difficulty; the second, meaning "because," is a conjunction that occurs with equal frequency, but it could not be read. Shown the word *stone,* an English-speaking patient may respond "rock." Coltheart (1979) reports the response to *Holland* as being "It's a country . . . not Europe . . . no . . . not Germany . . . it's small . . . it was captured . . . Belgium . . . that's it, Belgium" (p. 369). In addition to grammatical function words, abstract words (e.g., *origin, custom, charm,* no matter how common) are read far less well than concrete words (e.g., *soldier, custard, face*). Typically, comprehension (in general terms) is preserved, but the patient cannot pronounce or name words. The words can be copied, and, when given equal numbers of words and nonword letter strings like *tife,* the patient is usually able to decide correctly which are words and which are nonwords. Perhaps the greatest impairment is in the patient's ability to convert letters to sounds—that is, to employ grapheme-to-phoneme correspondence rules, the second of the two possible routes used to recognize words. The patient cannot pronounce aloud even the simplest of pronounceable nonsense words, such as *rud* or *glem.* He cannot judge that *fail* and *sale* rhyme, but, relying on the visual similarity, decides that *sew* and *few* do, when of course they do not. Nor can he say whether pseudohomophones (e.g., *brane, gote, caip, hurd*—words that sound like but do not look like real words) do in fact sound like real words. Yet, although normal subjects are slightly slower to reject these pseudohomophones as nonwords as compared with "true" nonwords, such as *frane, gofe, caib, lurd,* presumably being misled to some extent by the phonology of the pseudohomophones, deep dyslexics can reject both categories with equal facility.

The fact that deep dyslexics make paralexic errors, coming up with words of related meaning, suggests that they do in fact know a lot about what they are inspecting. (They even do something similar with the class of words they find hardest to read, the function words: They may read *to* as *which, or* as *with,* etc.) They know a lot about the word's meaning and/or usage, but less about its sound or phonology. Their paralexic errors are very similar to normal subjects' free associations, suggesting an inability to suppress competing semantic errors. This failure can be helped by, for example, putting the difficult item into a carrier phrase to constrain the context. Thus, mistakes like reading *May* as "June," *green* as "red," or *holly* as "ivy" occur far less often if written in the form Miss May, or Mr. Green. Syntactic context also helps with function words; they can be incorporated into common redundant phrases, such as *from heaven* or *off guard.* Interestingly, deep dyslexics seem to employ cross-cueing strategies of the sort described earlier with commissurotomized patients (Chapter Five), suggesting the involvement of right hemisphere strategies. If the name of a month, day, or letter is given, they may be unable to name it correctly, instead giving the name of *another* month, day, or letter, unless they are allowed serially to name aloud the days, months, or alphabet. They then stop and exclaim "That's right" when they encounter the correct one.

To explain these findings, Coltheart (1979, 1980a, b) proposes that phonological access and the left hemisphere's normal reading mechanisms are entirely inactivated. The right hemisphere accesses the meaning, in broad general terms, from the printed word where this is possible or easy (e.g., for nouns, high-frequency concrete words) and communicates the result in semantic terms to the (vocal) left hemisphere for naming. Since orthographic and phonological information is missing (to judge by the nature of the errors made by the patient), only semantic information is available to the left hemisphere, which then retrieves the word's (or a semantically closely related word's) pronunciation for the vocal response. Indeed the semantic information available to the left will tend to be insufficient to distinguish between synonyms or even between closely related but distinct words (e.g., *canary* and *parrot*). Since abstract words and function words possess a far poorer network of semantic associations, often very little is available to the left hemisphere except, perhaps, just the idea that a function word (which after all merely serves to indicate how to assemble the meaning of individual content words) or an abstract word had been presented. Indeed, one can even speculate whether, at least in reading, the left hemisphere (for reasons we discuss in Chapter Nine) mediates the orthographic, phonological, and syntactic aspects, while the right hemisphere is normally the actual seat of our semantic associative network.

Most of us probably employ both modes of lexical access, the direct route (which works particularly well with our irregular English phonology) and the phonological-recoding route, which is necessary whenever we encounter novel or unfamiliar items and, maybe, abstract and function words. We probably also need this second route to check that we have accessed the *exact* rather than a synonymous or a related meaning and to retain a phonological trace long enough to extract the sense from a whole string of words in a phrase or sentence. Some of the effects reported with deep dyslexics are also apparent, under special conditions, with normal subjects. Marcel and Patterson (1978) found that if briefly flashed words were backward masked and followed by another word of associated or unrelated meaning, even though subjects were quite unaware of the existence of the first word, its associated meaning would facilitate the report of the second word. They also reported semantic paralexias in normal people with backward masking. J. L. Bradshaw (1974) found that laterally presented and unreported words nevertheless biased the perceived meaning of a centrally presented homograph (a word with two or more possible meanings, such as *bank* or *box*). D. E. Meyer and Schvaneveldt (1971) reported that subjects were faster at processing a word when it was immediately preceded by a word of related meaning than when it was preceded by an unrelated word.

Finally, we should make two other observations. First, deep dyslexics will all have originally learned to read with an intact phonological system, which is now inactivated. Congenitally deaf children *can* learn to read without a phonological system (being deaf); one should perhaps look at these people for evidence of unusual types of error. Second, childhood developmental dyslexia (see Chapter Thirteen) may possibly also stem from lack of a phonological route. It is said that in Chinese, where a largely ideographic script makes phonology relatively unimportant, dyslexia is uncommon (see Chapter Fourteen). There is evidence, moreover, that Western dyslexic children can be taught to read a form of Chinese (Rozin, Poritsky, & Sotsky, 1971).

Japanese *Kana* and *Kanji*

The Japanese orthography is unique in that it uses in combination two types of nonalphabetical symbols, *kana* (phonetic symbols for syllables) and *kanji* (essentially nonphonetic, logographic, or ideographic symbols representing lexical morphemes) (Sasanuma, 1980). *Kanji* characters are usually more complex in configuration than *kana* and are usually employed to represent the base form of nouns, verbs, and adjectives, though these words can always be represented phonetically in *kana* also. All grammatical morphemes, such as the inflectional endings of verbs and adjectives and various kinds of function words, are written only in *kana.* Thus *kanji* characters represent the semantic building blocks in the sentence and stand out as bold figures against the background of *kana* symbols. There are two sets of *kana, hiragana* (cursive *kana*) and *katakana* (square *kana*), roughly equivalent to our lower and uppercase script. The *kana* characters each have a one-to-one correspondence with a syllable; most *kanji* characters have several alternative readings, depending on semantic or morphological context (Sasanuma, 1980).

As a result of the dual nature of this orthography, various types of dissociation may be seen in normal and brain-damaged subjects. With normal subjects, the left hemisphere (RVF) is typically better than the right (LVF) at dealing with *kana*, while the right hemisphere is better than the left at dealing with *kanji* (Hatta, 1977b, 1978a; Sasanuma, Itoh, Mori, & Kobayashi, 1977). Aphasic patients (presumably with left hemisphere damage), many of whom exhibit a selective impairment of *kana* processing, often have a relatively well-preserved or almost intact ability to process *kanji*. On the other hand, there are some rare patients who show a selective impairment of *kanji* processing with a remarkable preservation of *kana* processing (see Sasanuma, 1980, for review). Moreover, it would appear from error analyses that the strategies used for decoding the two types of symbols are different: a strategy of direct visual access to meaning for *kanji* and an indirect or phonological (grapheme-to-phoneme conversion) strategy for *kana*. Unfortunately, there is as yet no reported evidence of a selective impairment of *kanji* processing consequent on right hemisphere lesions alone. This may be because few Japanese clinical studies to date have looked separately at the two types of script in the context of the two kinds of lesions and because right hemisphere lesions (which are likely to damage *kanji* processing) tend to be less socially disrupting (in terms of expressive speech) and so are less likely to receive clinical attention.

Normal Western Subjects: Different Classes of Verbal Material and the Right Hemisphere

In dichotic listening experiments, a large REA is typically found for perceiving initial stop consonants, an intermediate REA for liquids, semivowels, and fricatives, and little or no ear differences for steady-state vowels (Shankweiler & Studdert-Kennedy, 1967; Studdert-Kennedy & Shankweiler, 1970; Haggard, 1971; Darwin, 1971; J. E. Cutting, 1974; Klisz, 1980). Other linguistic features of speech, such as intonation contour and pitch processing, are often better handled by the right hemisphere (Curry, 1968; Schulhoff & Goodglass, 1969; Zurif & Mendelsohn, 1972; Zurif, 1974; Van Lancker, 1975).

In the visual modality, a LVF superiority is typically reported when subjects judge pairs of letters in terms of their physical characteristics (i.e., make physical identity matches such as *AA* or *cc*) rather than in terms of what they stand for or their nominal identity (e.g., *Aa, Bb*), in which case the normal RVF superiority appears (Geffen, Bradshaw, & Nettleton, 1972). Similar findings were reported by Wilkins and Stewart (1974) in terms of the time course needed to generate phonological codes (the longer the interval between successive members of a pair of letters, the more likely that the phonologically based RVF (left hemisphere) superiority will appear). A LVF (right hemisphere) superiority is more likely to appear when subjects process letters in florid or unusual scripts (Bryden & Allard, 1976). J. L. Bradshaw and Mapp (1982) found that words written in a cursive script were associated with weak or nonsignificant RVF superiorities compared with those in normal upper or lower case. Presumably a visuospatial preprocessing component from the right hemisphere was required for cursive script. Similar effects occurred where judgments could be based on word shape, in terms of changes in the patterns of ascenders and descenders. Other studies that have demonstrated that the right hemisphere is involved in the initial processing of words, especially when conditions are difficult or unfamiliar or exposure durations are very brief, include those of Pirozzolo and Rayner (1977), G. J. Bradshaw and Hicks (1977), J. L. Bradshaw and Gates (1978). Likewise Jonides (1979) found a LVF superiority in a difficult letter detection task and the normal RVF superiority for an easy task. We have discussed similar findings (see, e.g., Goldberg & Costa, 1981) of a switch from a LVF superiority for difficult, unfamiliar material to a RVF superiority with familiar, easy material in Chapter Seven. Suffice to say, the right hemisphere may also take over the processing of simple verbal materials when the left is occupied or otherwise engaged with another primary task (Geffen et al., 1973).

It is often argued that although clinical and sodium amytal (Wada) tests demonstrate that perhaps 95 percent or more of dextrals have speech apparently located in the left hemisphere, tachistoscopic and dichotic studies show a much lower percentage (maybe around 75 percent). Some have claimed that this demonstrates either that such studies do not directly measure language lateralization or that the techniques are inherently inaccurate. However, it must be remembered that dichotic and tachistoscopic tasks normally measure only speech comprehension, not production; where vocal naming latencies to laterally presented words were measured, J. L. Bradshaw and Gates (1978) found RVF superiorities were larger than for other kinds of comprehensional task. Clinical tests, on the other hand, typically measure the ability to produce speech. In the clinic, dysphasia is of course far easier to quantify than comprehensional deficits, which can only be inferred. This being so, if speech production is indeed more strongly lateralized than speech perception, then there may in fact not be a discrepancy between clinical and normal studies; rather, each is tapping different aspects of speech.

We have seen that, for patients with deep dyslexia, abstract words are more difficult to read than concrete words. According to Richardson (1975, 1976) and Marcel and Patterson (1978) while concreteness and imageability are very highly correlated, imageability may be the more important or fundamental dimension. Various apparently successful attempts have been made to determine whether normal subjects show a greater left–right asymmetry for abstract or nonimageable nouns than for concrete or imageable ones (Day, 1977, 1979; H. D. Ellis & Shepherd,

1974; Hines, 1976, 1977; Marcel & Patterson, 1978). Others however have been unsuccessful (J. L. Bradshaw & Gates, 1978, Experiment 3; J. L. Bradshaw, Nettleton, & Taylor, 1981a; Orenstein & Meighan, 1976; Saffran, Bogyo, Schwartz, & Marin, 1980; Schmuller & Goodman, 1979). Several points should be remembered. Successful replications are always more likely to get published than unsuccessful ones. Day used an unnatural, unfamiliar, difficult format of vertical presentation for his words to avoid the possibility of left-to-right scanning contaminating the data (an unnecessary precaution; see J. L. Bradshaw, Nettleton, & Taylor, 1981b). Patterson (1979) claims that acquired dyslexics—whose apparent loss of ability to process low-frequency, abstract, nonimageable, or function words without the loss of ability to cope with high-frequency, concrete, or imageable words started the whole controversy—*can* successfully perform lexical decisions on the first class of words. Their problem is *not* one of saying if they *are* words or even of necessarily extracting *meaning*, but one of actually *naming*. If this is true, we should not expect to find the two types of word stimuli generating different laterality effects with lexical decisions. While differences might therefore be found with vocal naming, J. L. Bradshaw and Gates (1978, Experiment 3) were unable even then to demonstrate them. Moreover, Marcel and Patterson (1978) claim that masking is required to demonstrate the effect with normal subjects. We are therefore left with a problem. There is good clinical evidence for a right hemisphere contribution to the processing of high-frequency, concrete material; some grounds for suspecting that it may not be easily demonstrated with normal subjects (perhaps backward masking helps); and some apparently successful and some quite unsuccessful demonstrations of this effect with normal subjects. Further research is obviously warranted, with attention given perhaps to such methodological factors as masking conditions, unilateral or bilateral presentations, horizontal or vertical format, speed or accuracy measure, discriminative (word–nonword) or go–no-go responding, bimanual or unimanual responding, and vocal-identificatory or manual-discriminatory responding. This list is not exhaustive, but it can perhaps be tentatively concluded that with normal subjects the effect is more likely to appear under conditions of perceptual load or difficulty.

Finally, it is interesting to note that Warrington (1981) has described for the first time a form of acquired dyslexia that is *complementary* to loss of the ability to read abstract, nonimageable words. She found that her (single) patient was specifically unable to read *concrete* words, though the patient had a left hemisphere lesion and a phonological impairment otherwise similar to that of deep dyslexics. She argues that this finding goes against the idea of a concrete word processor in the right hemisphere, and that the phenomena of deep dyslexia in general and her own case in particular are just examples of category specificity in the organization of the semantic systems subserving reading. This would of course account for the frequently reported inabilities to obtain reduced RVF superiorities with normal subjects for concrete, imageable words.

Does the Right Hemisphere Contribute
to Arithmetic Processes, Bilingualism, Stuttering,
and Language Processes in the Congenitally Deaf?

Arithmetic and the right hemisphere. There are repeated suggestions in both the clinical and the normal literature that there might be something unusual about numbers and arithmetic processing, with the right hemisphere perhaps making a contribution. Bogen (1979) notes that commissurotomy patients tend to have difficulty in performing arithmetic problems with pencil and paper and implies that this could stem from a separation of the right hand from the right hemisphere, where aspects of the spatial layout necessary for such problems are elaborated. Teng and Sperry (1973) and E. Zaidel (1976), also working with commissurotomy patients, also conclude that there is some, if slight, evidence for a right hemisphere involvement in dealing with numerals. Saffran et al. (1980) also wonder if there is an affinity between the right hemisphere and number processing. In the clinical field, Levin (1979) divides the acalculias (acquired disorder of calculation) into three categories. In two (acalculia secondary to alexia, and pure anarithmetria) he claims the left hemisphere is largely involved, and only in the third (spatial acalculia) is there a right hemisphere component. In this syndrome numbers are improperly arranged and aligned in columns during the initial stages of computation. Studies with normal subjects, employing lateralized, tachistoscopically presented numerical stimuli for simple computation, difference judgments, and so on tend to invoke right hemisphere superiorities if not actual mechanisms (Dimond & Beaumont, 1972c; Qureshi & Dimond, 1979; Katz, 1980). Several electroencephalographic studies, however, indicate a predominantly left hemisphere involvement during calculation: for example, Butler and Glass (1974a), using the contingent negative variation; and Butler and Glass (1974b), Dumas and Morgan (1975), and Nava, Butler, and Glass (1975), measuring the amount of alpha suppression. Of course, these effects may have reflected the verbal and reading component. In summary, a contribution from the right hemisphere during calculation seems likely.

Bilingualism. Is there any evidence that polyglots have different localization of language functions for the languages they acquired later? Two studies with normals suggest the possibility of some degree of right hemisphere involvement with a second language. Silverberg, Bentin, Gaziel, Obler, and Albert (1979) found evidence of a LVF (right hemisphere) superiority in Hebrew-speaking children acquiring reading skills of their new language (English); as the child became more experienced, this then gave way to the normal RVF superiority. This phenomenon could, of course, simply reflect right hemisphere preprocessing of novel, unfamiliar characters (cf. Bryden & Allard, 1976). Walters and Zatorre (1978), working with adult English-Spanish bilinguals, found a RVF superiority for word identification in either language, though with a possible trend towards more bilateralization.

Others, however, from the clinical viewpoint, claim that all languages are normally equally represented in the language-dominant hemisphere. Thus G. A. Ojemann and Whitaker (1978b), reporting on brain stimulation studies on bilinguals, found that the pattern of organization of the two languages was largely similar, though *within* a given area there was sometimes a tendency for those sites concerned with a given language to cluster together. As they observe, this could be a function of processing strategies associated with that language, which in turn could depend on familiarity with it, whether it was used largely for comprehension and listening or for production, whether or not the subject was able to read and write it, and so on. They also noted a tendency for a subject's second language to be represented in a rather wider area of cortex than the primary language, suggesting that during acquisition of a language a larger number of neurons may be involved, with a reduction as proficiency increases. Such an account could also explain an initial, temporary, right hemisphere involvement during the early stages of acquisition of a second language, when in any case *comprehensional* processes (which are probably more bilaterally represented than *expressive*) receive more emphasis.

A number of factors are generally recognized as contributing to how and where a language is organized in the brain. These include such questions as the degree of proficiency in a given language (for expressive speech, understanding, reading, and writing), the age of acquisition (before or after any critical periods, see Chapter Twelve), whether the second language was acquired "naturally" or by instruction, whether it was acquired together with or after the other, and so on (Seliger, 1978). According to Whitaker (1978) such factors, coupled with amnesia studies showing that memories are apparently time-tagged in some way, leading to selective amnesias for certain periods in life, can account for such curiosities as an aphasic first recovering such an unlikely language as Classical Greek—perhaps because the patient's experience with it was largely or exclusively *visual.* Similar conclusions are reached by Vaid and Genesee (1980) in their comprehensive review on the neuropsychology of bilingualism. They argue that a right hemisphere involvement will be more likely the later a second language is learned and the more informal the exposure to it; possibly right hemisphere involvement is also more likely in the earlier stages of acquisition. The more similar the conditions of first and second language acquisition, the greater the likelihood that bilinguals will show comparable patterns of hemispheric involvement in processing their two languages.

In summary, we believe with Caramazza and Broner (1979), and Gordon (1980c), that the second language in bilinguals (and third or later language in polyglots) is represented in the brain in much the same way as the first, unless there were any abnormalities in the way the language was acquired or used. Only then, and only under abnormal circumstances at that, would there be any reason to suppose there would be a significant involvement of the right hemisphere.

Congenital deafness. A number of studies suggest reduced asymmetries for written letters and words in the congenitally deaf (e.g., McKeever, Hoemann, Florian, & Van Deventer, 1976; Manning, Goble, Markman, & La Breche, 1977;

Poizner & Lane, 1979; Scholes & Fischler, 1979). Other studies have found a LVF (right hemisphere) superiority when such people process the manual signs used by the deaf (e.g., McKeever et al., 1976; Poizner & Lane, 1979; Ross, Pergament, & Anisfield, 1979). As Cutting (1980) points out, such signs have a complex nature and origin and in many cases are quite different from and in no way parasitic upon the spoken languages around them. They all have a considerable spatial component and employ an essentially simultaneous rather than a sequential (as in speech) mode of display. This factor could possibly account for the apparent right hemisphere involvement in signing.

In another carefully controlled study, however, Virostek and Cutting (1979) found that the "true" congenital deaf (i.e., those born of deaf parents, unlike those employed in the other studies) give RVF superiorities for handshapes that are designated alphabetical and a LVF superiority for *illegal* signs, *hearing* signers giving a LVF superiority for *both* types of sign. The right hemisphere spatial contribution apparently does not extend to *alphabetic* signs in the truly congenitally deaf. They conclude that auditory experience is unnecessary for the normal development of left hemisphere language specialization, that lateral specialization for language is generally similar for deaf native signers and nondeaf native speakers of oral language, and that other studies are to be criticized for poor control of stimuli, stimulus counterbalancing, and choice of subjects. (To these criticisms Poizner and Lane, 1979, add some more, viz., lack of control over use of manual handshapes versus American Sign Language signs, use of static rather than "natural" moving signs, legal and illegal signs, subject's experience with signing, etc.) Virostek and Cutting's conclusion (that the deaf are left lateralized for language) is also compatible with the findings of Sarno, Swisher, and Sarno (1969; a congenitally deaf man experienced sign language dysphasia after left hemisphere lesions), and of Poizner, Battison, and Lane (1979). In this latter study, both the congenitally deaf and the hearing gave a RVF superiority to written words; the deaf gave a LVF superiority to static signs and no field differences to moving signs, presumably because of left hemisphere involvement in movement sequencing.

Signs, of course, are not normally encountered in a static format, when the right hemisphere spatial component may dominate. Similar findings (a left-hand or right hemisphere superiority) are found when the congenitally blind read Braille (Harris, 1980b). Again, one must appeal to the spatial preprocessing element. In the case of the deaf, we must ask whether the reduced left hemisphere superiority for written letters and words, which appears in some studies but not others, is a real phenomenon. Until this question is answered, we must conclude that the issue of possibly reduced lateralization in the congenitally deaf for *visually* displayed verbal material (alphabetic letters or signs), for whatever reason (the spatial component, or visual preprocessing), is as yet unresolved.

Stuttering. There are likely to be a number of different causative factors involved in stuttering, just as there are in many other clinical syndromes. However, as Corballis (1981) points out, it was once widely believed that interhemispheric conflict, due to poorly established cerebral dominance, might be one such causative factor. Despite its subsequently falling into disrepute, this factor has recently been revived. Thus R. K. Jones (1966) described a small group of stutterers who were found by the Wada test (which was applied for quite unrelated reasons) to have bilateral speech representation. Following unilateral surgery, they were apparently cured of stuttering and were found to have unilateral control of speech in the intact hemisphere. Corballis cites a number of similar results that have been reported since then, together with other evidence that stutterers as a group may have reduced or reversed asymmetry on various measures of lateralization. Finally Wood, Stump, McKeehan, Sheldon, and Proctor (1980) found that there was greater simultaneous activity (using regional blood flow measures) in Broca's area of the right hemisphere and Wernicke's area of the left while the patient was stuttering, but when the patients were given haloperidol to prevent their stuttering, the greater activity in the frontal regions now also occurred in the left hemisphere. However, a very recent study (Pinsky & McAdam, 1980) measuring laterality effects both by means of the EEG and the REA in dichotic listening found that stutterers were no less lateralized than nonstutterers. This issue is not yet fully resolved, but we shall see in Chapter Thirteen that in the case of developmental dyslexia, there is nowadays very little evidence for the proposition of a reduction in cerebral asymmetry.

Summary and Conclusions

Left hemisphere dominance for language is most pronounced with dextrals, males, adults, and the expressive (rather than comprehensional) aspects of speech. Nevertheless, the right hemisphere plays a not-inconsiderable role in mediating language-related behavior, though there are interpretational problems whether clinical, normal, or commissurotomy subjects are studied.

The Wada (amytal) test tells us more about the lateralization of speech production than speech comprehension, which has been little studied under Wada testing. The anaesthetic effect, however, is short-lived and can tell us little about the likely chronic effects of such unilateral suppression. Because the test is also disturbing to the patient and somewhat hazardous, it can be employed only in situations where preexisting neurological anomalies are likely. It does, however, demonstrate that the right hemisphere can become a source of aphasic speech after left hemisphere injury.

With commissurotomy patients there is always the possibility that massive cerebral reorganization has occurred as a consequence of preexisting epilepsy of long standing. The effects of surgical trauma and the need for artificial (e.g., tachistoscopic) procedures can also cloud the picture. Again these studies give little evidence of expressive ability in the isolated right hemisphere, though appropriate nonverbal testing procedures, particularly the more recent ones, demonstrate the hemisphere's considerable powers of comprehension, both visual and aural, for all grammatical classes of word. Earlier commissurotomy studies may have employed inappropriate testing procedures. There is some evidence that writing is initiated by the right hemisphere, particularly with young adults, though possibly, as with articulatory expression, it may normally be subject to the inhibitory influences of the left hemisphere. The right hemisphere is particularly deficient in syntactic and phonological processing, for example, in recognizing rhymes. Having a possibly very restricted verbal short-term memory, it nevertheless possesses an extensive lexicon, perhaps equivalent to that of a child at puberty. In recent commissurotomy studies reading appears to involve direct access rather than phonological coding. Thus the right hemisphere may act in an essentially supportive role to the left with respect to language.

Interpretations of lesion studies are subject to problems of inhibitory and possibly even facilitatory influences at an interhemispheric level and to problems of plastic reorganization and compensatory functioning both within and between hemispheres, especially with young individuals, although early lesions that do not modify hand preferences do not seem to change the side of language mediation. The left hemisphere tends to become and remain dominant for speech production, despite gross damage in early years, suggesting that reorganization may take place at a largely *intra*hemispheric level. The greatest likelihood of an *inter*hemispheric shift is with respect to speech comprehension. Right hemisphere damage has few obvious effects on language functions, though careful testing (which has been little employed in this context) may reveal subtle deficits, for example, in vocabulary, verbal creativity and fluency, word finding, use of automatic phrases, articulation, intonation, and prosody in spontaneous expression.

The effects of hemispherectomies (which, strictly speaking, are merely extensive decortications) depend on when the operation was performed (in infancy or adulthood) and when the individual is tested. Little or no premorbid control data is normally available, which is unfortunate since hemispherectomy studies are theoretically the easiest to interpret, given the absence of interhemispheric facilitatory or inhibitory influences. Right hemispherectomy may possibly lead to certain subtle deficits in syntactic comprehension. Left hemispherectomy is rarely performed with adults; although there are very occasional accounts of partial recovery, left hemispherectomy usually results in gross impairments of propositional speech and verbal short-term memory, with relatively unimpaired comprehension and, often, preservation of the capacity to sing. When left hemispherectomies are performed in infancy, the right hemisphere generally assumes control of most language functions, though careful testing in adulthood reveals the limits of such equipotentiality: There often appear to be subtle deficiencies for abstract linguistic functioning, syntax, and phonology, but exceptions do occur.

There are two routes to word comprehension in reading: the direct access route, which of course cannot function for nonwords or novel words, and a phonological route, which is of little help with words of irregular spelling or pronunciation. Phonological access and the left hemisphere's normal reading mechanisms may be inactivated in the syndrome of deep dyslexia. Individuals suffering from this syndrome appear to retain the ability to comprehend semantic aspects, though perhaps not enough to distinguish between synonyms and to inhibit the production of typically paralexic errors. They are best at reading high-frequency, concrete, imageable nouns and worst at reading grammatical function words, which have no specific referent and play a largely syntactic role. Normal subjects show some of these effects under conditions of backward masking—a preservation of meaning with loss of orthographic and phonological information. However, attempts to demonstrate a greater RVF (left hemisphere) superiority for low-frequency, abstract, or nonimageable words have not always been successful. Findings may depend on how stimuli are presented (with or without masking) and what the subject is required to do (name the items or perform lexical or semantic decisions on them).

While normal subjects do show evidence of a double dissociation in processing Japanese *kana* and *kanji,* with *kana* associated with a RVF superiority and *kanji* with LVF superiority, there is as yet no strong evidence in the clinical field of right hemisphere lesions selectively affecting the recognition of *kanji* characters. Normal subjects show a large REA for stop consonants under dichotic listening and often a LEA for unencoded, steady-state vowels. They show a LVF for preprocessing difficult, unfamiliar, or degraded letters or words and for judgments based on the physical aspects of verbal stimuli.

There is some evidence of a right hemisphere contribution to the mediation of arithmetic processes and possibly also in the second or later language of bilinguals or polyglots. The latter claim, however, could be a consequence of the comparative unfamiliarity of a nonpreferred language, whose written words demand a preprocessing contribution from the right hemisphere. Differences may also be tied to when and how the languages were acquired and the extent to which visual or phonological aspects predominate. The current view is that normally all languages are equally represented and similarly organized in the dominant hemisphere.

There is some evidence in the congenitally deaf of reduced asymmetries for written letters and words and a LVF superiority in processing manual signs, though the latter could be due to the considerable spatial component involved in signing, similar to the left-hand superiority in reading Braille. Other studies, however, have found a normal RVF superiority for correctly formed alphabetical signs and a LVF superiority only for the attempted processing of illegal ones. Auditory experience is probably unnecessary for the normal development of language specialization in the left hemisphere. Lateral specialization, moreover, is probably generally similar for both the hearing and the congenitally deaf; any apparent differences between these two groups seem to be due to poor experimental controls.

There is a long tradition, recently revived, that stuttering may in some cases stem from interhemispheric conflict and poorly established cerebral dominance, stutterers as a group having reduced or reversed asymmetries. Not all agree, and the issue is as yet unresolved.

We can conclude that the right hemisphere possesses very considerable powers of comprehension—more at the level of semantics and connotative meaning, less at the syntactic or phonological level—with extremely restricted expressive competence. The latent linguistic powers of the right hemisphere are likely to be expressed most clearly when misadventure befalls the left hemisphere early in life, with females and nondextrals, and with nonphonological and nonarticulatory materials and situations.

FURTHER READING

COLTHEART, M., PATTERSON, K., & MARSHALL, J. C. (Eds.). *Deep dyslexia*. London: Routledge & Kegan Paul, 1980.

NEBES, R. D. Direct examination of cognitive function in the right and left hemispheres. In M. Kinsbourne (Ed.), *Asymmetrical function of the brain*. Cambridge: Cambridge University Press, 1978.

SEARLEMAN, A. A review of right hemisphere linguistic capabilities. *Psychological Bulletin*, 1977, *84*, 503–528.

ZAIDEL, E. Auditory language comprehension in the right hemisphere following cerebral commissurotomy and hemispherectomy: A comparison with child language and aphasia. In A. Caramazza & E. B. Zurif (Eds.), *Language acquisition and language breakdown: Parallels and divergencies*. Baltimore: John Hopkins University Press, 1978.

CHAPTER NINE
The Analytic–Holistic Processing Distinction and Left Hemisphere Segmental Processing

We have treated human cerebral asymmetry so far largely in terms of a verbal–nonverbal dichotomy, which is perhaps more marked at the motor or expressive level; we have hinted at the possibility of a more fundamental distinction, such as an analytic–holistic processing dichotomy, but until now have not considered this possibility in any depth. Before doing so we shall review the evidence for the traditional verbal–nonverbal distinction.

The Verbal-Nonverbal Dichotomy

Apart from the laterality research with normal subjects and the long tradition of work with clinical and commissurotomy patients already reviewed, there are two other lines of research, quite independent of each other and of the work on human cerebral asymmetry, that support the idea of a verbal-nonverbal dichotomy. Intelligence testing theory has long proposed the existence of two major clusters of abilities, *verbal* and *performance*; the latter generally subsumes abilities requiring pattern and space perception, shape, form, and geometry.

The other line of research concerns the dual encoding hypothesis (e.g., Paivio, 1971) in memory theory. It is used to explain apparent differences in coding and memory functions for verbal and imaginal material. The two types of material are said to be represented and processed in two separate and functionally independent though interconnected symbolic systems. The pictorial, or imagery, system is said to operate in a direct analogue fashion, and its output has a synchronous and spatial character permitting dynamic transformations in terms of visual and spatial attributes such as size, location, orientation, rotation, reflection, distortion, deletion, and substitution of the imagined objects. The other system is specialized for dealing with linguistic and sequential information for generating speech. Evidence for the dual encoding hypothesis comes from findings that verbal and pictorial information may be independently acquired, coded, stored, and retrieved, with minimal mutual interference and independent and idiosyncratic forgetting functions (see R. E. Anderson, 1976; Paivio, 1971; J. L. Sherman, Kulhavy, & Burns, 1976). J. R. Anderson (1978; see also Wickelgren, 1975) asks whether the picture metaphor is the only valid interpretation of the image aspect. He concludes that arguments in favor of an underlying propositional representation of pictures and images (which would make the imaginal system operate similarly, if not identically, to the verbal system) are not compelling, though empirically it may never prove possible to finally decide between an underlying representation in imaginal or propositional terms. In some ways the two types of representation might always prove indistinguishable in their explanatory and predictive capacities, and like the wave–particle theories of light, under certain circumstances one may merely prove to be more useful than the other. It is of interest that proponents of the idea that the imaginal mode of thinking is nonpropositional have recently come to invoke the laterality findings, a somewhat circular state of affairs since the laterality studies themselves merely refer to the two modes of thought (verbal and imaginal) as labels for their own findings.

Perhaps the first evidence of inadequacy in a rigid verbal–nonverbal distinction and for a more fundamental mode of specialization came from clinical observations of patients' drawing abilities and their perception of space. Patients with left hemisphere lesions seemed to have problems in sequential organization, where objects are sorted by conceptual or abstract categories, and their drawings showed oversimplification or lack of detail, though they retained the general outline or shape. Lesions on the right side apparently led to overattention to details, a lack of awareness of overall organization or form relationships, and problems in dealing with maps, appreciating spatial wholes, perspective, and closure (see Chapter Four).

Gestalt functions of the right hemisphere.   Nebes (1978) reviewed his earlier findings that the right hemisphere is superior at perceiving the relationship between component parts and the whole configuration and in performing spatial transformations of the visual input. He believes that the right hemisphere is responsible for forming, from the incomplete sensory information, the spatial and cognitive map of our surroundings within which behavior is planned and organized. From his observations of the commissurotomy patients, Nebes claims that the ability to form a complete gestalt (e.g., a circle) from incomplete information (e.g., arcs of a circle) is a right hemisphere function and the ability to discover or isolate a shape within an irrelevant background is a function of the left hemisphere. Other right hemisphere functions involve the accurate perception and memory of stimuli that cannot easily be verbally labeled, or that are too complex or similar to specify or discriminate in words. The left hemisphere tends to make *conceptually* similar matches, the right hemisphere *structurally* similar ones, though the right can indeed also make judgments in terms of usage (e.g., matching a cigarette to an ashtray). Such findings with commissurotomy patients (see Chapter Five) enable us to conclude that the left hemisphere employs an analytic strategy to recognize faces and complex shapes, while the right hemisphere may immediately apprehend complex configurations as a gestalt.

Some Definitions
of Analytic-Holistic Modes of Processing

At this point we should try to clarify what is apparently being meant by such terms as *analytic, holistic, global, gestalt,* and so on. These ideas have been developing over a period of time, in a number of different areas and laboratories, and this has led to a certain "slipperiness" in usage. The term *analytic* properly applies to perceptual processing, rather than, for example, to the preparation of a response sequence, in the context of a segmental breakdown of a visual array or an auditory grouping into separate components, features, or elements. In theory at least, such a breakdown may be performed either serially and sequentially or in parallel. In contrast, *global, holistic,* or *gestalt* processing can be viewed as a more immediate and possibly primitive mode of apprehension; it places more emphasis on the whole configuration and on the patterns of interrelationships between, and otherwise independent of, the component parts. W. R. Garner (1978), without reference at all to the laterality literature, argues for two classes of stimulus properties, component and holistic. The component class he subdivides into dimensions (e.g., brightness, loudness, form) and features (e.g., presence of a horizontal line, an intersection, and so on). The holistic class of stimulus properties he subdivides into "simple wholes" (e.g., "blob processing," where an entity is not or cannot meaningfully be further subdivided or analyzed), "templates" (the simplest "canonical" or idealized form of a configuration) and "configurations" (where the whole constitutes something over and above the sum of the individual component elements). Likewise Neisser, in the context of thought and cognition and again without reference to the field of cerebral asymmetry, noted that

> Historically, psychology has long recognized the existence of two different forms of mental organization. The distinction has been given many names. . . . to list them together so casually may be misleading. . . . Nevertheless a common thread runs through the dichotomies. (1967, p. 297)

With respect to visual, auditory, and possibly tactile information processing, we would argue that the common thread is some such distinction as the following: On the one hand, is the array or pattern to be processed "as is," without further analysis or reference to component features or elements? Is it to be processed in terms of an emergent whole that is more than the sum of its component elements and that reflects patterns of interrelationships between and independent of those elements? On the other hand, is the configuration to be recognized by breaking it down into smaller components, elements, or distinctive features? Such a description is at best an attempt to capture the ideas' elusive connotations.

Visual Studies: Faces

We have reviewed the evidence for a LVF (right hemisphere) superiority in the processing of faces, whether photographed, IdentiKit, or schematically drawn, in Chapter Six. This superiority holds when normal subjects have to match a laterally presented test face to a stored representation of a target face when nontarget faces differ in all possible aspects from the target. However, when nontarget faces that are very similar to the target, differing from them by only one single feature, are used, a RVF (left hemisphere) superiority typically appears (K. Patterson & Bradshaw, 1975; J. L. Bradshaw, Taylor, Patterson, & Nettleton, 1980). Moreover, in a recent series of experiments using both facelike and meaningful nonfacelike (bugs) stimuli, J. L. Bradshaw and Sherlock (1982) imposed either an analytic or a holistic mode of processing on the same laterally presented stimuli. We varied the spatial interrelationships between and independent of the individual feature elements themselves, and we also varied the shapes of the component features independently of the above patterns of spatial interrelationships. In the same ensemble of stimuli, subjects could use only one or the other aspect to perform correct discriminations, and thus were forced to adopt either a holistic or an analytic mode of processing. The predicted LVF (right hemisphere) superiority appeared for holistically processed faces and bugs, and a RVF (left hemisphere) superiority appeared *for the same set of stimuli* when the subjects were set to attend to the characteristic features or elements, rather than to the overall configuration. Interestingly, such effects were generally stronger when the subject was practiced or familiar with the stimuli, later in a stimulus sequence, or in the second of two consecutive tasks, suggesting once more the importance of the development of an appropriate and consistent processing set before these directional asymmetries can fully emerge.

The Serial-Parallel Distinction

Closely related to the analytic-holistic distinction is that of serial-parallel processing (G. Cohen, 1973). On the basis of admittedly somewhat confusing and unsatisfactory results, Cohen argued that right hemisphere processing time is less dependent on the number of features that make up a configuration, and left hemisphere processing time is likely to increase as the number of discriminating and relevant features increases. Her original thesis, that the left hemisphere is a serial analyzer whose reaction-time slope increases as a function of the number of items, while the right is not so affected, gained strong support from Ohgishi (1978) using letter stimuli. M. J. White and White (1975), however, using both configurational and letter stimuli found no evidence for an increase in reaction time with increasing number of stimuli for either left or right presentations and concluded that, at least in their tasks, both hemispheres exhibited parallel processing. Two other studies (Polich, 1980; and Umiltà, Salmaso, Bagnara, & Simion, 1979) were unable to replicate Cohen's results, though in different aspects. Short of a detailed analysis of task-demand characteristics, it is not easy to account for such discrepancies.

We noted earlier that support for the verbal–nonverbal dichotomy came from the observations, outside of the laterality context, that encoding and memory functions may apparently dichotomize into verbal versus imaginal. Again, outside of the laterality context, there is a fairly long tradition of appealing to two separate processors (operating in parallel) for same–different judgments: a fast identity matcher for judgments "same" and a slower, serial analytic one that can detect differences (see Bamber, 1969; Beller, 1970; Bindra, Donderi, & Nishisato, 1968; Egeth, 1966; Keuss, 1977; Krueger, 1970). We have in the past (J. L. Bradshaw, Gates, & Patterson, 1976; K. Patterson & Bradshaw, 1975) from a review of our own and others' findings noted that the superiority of the right hemisphere is quantitative rather than qualitative and is most apparent under conditions of rapid identity matching. On the other hand involvement of the left hemisphere in visuospatial processing apparently reflects a slower, more detailed *analysis* of a configuration into its component elements and may typically lead to judgments of difference. We found with arrays of discrete elements in an easy task where "same" judgments are made faster than "different" judgments that "same" judgments tend more often to be mediated by the right hemisphere and "different" judgments by the left. With integrated configurations like faces, where nontargets differ completely from targets, a general right hemisphere superiority appears. Where such configurations can only be compared on the basis of separate or single features (because of extreme similarity or difficulty), the left hemisphere tends to be superior for both judgments. Where such stimuli are not seen as configurational or where the storage load is increased by continually changing the target item, a hemisphere-by-judgment interaction typically appears, with the right superior for "same" judgments and the left for "different" judgments. However, we should perhaps note that G. Cohen's (1973) original serial–parallel distinction may not be as useful as the more general analytic-holistic one since, in theory at least, parallel processing may still be a consequence of an analysis of a configuration into its component elements, with each element processed concurrently with its partners, though *not* in a holistic, global manner.

Auditory Studies:
Musical Sequences and Melodies

We have already seen (Chapter Six) that a LEA typically appears for judgments involving sound intensity, short durations, musical chords, timbre, melodies, environmental sounds, nonverbal vocalizations, sonar signals, and emotional tones or intonation patterns. Right temporal lobectomies damage performance on the Timbre and Tonal Memory subtest of the *Seashore Test of Musical Abilities* (B. Milner, 1962) and the recognition of orchestrated melodies (Shankweiler, 1966). Using the Wada amytal technique, Bogen and Gordon (1971) concluded that the right hemisphere generally mediates musical processing. Gordon (1974), reviewing the evidence that excision of the right temporal lobe impairs such musical abilities as tonal memory and timbre, noted that there is a dissociation between the ability to sing but not say the words (with left hemisphere excisions) and the opposite syndrome (after right hemisphere excisions) and concluded that the right hemisphere plays a major role in singing.

Until about thirty years ago, deficits in musical perception or production were largely thought to be linked to aphasia and left hemisphere syndromes; recently more attention has been paid to the right hemisphere (for reviews see Benton, 1977; Damasio & Damasio, 1977; Gates & Bradshaw, 1977a; Wyke, 1977). In the last few years the sequential nature of auditory information in music has been seen as posing a problem for exclusive right hemisphere mediation. Since auditory stimuli may be integrated over time in the way that visual stimuli are integrated over space to form perceptual wholes, two developments have occurred. One is the hypothesis of the alternative more fundamental dichotomy, the analytic–holistic distinction. The other is an increasing emphasis on bihemispheric mediation of musical function, and an attempt to make a finer-grained analysis of music into its possible discrete component elements, not all of which may be lateralized in the same way, rather than treating it as a unitary whole.

Shanon (1980), using musicians as subjects, found a left hemisphere advantage for performing *complex* musical tasks. Gates and Bradshaw (1977b) investigated the detection of pitch, rhythm, and harmony changes in music perception. While reaction times did not differ between ears for the detection of a changed note in either a single-line melody or a five-note whole tone sequence, the right ear proved the more accurate. In detecting rhythm changes in a five-note sequence, the left ear proved the faster and the right more accurate. No ear differences were apparent in the detection of harmony changes. The right ear proved more sensitive (d') in recognizing excerpts from unfamiliar melodies, and the left for recognizing excerpts from familiar melodies. We may therefore conclude that, *overall,* musical functions are not strictly lateralized to the right hemisphere, though there may often be a considerable right hemisphere involvement. Varying degrees of right hemisphere mediation may appear for the perception of pitch, harmony, timbre, and intensity, particularly perhaps for more complex, structured, tuneful melodious combinations and as a function of competence and familiarity.

In this context according to a seminal paper by Bever and Chiarello (1974), listening strategies that influence laterality differences in music perception are a function of musical training. From their observation that in a melody recognition task a LEA appears for nonmusicians and a REA for experienced musicians, they argued that educated listeners "have learned to perceive a melody as an articulated set of relations among components," while naive listeners "focus on the overall melodic contour" (p. 138). Bever reported exactly comparable findings in a later study (Kellar & Bever, 1980). Again, instead of a left-hemisphere-verbal, right-hemisphere-nonverbal dichotomy, we see LEAs and REAs in a nonverbal (musical) task as a joint function of expertise and mode of processing.

The idea that melody perception is a *gestalt* (i.e., holistic) phenomenon for naive listeners (who thus focus upon the overall melodic contour) while for musically experienced listeners the melody is perceived as an articulated set of component elements rather than as a unitary whole is not a new one. Thus Bever (1980) cites Werner (1948) and L. B. Meyer (1956), two musical authorities who were writing long before the analytic–holistic issue arose in neuropsychology.

Other support for Bever's findings of a REA for musicians and a LEA for nonmusicians comes from the work of Gordon (1975, 1978a), P. Johnson (1977), Davidson and Schwartz (1977), Hirshkowitz, Earle, and Paley (1978). R. C. Johnson, Bowers, Gamble, Lyons, Presbrey, and Vetter (1977) argued that it was not so much a matter of musical expertise *per se* but rather the ability to *transcribe* music that differentiated the subjects in terms of directional ear superiority. Gaede, Parsons, and Bertera (1978) found instead that it was musical *aptitude* that was all-important.

Studies in frank opposition to the direction of Bever and Chiarello's ear-by-expertise interaction have been reported; for example, a LEA for musicians and a REA for nonmusicians have been noted by Darwin (1969), Doehring and Ling (1971), Locke and Kellar (1973), and McDonough (1973). Moreover, as Gates and Bradshaw (1977b) point out, a right hemisphere superiority has been demonstrated with musicians by Bartholomeus (1974) and Kimura (1967). It may not be musical training, expertise, or talent that determines laterality effects but rather *how* the subject attends to music, regardless of these factors. Similar task requirements may induce similar processing strategies in both experienced and naive listeners, and the effects of different task requirements themselves may be determined by the subject's familiarity with the stimulus material itself.

Left Hemisphere Superiority for the Discrimination
of Duration, Temporal Order, Sequencing, and Rhythm

As we have just seen, the left hemisphere is functionally important for musical abilities that share properties with speech, such as temporal order, duration, simultaneity, and rhythm (Gates & Bradshaw, 1977a; Krashen, 1973a). Carmon (1978) and Natale (1977) review the extensive clinical evidence in support of this position and conclude that the left hemisphere is responsible for the sequential processing and temporal resolution of information, since lesions here typically result in the patients' needing more time to perceive order and sequencing, irrespective of spatial complexity. Right hemisphere lesions impair perception only in relation to spatial complexity of patterns rather than with respect to the perception of sequences. The prototypical picture of left hemisphere mediation of judgments of sequencing and temporal order (Divenyi & Efron, 1979; Efron, 1963a, b; Mills & Rollman, 1980), however, is said by Tallal (1976) to reflect capacities to process rapidly changing acoustic information and the ability to discriminate two sounds from one when they are very closely contiguous.

With normal subjects, Halperin, Nachshon, and Carmon (1973) found that while the left ear was superior for simple tonal sequences (long and short), the right ear was superior for more complex sequences, when the number of temporal transitions became important. G. M. Robinson and Solomon (1974) obtained a similar REA using dichotic pairs of rhythmic pure tones. Papçun, Krashen, Terbeek, Remington, and Harshman (1974) using morse code found that skilled operators gave a REA for both complex and simple sequences, but naive subjects gave a LEA for complex sequences. Deutsch and Roll (1976) also obtained a preference for right ear report with a dichotic tonal sequence where three 800 Hz tones were followed by two 400 Hz tones on one channel, with three 400 Hz tones followed by two 800 Hz tones on the other, all of the same duration and interstimulus interval. Natale (1977) found a REA superiority in the report of nonverbal rhythmic sequences, particularly for the more complex sequences and for the more dextral subjects. (He also concluded that this left hemisphere specialization for the temporal resolution of rhythmic sequences is part of a preliminary stage in the analysis-by-synthesis perception of speech, taking advantage of the fact that such patterns have a trajectory that can be tracked without constant monitoring.) Mills and Rollman (1979) obtained a REA for the discrimination of duration (unconfounded with the perception of temporal order, as in all the studies described above), but only when the intervals were of 50 msec or less. They noted that this duration is of the same order of magnitude as that required for achieving the perceptual distinctiveness of phonemes and speculated that both phenomena may depend on a specialized timing mechanism in the left hemisphere (the right sufficing for the gestalt apprehension of speech at the level of the syllable or whole word). J. Schwartz and Tallal (1980) found that the left hemisphere superiority for processing stop consonants diminishes as they are slowed down while still preserving their phonemic character. They concluded that the basis for left hemisphere superiority for language may be its greater ability to process rapidly changing acoustic spectra, such as formant transitions in consonant phonemes, and that it is this ability, rather than the linguistic or verbal nature of the stimuli, that generates the REA.

In a similar vein, Vroon, Timmers, and Tempelaars (1977) found that the left hemisphere is better at estimating simple reaction times, predicting time of arrival, and detecting short interruptions with *auditory* though not with *visual* stimuli. They concluded that the left is better able to discover the internal structure of a time series. A. E. Davis and Wada (1977a), on the basis of spectral analyses of visual and auditory evoked potentials to groups of flashes and clicks, concluded that the left hemisphere analyzes temporally ordered information and the right processes spatially distributed information. Finally Gordon (1978b) found a REA in a dichotic test of melodies differing only in rhythm and concluded that the left hemisphere is concerned with the sequential, temporal aspects of the time dimension.

With tactile tasks essentially similar observations appear. Nachshon and

Carmon (1975) studied hand preferences in the sequential localization of touched fingers. While bimanual (dichaptic) rather than unimanual stimulation was necessary to generate hand differences, the right hand proved better on tasks requiring temporal analysis and the left on tasks where spatial relationships were most significant. Bakker and Van de Kleij (1978) managed to obtain lateral differences similar to the above in the localization of touched fingers under both dichaptic and unimanual stimulation (cf. Hatta, 1978b).

Limbs, Hands, and Fingers: Motor Control

Observations of clinical patients and experiments with normal subjects converge to indicate a role of the left hemisphere in controlling fine, sequential, manipulative movements of the limbs, hands, and fingers, both bilaterally and with the right (preferred) hand. Kimura (1977) found that patients with left hemisphere damage, aphasic or not, were impaired in the acquisition and performance of manual skills requiring several hand movements. She claims that the left hemisphere's function is the control of changes in limb or articulatory posture, and its complex verbal and praxic functions derive from such control. She reviews the evidence that left hemisphere preeminence is in terms of motor control rather than verbal processes, with deficits as diverse as pursuit rotor tasks, rapidity of targeting limb movements, and copying of meaningless gestures associated with left hemisphere damage. She also reviews her work with normal subjects (Lomas & Kimura, 1976), demonstrating an impairment of sequential finger and arm movements by concurrent speaking. This is interpreted as indicating an inability by the left hemisphere to allocate attentional capacity to both articulatory and limb positioning *together* and *independently*—though *dependent* limb movement of the right hand may occur during speech in *synchrony* with articulation (Kimura, 1973b).

In summary, Kimura suggests that it is the rapid positioning of a limb or its parts in terms of kinesthetic control towards internalized representations of target loci that are lateralized to the left hemisphere, as are the control processes governing the oral musculature. This would have the slightly paradoxical consequence of implying that the left hemisphere also is specialized in terms of spatial information —not, perhaps, the relatively static exteroceptive visuospatial functions of the right, but rather the dynamic, kinesthetic-interoceptive, temporally dependent targeting of the limbs (and articulators) in terms of the body schema (cf. LeDoux, Wilson, & Gazzaniga, 1977). Summers and Sharp (1979) develop these ideas to their logical conclusion in their claim that both hemispheres are involved in the control of sequential movements, the left with respect to organization into correct sequential order, the right for exactly locating the limbs and fingers in body space.

Other evidence (clinical and normal) that the left hemisphere is specialized in the control of fine, precise, bilateral coordination of the limbs, hands, and fingers while the right is responsible for accurate spatial localization and the tactile perception of spatial relationships may be found in Whitaker and Ojemann (1977), Wolff

(1977), Wolff and Hurwitz (1976), Wolff, Hurwitz, and Moss (1977, they noted that there may be some dissociation between language and serial motor organization in sinistrals), and G. Young (1977). Kimura and Archibald (1974) found that patients with left hemisphere damage were impaired in copying visually presented hand movements; they also found some evidence of a dissociation between linguistic and limb gestures, in that aphasics tended to lose articulator control in complex, voluntary *nonverbal* movements (yawning, teeth chattering, whistling), independently of limb control, while apraxics tended to lose the ability to perform meaningful and meaningless limb movements, independent of speech.

Left Hemisphere Control of the Articulatory Mechanisms: The Sussman Paradigm

Sussman (see MacNeilage, Sussman, & Stolz, 1975; Sussman, 1977; Sussman & Westbury, 1978) pioneered a pursuit auditory tracking task whereby the subject monitors in one ear a tone that continuously and randomly changes in either frequency or intensity. He or she then matches this tone to another (the cursor) presented to the other ear, by continuously controlling the latter tone through unidimensional movements of some part of the body (tongue, jaw, lips, or hand). Sussman found that performance (with intensity rather than frequency control) was best when the target tone went to the left ear and the cursor to the right, though this REA was weakest with control by respiratory or hand movements, leading to the conclusion that the speech musculature proper is more relevant to lateralized sensorimotor integrations. However, in Sussman and Westbury's latest study (1978) they did succeed in obtaining a significant REA under conditions of right-hand tracking, which they claim supports the Kimura (see previous section) position of a left hemisphere dominance in controlling *all* coordinated movements, limb as well as oral-facial. In general, Sussman and coworkers conclude that the left hemisphere is specialized for the sensorimotor integration of speech-related movements and their auditory concomitants and for the complex sequential programming of changing oral-facial configurations from one target position to another. Conclusions such as this would predict that left hemisphere lesions should result in a decrement in ability to imitate nonverbal oral movements. Mateer (1978) found that errors of perseveration did appear, with searching movements as if the patient was unsure when the designated target position had been obtained.

We can conclude, therefore, that the left hemisphere is closely involved in time-dependent praxic movements of the limbs, hand, and fingers and in the achievement of target oral configurations (even when unrelated to phoneme production), all in terms of a sequentially ordered kinesthetic-proprioceptive body schema. Such a conclusion was in fact reached in the first decade of the twentieth century by Liepmann (cited by Heilman, 1979a), who proposed that left hemisphere lesions lead to general apraxia and disorders of sequences of skilled movements rather than disorders of symbolic behavior.

The concept of analytic *perceptual* processing seems to have arisen largely independently of the idea of the segmental control of *motor* processes. It could well be that the perceptual aspect is biologically secondary to the left hemisphere's mediation of such motor processes. This would account for the common finding that lateralization is more pronounced at motor than at perceptual levels, whether for speech (see the previous chapter) or for "perceptual-spatial" tasks (LeDoux et al., 1977). The segmental aspects of perception are perhaps tied to the left hemisphere through the latter's prior involvement in motor sequencing and segmentation in general. If different zones of the left hemisphere have different properties, they perhaps all have some aspect of segmentation in common, and according to the view now being put forward, different aspects of speech and language (phonology, syntax, and lexical processing) might map onto these areas.

Dysphasia and Dyslexia:
The Role of the Left Hemisphere

We have just reviewed the evidence that overt left hemisphere lesions are associated with defects of oral control and articulation. Even when no actual evidence of such lesions exists and they must be inferred, speech disturbances, developmental dysphasia, and "aphasoid performance" have long been associated with impairments in the perception of the temporal order of auditory stimuli, nonverbal as well as verbal (see Benton, 1977, 1978). Tallal and Piercy (1978), however, claim that the undisputed impairments in auditory serial memory for temporal sequences shown by dysphasic children may in turn be reduced to difficulties in making fine temporal discriminations and to defective processing of rapidly changing acoustic information. Thus, in a recent study Tallal, Stark, Kallman, and Mellits (1980) showed that it is the rate of change in the critical components in the acoustic spectra of speech rather than the verbal nature of the stimuli *per se* that determines the grossly impaired discriminatory performance of such children. Many etiologies have been proposed for developmental dyslexia, as for developmental dysphasia, and other aspects will be considered in a later chapter (Chapter Thirteen), but breakdowns in sequencing, time sense, temporal order, and rhythm are commonly reported (Birch & Belmont, 1964; Bradley & Bryant, 1978; Corkin, 1974; Holmes & McKeever, 1979; Jorm, 1979; Zurif & Carson, 1970).

Semmes's Focal–Diffuse Distinction

Closely related to the analytic–holistic dichotomy is the concept of Semmes (1968) who argued from her observations of clinical patients that sensory and motor capacities are more focally represented in the left hemisphere and more diffusely in the right—analogous, perhaps, to the more one-to-one linkage of foveal cones to bipolar and ganglion cells, and the convergence of rods in the periphery onto higher order cells. She claimed that right hemisphere damage (outside of the primary projection areas) leads to impairment in motor performance similar to the effects of damage to the projection areas; in the left hemisphere such decrements in performance are found only after damage to the specific projection areas. Moreover, damage to a specific area of the focally organized left hemisphere typically leads to specific function loss; damage great enough to disrupt one function in the more diffusely organized right hemisphere tends to disrupt other functions as well. She argued, therefore, that the left hemisphere is consequently superior at tasks requiring fine spatial or temporal acuity, such as manual skills or speech; the more diffusely organized right hemisphere performs the more integrative functions such as spatial abilities.

Though Dimond at no time relates his ideas to those of Semmes, his (1979a, b) claim of a right hemisphere superiority for vigilance tasks in commissurotomy cases (see Chapter Seven), with the right hemisphere better able to maintain sustained attention and the left selective or focal attention, is undoubtedly in the same tradition. Semmes argues that such a diffuse (right hemisphere) organization may be the natural state for infrahuman species, which lack speech and rely on spatial and topographical skills, which in turn depend on a convergence of unlike elements (visual, kinesthetic, vestibular, etc., information) combining in such a way as to create through experience a single supramodal space. Left hemisphere specialization for manual dexterity and language is therefore seen as the more specialized and advanced, being superimposed (unilaterally) on what might be seen as two primitive right hemispheres. The future success or failure of Semmes's interpretation will depend on whether others will be able to replicate her lesion studies (which, curiously, no one has seen fit to do during the last ten years). However, a recent piece of supporting evidence comes from R. C. Gur, Packer, Hungerbuhler, Reivich, Obrist, Amarnek, and Sackeim (1980), who found that there was more gray matter, relative to white, in the left than in the right hemisphere (and especially in frontal and precentral regions). They concluded that this is in accord with the hypothesis that the left hemisphere tends to mediate processing within discrete regions and the right hemisphere between them.

Conclusions So Far

The most traditional account of hemispheric asymmetry characterizes it in terms of a verbal–nonverbal dichotomy. Studies involving brain-injured and commissurotomy patients and normal subjects have all emphasized the role played by the left hemisphere in mediating language, more particularly perhaps at the motor than at the receptive level. A REA is found for all manner of verbal materials, meaningful or not, and even for tonal quality if it is linguistically relevant; a LEA is found for simple, nonverbal acoustic stimuli such as judgments involving pitch, harmony, intensity, timbre, musical chords, melodies (under certain circumstances), environmental sounds, nonverbal vocalizations, sonar signals, emotional tones, and intonation patterns. Additional support for the hypothesis comes from the concepts developed independently in memory theory of a dual-encoding system, verbal and imaginal; some theorists, however, are questioning whether imaginal contents may themselves ultimately be coded in propositional form. Further support comes from the proposed verbal–performance dichotomy in intelligence testing. Finally, ear and visual field superiorities can be made to reverse, for the same subjects and stimuli, as a function of imposed or adopted set or strategy, suggesting that it is not so much the stimuli themselves as how they are processed that is important.

Problems for the simple verbal–nonverbal dichotomy appear when it is found that the right hemisphere possesses considerable linguistic powers, more strongly receptive perhaps than expressive; that the left hemisphere is superior in certain visuospatial tasks that are best performed by a strategy involving an analytic extraction of significant or distinguishing features or elements; and that the right hemisphere is not always, or in all aspects, dominant for music, particularly where the sequential or temporally extended nature of the auditory stimuli are important, as in judgments involving temporal order, durations, simultaneity, rhythm, or categorical perception. Moreover, studies with both clinical patients and normal subjects have indicated that the left hemisphere may be uniquely specialized in terms of temporal order, sequencing, and segmentation, at both sensory and motor levels, in the latter case for the control of rapid sequential changes in limb, hand, finger, or articulator positioning. Thus, the left hemisphere may act as a dynamic, kinesthetic-interoceptive, temporally dependent control system for target acquisition within the body schema while the right acts in terms of static, exteroceptive, visuospatial functions largely outside of body space. Additional and independently derived support for such a concept comes from work with dysphasic and dyslexic children, for whom there now appears to have been a long natural history of deficits in perceiving the temporal order of nonverbal auditory stimuli. Accordingly, the left hemisphere mediation of language may possibly not depend on its *symbolic* or even largely *phonological* attributes, but rather on the need for *analytic,* time-dependent, and sequential coding to occur, both at receptive and, more particularly, expressive levels.

We are now faced with a major problem. The left hemisphere undoubtedly does mediate language processes: All the evidence from asymmetries in brain morphology and the effects of clinical lesions support such a position. Does it mediate them *because* of a prior analytic or segmental specialization of the left hemisphere? (That is, at some time in the evolutionary history of humans or even in the ontogenetic history of the individual, were language mechanisms attracted to and subjected to further neural development in the left hemisphere because of its prior analytic-segmental specialization?) This position would view the left hemisphere as being adapted not for symbolic functions *per se,* but rather for the execution of some categories of motor activity that happened to lend themselves readily to communication. Alternatively, are *all* the apparent left hemisphere language superiorities *really* just manifestations of the left hemisphere's processing analytically and sequentially? Certainly, there seems to be plenty of evidence for analytic or segmental left hemisphere superiorities *independent* of any phonological or verbal component. However, some (e.g., Studdert-Kennedy, 1970; Springer, 1979) argue strongly for the primacy of speech and verbal processes with respect to left hemisphere dominance, in particular the unilateral *motor* control of the speech apparatus. Speech, they say, is a species-specific capacity representing a "quantum jump in evolution"; it is therefore mediated by a specialized left hemisphere mechanism to cope both with the limited resolving power of the human ear and the lack of acoustic invariance in the speech signal. Such a mechanism is held to be responsible, on the one hand, for the phonological or sound system that specifies the elemental speech sounds and applies rules for their combination into meaningful words and, on the other, for the rules of syntax for combining such words into phrases or sentences.

Apart from the specific question of whether a specialization for language processes or, alternatively, for analytic segmental processing underlies left hemisphere superiorities for mediating verbal stimuli, there is currently another related, more general, but no less vigorous controversy over whether there is something "special" about speech. Does speech perception depend wholly, in part, or not at all on a speech synthesizer (the analysis-by-synthesis account; see Wanner, Teyler, & Thompson, 1977, for review) or on feature detectors finely tuned to restricted ranges of acoustic information in the speech signal (Studdert-Kennedy, 1980a)? Is there a specialist processor (wherever located) to deal with the nonvariance in and the encodedness of the speech signal, and does it operate by means of acoustic feature or property detectors and categorical perception? Some, as we have seen, claim that categorical perception is neither peculiar to speech (nor even the auditory modality) nor necessary for speech perception (Studdert-Kennedy, 1980b). Others go even further, denying that there is anything special about perceiving in the speech mode, claiming that all aspects previously thought to be unique to speech can and do occur in music (J. E. Cutting, 1979), and arguing that speech analysis by the left hemisphere is merely part of a much more general system for segmenting sequential acoustic input (Allard & Scott, 1975; Schouten, 1980). Indeed, as we saw in Chapter Eight, the right hemisphere may be far from irrelevant for the mediation of language functions. Dennis, Lovett, and Wiegel-Crump (1981) noted with infantile hemidecorticates tested as adults that while the left hemisphere is superior for morphophonemic processing, the right is superior at the logographic level (of *extra*phonological reading and comprehension). According to Perecman and Kellar (1981), patients with left hemisphere lesions cannot perform discriminations on the basis of place of articulation (e.g., /b/ versus /d/, /p/ versus /t/, /d/ versus /g/, /t/ versus /k/, and so on, where voicing is kept constant but articulator position is varied); these patients, however, *can* perform such discriminations on the basis of *voicing* (e.g., /b/ versus /p/, /d/ versus /t/, and /g/ versus /k/, where only the voiced aspect is varied). This suggests that one of the fundamental distinctive features that differentiates between the speech sounds we make, voicing, may be mediated by the right hemisphere. Molfese (1980), in his review of his auditory evoked response (AER) work on voice onset time (VOT) perception (see Chapter

Twelve), claims that VOT (which is an important cue for discriminating between voiced and unvoiced consonants) is mediated by the right hemisphere. He believes that the right hemisphere is also sensitive to such cues (i.e., simple onset asynchronies, cf. the work of Sidtis, 1980, 1981, reviewed in Chapter Six, on right hemisphere mediation of steady-state harmonic information of complex tones) in *nonspeech* acoustic stimuli. Likewise, the left hemisphere, sensitive to *rapidly changing* formant transition cues that permit place of articulation to be identified for consonants, is according to Molfese similarly sensitive to such cues outside the speech context. He concludes that hemisphere differences long ascribed to speech perception may be due to the differential distribution of specific acoustic processing mechanisms between the two hemispheres and that these differences are not limited to speech processing.

The often acrimonious debate on the uniqueness of speech processing mechanisms is yet to be resolved, but we should note that clinicians, more than experimental neuropsychologists, seem to favor the old material-specific hypothesis that the verbal–nonverbal nature of the stimulus or task is what is important. Thus Kim, Royer, Boustelle, and Boller (1980) argue that left hemisphere lesions hit *verbal* sequencing and right hemisphere damage decrements *nonverbal* sequencing. E. Zaidel (personal communication) also believes that a left hemisphere language specialization is indeed the key, but only for the computational and combinatorial algorithms that characterize abstract syntax and phonology. It is, he says, an open question whether this linguistic specialization *precedes* or depends on a prior cognitive segmental-analytic ability.

Evolutionary Issues:
A Hierarchy of Questions on the Evolution
of Tool Use, Handedness, and Language

Why is the mapping of sensory and motor relationships on the brain organized in a crossed or contralateral pattern in vertebrates? The far more "obvious" *uncrossed* or ipsilateral relationship is perfectly possible and works very well in, for example, the cephalopods (squids, octopus, cuttlefish), many of which have brains equaling the vertebrates' in complexity (J. Z. Young, 1976). Kinsbourne (1978) notes that the central neuraxis is ventral in invertebrates and dorsal in vertebrates, with a similar reversal of inward- and outward-flowing blood supplies between the two phyla, and speculates that both these differences and the general issue of contralateral representation in vertebrates can be resolved if we postulate an 180° torsional rotation in an early ancestor. An alternative proposal (see Sarnat & Netsky, 1974) is that primordial defensive reflexes in vertebrate precursors resembling Amphioxus required that tactile stimulation from one side of the body elicit muscle contraction on the opposite side, and the crossovers were thus built into the vertebrate system from the beginning.

Locomoting animals need paired, equally strong control centers to avoid the development of turning biases in a left-right unbiased world (Corballis & Beale, 1976). Such lateral symmetry may be lost if animals return, phylogenetically or ontogenetically, to a sedentary life style (e.g., tunicates, barnacles). Therefore, it is probably no accident that asymmetries are most apparent at *cognitive* levels, where they cannot lead to the maladaptive development of turning biases or of unilateral sensory neglect. Cognitive functions are most highly developed in humans, who most clearly demonstrate asymmetrical functioning.

What is the advantage of cognitive and motor asymmetry in humans? Does it avoid redundant duplication of functions, thus increasing cognitive capacity within a limited processing space (J. Levy, 1977b)? Yet, the amount of laterally specialized neural tissue relative to the rest of the symmetrical brain mass is not large. Does it permit the isolation of analytic thought processes from interference from the possibly more primitive modes of holistic thought? There is no reason to suppose that *interhemispheric* isolation should be any more effective than *intrahemispheric* isolation, at least at the *cognitive* level. At the *motor* level does such segregation permit undivided executive control over the unpaired articulators to be maintained by a single leading hemisphere? Competition for motor outflow to our single speech system could be disadvantageous; indeed, there is some evidence (Corballis, 1981) that some forms of stuttering might arise from bihemispheric representation of language. However, the musculature of the neck, eyes, and trunk does not apparently suffer from such divided bilateral control (Whitaker & Ojemann, 1977), though there the rate of information transmission is far lower. Does such cognitive and motor asymmetry permit the development of a division of labor between the hands, so that one hand can perform a holding function and the other a manipulating or operational role? Intuitively, this perhaps seems the most likely candidate and will be considered further in the context of lateralization of the *population* rather than of just the *individual*.

Another possible reason for asymmetry, at least at the *cognitive* level, is that we can thereby more readily perform discriminations of mirror-image stimuli, a problem that is difficult enough for humans and *almost* impossible for most other species of animals (see Chapters One and Thirteen). Even we have great difficulty in learning to turn right (or left) on command or to discriminate between mirror-image shapes. The former task involves correctly assigning one of a pair of mirror-image responses to an asymmetrical stimulus (left or right). The latter, where an asymmetrical response (yes or no) has to be assigned to mirror stimuli (e.g., the lines / and \, or the letters *b, d; p, q*) is difficult for most children and some adults (see, e.g., J. L. Bradshaw, Bradley, & Patterson, 1976; Corballis & Beale, 1976). Only humans, perhaps, with their arbitrary distinctions of directionality, need to be able to perform such *discriminations*. For other members of the animal kingdom it is far more useful to be able to perform stimulus *generalization*, whereby mirror-image stimuli are instead treated as functionally identical, that is, as different manifestations of the same object viewed from a different angle. That physiological asymmetry can act as a substrate on which mirror stimuli (/ and \) can be discriminated was demonstrated by an experiment in which some pigeons managed to perform the discrimination successfully by tilting their heads to one side, thus converting the stimuli to horizontal and vertical lines (Corballis & Beale, 1970b). This strategy, of course, only works if the head is always tilted to the *same* side, thus converting / and \ into | and — if the head is tilted to the right, or vice versa if to the left. The bird can only remember to tilt its head the same way each time if it is somehow asymmetrical to start with. The same applies to humans, again perhaps emphasizing the fact that in such contexts memory functions are more important than purely perceptual functions.

The ultimate origin, however, of asymmetries in the animal kingdom, including humans, still remains to be resolved. As we shall see in Chapter Ten, one possible explanation is that of Corballis and Morgan (1978) that such asymmetries are under the influence of a left-right maturational gradient coded into the cytoplasm rather than the genes, a gradient possibly based on asymmetries in the molecular structure of living matter. This explanation, however, is not widely accepted.

Why are the manifestations of lateral asymmetry so weak that often they can be demonstrated only through an unusual information load (e.g., Moscovitch, 1979; see also Chapter Seven) or complex cognitive or motor tasks (e.g., writing or tool use) in humans, or through unusual modes of rearing, treatment, or handling in other vertebrates (Denenberg, 1981)? Is it because the biochemical or cytoplasmic asymmetries (Corballis & Morgan, 1978) are *themselves* weak, or because the evolution of lateralization is as yet incomplete? If it is for the latter reason, then it is remarkable that so many species are independently embarking on an asymmetrical future. Are the manifestations weak so that in the event of injury an emergency back-up system is still available on the other side? Although the least lateralized individuals should then be at an advantage if they sustained a unilateral injury, in normal health they should be at a corresponding disadvantage. This may in fact be the case with human sinistrals (see Chapter Ten), though not apparently with females, who *also* tend to be less lateralized (McGlone, 1980; see also Chapter Eleven). The effects are possibly too subtle and small for evolutionary significance.

Are there *costs* associated with stronger lateralization, such as turning biases and a tendency to unilateral hemineglect? This would be less serious for predator species, like humans, who are the most strongly lateralized of all. Is there any evidence that lateral asymmetries are generally stronger in predator species than in prey species? What other *costs,* such as cognitive inflexibility or a reduction in the possible extent of interhemispheric cooperation, might follow strong lateralization? Conversely, are there *benefits*? Does strong lateralization reduce the danger from interhemispheric competition, interference, and "crowding" of functions? Does the group, society, or species somehow benefit from being composed of both weakly and strongly lateralized individuals, just as Kolakowski and Malina (1974) suggest that society might benefit from a sexual dimorphism in terms of opposing cognitive specializations? These and many similar questions remain largely unanswered.

Why should a *population* be lateralized, with most humans right-handed and left-brained for language? Is it again a consequence of Corballis and Morgan's (1978) cytoplasmic and molecular asymmetries? If so, why is there apparently a hereditary component for handedness in humans (see Chapter Ten) but apparently not in other vertebrates, even though as individuals they may show strong paw preferences (see Chapter Two)? Moreover, a biochemical explanation would require that *nonhuman* populations should *also* be lateralized. Is there an evolutionary advantage for a relatively uniform pattern of handedness in humans? Shared tool use is an obvious candidate, with a respectable evolutionary history, even to the extent that simple hand scrapers work better if they have the indentations for grip made to fit a given hand. Indeed, there are no other obvious respects in which a dextral and a sinistral individual would interact less efficiently (except possibly in team games and warfare) than two dextrals (or two sinistrals). Does this suggest that shared tool use (together with manual specialization) is the true source of the unique degree and manifestation of human asymmetry? If so, it supports the idea that tool use antedates spoken language (possibly with gesture as an evolutionary intermediary on which we still readily fall back in the event of stress, deafness, or incomprehension; see, e.g., Hewes, 1973), with language lateralization being *built on* and *secondary to* a left hemisphere mediation of segmental, time-dependent processes. The opposite argument, that language (and specialized modes of cognition and thought) developed as an inevitable concomitant of increasing cortical development, which was demanded by a need for survival in the new ecological niche created by glaciation and requiring social cooperative hunting and butchering, would not require the lateralization of the population (see, e.g., Parker & Gibson, 1979).

There are therefore two possible scenarios—that tool use, manual gesture, right-handedness, and cerebral lateralization antedated and determined speech, or that spoken language came first. Unfortunately, behaviors do not fossilize. There are no fossil phonemes, no petrified grammars; our only legacies are tools, art, bones, and potsherds. As Dingwall (1979) points out, the question of the origin of language was so much "done to death" that it was twice banned from discussion by the Société de Linguistique de Paris (in 1866 and 1911). It is only the recent growth of a large number of relevant interdisciplinary studies (paleontology, anthropology, neurology, linguistics, experimental psycholinguistics, ethology, zoology, biochemistry, and so on) that has again made the question respectable. Paradoxically, the *biochemical* evidence on the extremely close relatedness of humans and the chimpanzees (though both species are of course *evolved* descendants from a single common ancestor) continually pushes forward the split between humans and apes, while the *archaeological* data seem to be pushing back the common ancestry. Much of the answer will depend on how humans are defined as a species, and how the fossil record is eventually interpreted.

Falk (1980) supports the second of the above two scenarios (that spoken language came first), based on an analysis of homologous areas of monkey and human cortex (see Chapter Two). However, his view is surely mistaken. Our language is almost entirely cortically controlled, while primate vocalization of affect is essentially limbic, and even chimpanzees have no need of a structure such as Broca's area (which does not control sound production itself but rather the way in which sounds are assembled into sequences). This is because the species-specific calls of chimpanzees are not constructed by varying the sequential order of elementary units (Passingham, quoted by Isaac, 1980; for consideration of the opposite viewpoint, see Marin, Schwartz, & Saffran, 1979).

Current thinking considers that bipedal locomotion was adopted 3 to 4 million years ago, freeing the hands for making and using tools (Curtis, quoted by Isaac, 1980), though according to Tobias (quoted by Isaac, 1980) this change occurred long before the fossil record gives any indications of major changes in brain form or size. The use of gestures might have preceded, succeeded, or accompanied the manufacture and use of tools. Certainly it is still a ready means of communication we fall back on after being deafened (whether late in life or before birth), when stressed, or when in a foreign country, and many species of living primates use gestures (manual and facial) naturally and freely (van Lawick-Goodall, 1971). It also provides natural precursors in the form of pointing and iconic symbolization for the arbitrary symbols of later developing speech.

However, gestures are slow and inefficient compared with speech; they cannot be seen in darkness, through the forest, or at a distance; they are not salient or attention-getting and cannot be made while wielding tools or weapons or carrying objects. These disadvantages may have led to the evolutionary development of cortical modulation of the earlier limbic-controlled vocalizations of affect. Facial gestures may have appeared as an intermediate stage, via grimacing and the consequent modulation of ongoing vocalization; the face, of course, has long been a means of both individual recognition and the communication of affect. Thus, face and articulatory gestures initially perhaps synergistically accompanied *manual* gestures and then came to replace them. It is certainly no accident that the cortical areas for hands, mouth, and ears are all adjacent to each other in humans, are all relatively much larger than the corresponding areas in apes, and all control syntactic organization and sequential ordering.

Did language develop only once (like the alphabet—see, e.g., Diringer, 1968; and Jensen, 1970—and possibly like life itself), or did it develop several times, only to abort before reaching its current form? On the basis of reconstruction of certain aspects of the Neanderthal vocal tract from fossil skeletal remains, there is doubt as to whether these near cousins of ours could have spoken (Lieberman, 1979). They *might* of course have produced different *sorts* of speech; humans with grossly damaged vocal tracts and even birds can certainly generate perfectly intelligible speech sounds. Are humans unique in possessing language? Do the cetaceans "speak"? If so, the very long distances (possibly many thousands of miles) over which whales are said to be able to communicate (Prince, 1980) owing to the special acoustic properties of seawater, would impose very long turn-around times for messages, possibly accounting for the nature and length of their recorded calls. Do chimpanzees "speak"? They can certainly be taught gestural communication, as the recent dramatic studies show (see, e.g., Terrace, 1980), though not everyone

functional differences between the hemispheres, such a conclusion could possibly be artifactual, from the facilitatory influences of information transmitted over intact commissures and ipsilateral pathways, blurring and smoothing over sharp underlying qualitative asymmetries. Certainly the apparently devastating effects of clinical lesions seem to support the model of exclusive hemispheric specialization (see Chapter Four), with laterality differences in normal subjects instead reflecting interhemispheric transmission time and/or signal degradation during such inter-hemispheric transmission (see Chapter Seven). Such devastating and apparently all-or-none clinical effects may *themselves* stem from the presence of intact com-missures, acting in an *inhibitory* rather than a facilitatory capacity. Numerous accounts in the clinical literature of severe aphasia after left hemisphere trauma report considerable alleviation after removal or disconnection of the damaged left hemisphere areas, which leaves the right hemisphere to perform its not-inconsid-erable verbal functions free from inhibitory influences from the left. In health these inhibitory influences might perhaps act to eliminate maladaptive bihemispheric competition. Certainly the evidence from the commissurotomy studies (where interhemispheric transmission—facilitatory or inhibitory—is perforce inoperative) emphasizes the continuum of function between the hemispheres and the quanti-tative and relative nature of functional differences; that is, each hemisphere is able to function in any processing mode open to the other but at different levels of competence and in different preferred directions.

Perhaps the only exception to such a viewpoint, which comes from the work with commissurotomy patients, may be the apparent inability of the right hemi-sphere to perform phonetic analyses in dichotic listening to stop consonants (see Chapters Five and Eight). But even here, as J. Schwartz and Tallal (1980) have shown, the left hemisphere superiority for processing stop consonants diminishes as they are slowed down while still preserving their phonemic character. Thus even this last bastion of left hemisphere absolute superiority may be crumbling, if it is just a matter of relative speeds (whether of input information or of processing). With normal subjects, conferring a signal-to-noise or a temporal advantage to the in-ferior ear or visual field does not erase or reverse the laterality effects, as would be predicted if laterality differences depended on interhemispheric transmission from quite incompetent to exclusively functional hemispheres (Weiss & House, 1973; Studdert-Kennedy, Shankweiler, & Schulman, 1970). Even the clinical studies often emphasize the phenomena of plasticity, mass action, and recovery of function, so the viewpoint of quantitative superiorities would seem to be the common-sense one. As both we (J. L. Bradshaw & Nettleton, 1981) and Bever (1980) have pointed out, an original quantitative asymmetry can give rise to the appearance of qualitative, all-or-nothing differences if the former quantitative asymmetry is large enough, if analytic processing requires more powerful process-ing capacity than holistic, and if the left hemisphere is more powerful computa-tionally than the right in its early development, whatever the reason may be for such ontogenetic differences.

The Analytic–Holistic Processing Dichotomy
and the Question of Cognitive Style

Bogen (1969b, 1975) came to the conclusion that the two "modes of thought," which philosophers have long propounded, can be characterized as propositional, versus appositional, relating respectively to the left and right hemispheres. The distinction, he believes, is not so much in the type of stimuli processed or responses initiated but rather in the *way* that information is processed. He introduces the concept of *hemisphericity,* whereby an individual is held to rely more on one mode of processing than another, with the propositional mode perhaps dominating more in intensely educated Western societies and a reverse tendency in nonliterate cultures that emphasize spatial skills (cf. Paredes & Hepburn, 1976).

Such considerations have led to an extensive literature on cognitive style and cerebral asymmetry (Arndt & Berger, 1978; K. P. O'Connor & Shaw, 1978; Zenhausen, 1978; Zoccolotti & Oltman, 1978). It has become popular to identify individuals as having a left or right cognitive mode according to the extent that they exhibit characteristics associated with the left or right hemisphere. People who tend to be verbal and analytic are often assumed to use their left hemisphere more extensively or effectively; the reverse is assumed for people who favor spatial and holistic approaches. People are held to be characterized by the degree, nature, and direction of functional hemispheric specialization they exhibit in information processing and preference behavior. Cognitive styles are viewed as reflecting not only individual differences in perceptual processes, but also intellectual, social-interpersonal, and general personality variables. However, such views have often tended to lead to speculative generalizations and unsubstantiated oversimplifications in the popular literature, relating all aspects of behavior, aesthetics, skills, and employment preferences to lateral differences in cerebral functioning. As Arndt and Berger (1978) point out, tests of cognitive mode may be quite adequate to characterize the individual's general approach to problem solving and his or her relative skill on spatial-holistic tasks compared to verbal-analytic tasks, but it is misleading to use cognitive mode to characterize people as being dominated by one hemisphere or the other.

While it is undoubtedly true that by virtue of cerebral specialization some cognitive processes are primarily controlled by one hemisphere, the other hemisphere is not thereby *incapable* of such activities. Especially in the immature individual the other hemisphere may well take over many of the functions of the damaged specialist hemisphere. When a hemisphere is removed, patients do not suddenly adopt a different cognitive style. The disconnected hemisphere in the commissurotomized patient does not indulge in a newly liberated cognitive style; rather, it adopts the same mental set that the person had before, merely less efficiently if the processing mode of the moment is one for which the other hemisphere is the more specialized. Thus we must distinguish between specialization for cognitive processes and the selection of a cognitive style. There is no systematic evidence that one hemisphere would choose to cope with a task in one style and the other in another. The individual as a whole surely has an idiosyncratic personality or cognitive style that is probably little affected by lateralized hemispheric damage. He or she is merely now less efficient at those functions that were mediated by the now-damaged hemisphere. It is far too simplistic to claim (cf. Ornstein, 1972) that an individual is either characterized by a left hemisphere analytic or right hemisphere holistic cognitive style, or that the individual selects one or the other mental set to solve problems that can be solved in either mode.

Summary and Conclusions

The verbal-nonverbal processing distinction has a long history, independent of laterality research, in intelligence testing and in the dual encoding hypothesis of memory theory. Recently, however, it has been shown that the (nonverbal) minor hemisphere has considerable powers of comprehension. Clinical studies have revealed that unilateral lesions differentially affect space perception, drawing, and block design: Damage to the left hemisphere is associated with inattention to detail, and damage to the right with lack of awareness of overall organization and interrelations between elements. Commissurotomy studies have also revealed a right hemisphere superiority in perceiving relationships between components and the nature of the total configuration, and a left hemisphere superiority in using an analytic strategy to recognize patterns.

Such considerations have led to a distinction between detailed analytic processing on the one hand and immediate holistic, global, or gestalt apprehension on the other. However, a certain "slipperiness" is associated with the definitions of these terms, and other related distinctions have been made, for example, Semmes's focal-diffuse and the serial-parallel processing distinction. Since analytic breakdown of a configuration into its components may be performed by either a serial or a parallel process, the serial-parallel distinction may be viewed at best as a less than satisfactory version of the analytic-holistic dichotomy. Holistic or gestalt perception may be seen as the more immediate and possibly more primitive mode of apprehension, of the whole configuration, and of the pattern of interrelationships between, and otherwise independent of, the component parts. Like the verbal-nonverbal distinction, the analytic-holistic distinction has also long been made independently of laterality research in the contexts of pattern recognition, listening to music, and modes of thought.

The distinction gains further support from findings of a LVF superiority in the recognition of faces and complex configurations, which gives way to a RVF superiority when the discrimination is difficult and a single critical feature has to be isolated. A LVF superiority is typically found for rapid global identity matching, and a RVF superiority for slower, serial, analytic, difference detection. In the auditory modality a LEA may occur for simple judgments of the acoustic properties of a stimulus and for the perception of pitch, harmony, timbre and intensity, but musical functions are not lateralized *per se* to the right hemisphere. Many aspects of music may be mediated by the left hemisphere, especially the more complex, rhythmic, and time-dependent aspects. The empirical outcome often will depend on *how* a subject *listens* to a piece, which in turn may depend on musical expertise. Nonmusicians who tend to focus on the overall melodic contour show a LEA in musical recognition tasks; musicians who perceive a melody as an articulated set of elements show a REA. These findings are not universally accepted, and some believe that other related factors, such as the ability to transcribe music, musical aptitude, or the general way attention is paid to the piece, may be more important.

In studies employing both clinical patients and normal subjects, a large REA (left hemisphere superiority) is typically found for the discrimination of duration, temporal order, sequencing, and rhythm, leading to the suggestion that there is a fundamental left hemisphere capacity for discriminating between rapidly changing acoustic signals, and that this capacity underlies the traditional verbal superiority of the left hemisphere. Similar studies of normal subjects, brain-damaged individuals, and dyslexic and dysphasic children have demonstrated an important left hemisphere superiority in controlling fine, sequential, manipulative movements of the limbs, hands, fingers, and articulators, in terms of kinesthetic control towards internalized representations of sequential target positions. Although the right hemisphere may be responsible for an awareness of spatial interrelationships, the left organizes movement into correct sequences. Such considerations may account for the fact that motor sequential or segmental aspects may be more strongly lateralized than the perceptual, particularly if they are the more fundamental.

If language mediation by the left hemisphere depends ultimately on its analytic, segmental capacities and if the superiorities of the right are simpler, less specialized, more primitive, and gained by default, there may be no true dichotomy of function. This may mean that RVF superiorities and REAs with verbal stimuli are not due to a specialized language processor in the left hemisphere but depend instead on that hemisphere's having to operate, with such stimuli, in a certain processing mode. Alternatively, the prior possession of such a processing mode may have "attracted" language mechanisms to the left hemisphere early in phylogenetic evolution or possibly even in ontogenetic development.

Still in dispute is whether there is a species-specific processor for speech in the left hemisphere, and whether there is something special about the perception of the encoded aspects of the speech signal. Some would argue that speech analysis by the left hemisphere is merely part of a more general system for segmenting the sequential acoustic input. Clinicians tend to favor the old material-specific hypothesis, but some experimentalists claim that there is nothing special about speech perception. We ourselves feel that the verbal–nonverbal distinction is commendable for its simplicity and convenience, and we shall continue to employ it wherever appropriate, for much of the rest of this book; however, it is not the most fundamental distinction. Moreover with respect to all distinctions—the verbal–nonverbal, the analytic–holistic, and the possibly parent capacity of the left hemisphere to mediate sequential, segmental processing—interhemispheric differences are relative, quantitative, and a matter of degree rather than qualitative or absolute. Apparent absolute superiorities in the clinical literature may stem from interhemispheric inhibitory influences.

Such considerations open up a series of evolutionary questions. Why is there a predominantly contralateral pattern of sensorimotor representation in vertebrates? Locomoting animals are likely to require left–right symmetry to avoid turning biases and hemineglect. Does this mean that asymmetries are more likely to occur for cognitive than for perceptual functions? What is the advantage of cognitive and motor asymmetry in humans? Does it avoid redundant duplication of functions in a limited processing space? Does it keep the two modes of thought isolated and independent? (Why should *inter*hemispheric separation achieve this any better than *intra*hemispheric?) Does hemispheric asymmetry avoid competition for the unpaired speech musculature? Does it permit a division of labor between the hands? Does it permit us to perform mirror-image *discriminations,* unlike laterally unspecialized animals, who make do with mirror-image *generalization?* Why is our lateralization relatively so weak, able to be demonstrated only with relatively complex cognitive or motor tasks? Is it because underlying biochemical asymmetries themselves are weak? Or does it provide an emergency back-up system in the event of injury to the preferred processor?

If lateralization is too strong, are there *costs,* such as cognitive inflexibility, a reduction in interhemispheric cooperation, turning biases, and hemineglect? Are such costs potentially less serious for predators, and hence for humans, who are the supreme predators and the strongest lateralized? Are there *benefits,* such as reduced cognitive "crowding," competition, and interference? Does *society* benefit if composed of a mixture of the strongly and weakly lateralized? Why is the human *population* lateralized? Because of its constituent individuals' underlying biochemical asymmetries? If so, why is handedness partially heritable only in humans, and why are nonhuman populations not also lateralized? Is the human population lateralized to permit shared tool use? Does that mean that tool use antedates language?

We believe that bipedal locomotion freed the hands for both tool use and gestural communication. This form of communication would have been of limited use in darkness, at a distance, or when the hands were otherwise occupied, so facial gestures could have led to the cortical modulation of the previous, apelike, limbically driven grunts of affect, so leading to true speech. Tool use is *almost* unique to humans, humans share gesture with the great apes, and speech is probably unique to humans. Only we possess all three capacities, and it is probably no accident that all three need a single controlling hemisphere for syntactic segmental organization, and all three occupy closely adjacent brain centers.

FURTHER READING

BEVER, T. G. Broca and Lashley were right: Cerebral dominance is an accident of growth. In D. Caplan (Ed.), *Biological studies of mental processing.* Cambridge, Mass.: MIT Press, 1980.

BRADSHAW, J. L., & NETTLETON, N. C. The nature of hemispheric specialization in man. *Behavioral and Brain Sciences,* 1981, *4,* 51–91.

HEWES, G. W. Language origin theories. In D. M. Rumbaugh (Ed.), *Language learning by a chimpanzee: The Lana project*. New York: Academic Press, 1977.

MORAIS, J. The two sides of cognition. Paper presented at the C.N.R.S. Conference, Paris, June 15–18, 1980.

MOSCOVITCH, M. Information processing and the cerebral hemispheres. In M. S. Gazzaniga (Ed.), *Handbook of behavioral neurobiology, Vol. 2: Neuropsychology*. New York: Plenum, 1979.

NEBES, R. D. Direct examination of cognitive function in the right and left hemispheres. In M. Kinsbourne (Ed.), *Asymmetrical function of the brain*. Cambridge: Cambridge University Press, 1978.

NOTTEBOHM, F. Origins and mechanisms in the establishment of cerebral dominance. In M. S. Gazzaniga (Ed.), *Handbook of behavioral neurobiology, Vol. 2: Neuropsychology*. New York: Plenum, 1979.

STUDDERT-KENNEDY, M. The beginnings of speech. In G. B. Barlow, K. Immelman, M. Main, & L. Petrinovich (Eds.), *Behavioral development: The Bielefeld interdisciplinary project*. Cambridge: Cambridge University Press, 1980.

TALLAL, P., & SCHWARTZ, J. Temporal processing, speech perception and cerebral asymmetry. *Trends in the Neurosciences*, 1980, *3*, 309–311.

CHAPTER TEN
Handedness: Behavioral and Genetic Accounts

According to Sir Cyril Burt (1937, cited in Harris, 1980a), left-handers "squint, . . . stammer, . . . shuffle and shamble, . . . flounder about like seals out of water. Awkward in the house, and clumsy in their games, they are fumblers and bunglers at whatever they do . . ." (p. 4). In Chapter One we saw how pejorative are many of the appellations applied to sinistrals, not least being *sinistral* itself, with all its connotations. The Italian criminologist Cesare Lombroso in 1903 claimed to find the jails full of left-handers, especially among the swindlers. According to him, in criminals the right lobe "predominates very much more often than in normal persons. While the healthy man thinks and feels with the left lobe, the abnormal wills, and feels more with the right—thinks 'crooked,' as the popular proverb has it" (cited in Harris, 1980a, p. 443). Andrew (1978) still finds that there are more sinistrals and people of deviant lateralization among offenders. On a less somber note, Subirana (1969) bemoans the great variability in lateralization and other neuropsychological and cognitive characteristics and claims that it exists solely to confound and dismay neurologists, and that sinistrals were put on earth to plague and complicate straightforward interpretations of human cortical functioning.

Dextrality in History and Prehistory

Not many other species of animal display reasonably consistent hand, paw, or claw preferences, though among *individuals* paw preferences may be idiosyncratic and strong (see Chapter Two). Certain species of parrot may be our only analogues in this respect. Human dextrality, however, has a long history and prehistory (see Chapter One; Hardyck & Petrinovich, 1977; Hicks & Kinsbourne, 1976a). Hardyck and Petrinovich point out that in the Bible there is not a single honorable reference to the left hand; honors, virtues, and powers are consistently ascribed to the right hand. In Matthew 25, for example, those on the King's right hand will inherit the kingdom of heaven, while those on his left hand will be cast into eternal fire. Coren and Porac (1977) assessed more than 12,000 photographs and reproductions of drawings, paintings, sculptures, tools, and weapons produced over the last 5,000 years, and out of 1,180 scorable instances they found that the right hand was used in 93 percent of cases, regardless of historical era or geographical location. Logically, one should be careful of concluding that this shows that a similar percentage of people prefer, and always have preferred, to use the right hand: Artists may themselves be idiosyncratic and unusual in their *own* hand preferences, as we shall see below, and may tend to reflect their own, possibly nonrepresentative preferences in their art. A painter might choose to represent in *every* instance what is merely a *statistical* preference in reality, rather than consciously or unconsciously matching the frequency of his own representations to that of objective reality.

Going further back into prehistory, most paleolithic tools and weapons seem to have been made by—and for—the right hand (Wilson, 1885; Mortillet, 1890), and a majority of prehistoric handprints are those of dextrals (Uhrbrock, 1973). The profiles of human and animal heads in cave paintings typically tend to face left (Wilson, 1885), a characteristic still evident in the work of modern right-handed artists (left-handed artists find it easier to draw profiles facing right). Likewise Cro-Magnon hand silhouettes are usually of the left hand (i.e., drawn by the right around the left; Magoun, 1966). Earlier still, the stone implements used by Peking man seem to fit the right hand better than the left (Black, Young, Pei, & de Chardin, 1933). Even *Australopithecus* seems to have been predominantly dextral, according to Dart (1949). He reached this conclusion from a forensic analysis of the side of injury to fossil baboon skulls found with the remains of this hominid in circumstances suggesting the baboons were prey.

Eye Dominance, Earedness, Handedness, and Footedness

Lateral dominance is most manifest, and probably strongest, in handedness (Porac & Coren, 1979a). However, it also occurs for foot, eye, and ear preferences in such situations as kicking a ball or stamping on a match (footedness); viewing through a telescope, microscope, or keyhole or sighting along a gun (eyedness); and pressing one or the other ear against a watch to hear a faint tick (earedness). Most of us to varying degrees are preferentially right-sided, but tests may be more or less confounded by the use of the preferred hand in manipulating such objects as telescope, gun, or watch. Preferences (see, e.g., Coren & Porac, 1980b) seem to be strongest for handedness (85 to 95 percent of us are dextrals), followed by footedness (80 percent), eyedness (65 to 70 percent), and earedness (55 to 60 percent). Peters and Petrie (1979) determined the leading leg in the stepping reflex in infants who were the offspring of dextral parents. Even infants as young as seventeen days generally advanced the right leg first. Peters and Petrie noted that in adults the left femur tends to be heavier, being used as a support while the person kicks, mounts, or stamps with the right. However, J. Levy and Levy (1978) found that dextral males have larger right feet and females larger left feet at all ages. They claimed that this relates to the fact that the left hemisphere of girls and the right hemisphere of boys is more developed than the other side of the brain (see Chapter Thirteen). Nevertheless, Pomerantz and Harris (1980) were only partially able to confirm the above findings, the effects being apparent only in their sample for fifteen-year-old boys and eleven-year-old girls (they tested boys and girls at ages seven, eleven, and fifteen years). In any case Vanden-Abeele (1980) argues for a distinction between such indices as footedness and "leggedness," and recommends further distinguishing between three possible uses and activities of our lower limbs:

1. *Posture* (which limb is preferred for load bearing when standing with weight on one leg or when kneeling)
2. *Operant behavior* (kicking, stamping, using a spade)
3. *Locomotion* (stepping forward)

He rightly concludes that the field of foot and leg preference needs clarification.

Turning to eye preference, perhaps the best survey of the field is that of Porac and Coren (1976). They point out that the dominant eye can be defined in a number of possible ways:

1. *Sighting tests:* The eye deliberately chosen to look through or along a microscope, keyhole, rifle, etc.
2. *Unconscious sight test:* The eye that "sees" both a distant view (on which the eyes are focused) and a close object (for example, a pencil held at arm's length between the viewer and the distant view). If the near image seen in one eye were not suppressed, parallax effects would cause the viewer to see two pencils, which does sometimes happen. The dominant eye can be determined by getting the subject to close first one then the other eye while focusing on the distant scene. If the pencil is seen to move when one eye is closed, the closed eye is dominant, since the image of the pencil seen by the other eye would have been suppressed while both eyes were open.
3. *Binocular rivalry tests:* Suppression of one eye in favor of the other occurs when the observer is stereoscopically presented (one item to each eye) with a nonfusable pair of stimuli, such as a grid of horizontal stripes to the left eye and a grid of vertical stripes to the right. Rather than appearing as a combination of the two displays in a single unified stable percept, the two monocular views alternate in consciousness as one suppresses the other, depending partly

on stimulus intensity and pattern aspects; when these are controlled, the pattern in consciousness indicates eye dominance.
4. *Acuity tests:* One eye is usually refractively superior to the other. As a "cause" or manifestation of eye dominance this is unlikely to be systematically or closely related to handedness, or indeed to the other indices.
5. *Motoric efficiency tests:* The dominant eye is the one that shows little or no deviation or phoria during changes in binocular fixation.

Porac and Coren (1976) find correlations between the above measures to be low and believe that all measure more or less different aspects. From a factor analysis they suggest three factors—sighting, sensory, and acuity dominance:

1. *Sighting dominance:* A preference measure, like handedness and footedness. This factor seems to be the best understood and measured. Porac and Coren find that 65 percent of the population are right-eyed, 32 percent left-eyed, and 3 percent show no consistent preference. Males and dextrals appear to be the more consistent, exactly as in measures of *cerebral* asymmetry. However, no clear correlation emerged between this factor and either visual field superiority (in laterality tasks) or hand preference (see also Birkett, 1979). This is perhaps not surprising: While we maintain a largely contralateral motor control of our limbs, the sensory fibers from our eyes are subject to semidecussation. Later, however, Gur and Gur (1977b) did claim an association between handedness and sighting dominance, but only for males.
2. *Sensory dominance:* In situations of ocular rivalry 48 percent of the population were found to be right-eyed, 32 percent left-eyed, and 19 percent ambiocular. Such ocular dominance could possibly serve to inhibit double images of objects before or beyond the point of fixation.
3. *Acuity dominance:* In tests of refractive resolution, eye superiorities were much more evenly distributed, and no clear correlations emerged with the other two factors, as might be expected. However, in their later paper Gur and Gur (1977b) did find an association between eye acuity and sighting dominance, but this time only for females.

When we look at other correlations involving foot, ear, eye, and hand preferences, Peters and Durding (1979) found a positive correlation between hand and foot *performance* (tapping rate) measures: Dextrals were superior with both right limbs and sinistrals with both left, though the effects were smaller in sinistrals. In separate studies, Porac and Coren (1979a), and Porac, Coren, Steiger, and Duncan (1980) found that all four indices (for hand, foot, eye, and ear preferences) intercorrelated; hand and foot had the highest correlation and eye and ear the lowest of all possible pairs. They concluded that there is probably no single causal mechanism to account for all the manifestations of lateral preference of limb and sense organ, and that human laterality is a multidimensional process. Searleman (1980), using a dichotic test with verbal stimuli, found that preferred footedness was the best predictor of language lateralization, compared with handedness, sighting dominance, hand posture used in writing (see the following section), and strength of handedness. Left-footed subjects had the highest incidence of a LEA, perhaps because cultural bias against left-footedness is less than against left-handedness.

Handedness: Preference and Performance

It is not as easy as it might at first seem to determine a person's handedness. The subject is often unaware, until tested, of his or her own ambilaterality, and the ultimate determination often depends largely on the testing instruments, techniques, and criteria employed, as well as the society from which the individual comes. Contemporary estimates of the incidence of sinistrality range from 1 to 30 percent, with a mode of around 10 percent (Hardyck & Petrinovich, 1977) and a higher incidence when less stringent criteria are employed. Writing hand, though relevant only to writing and often correlating poorly with other indices, is one of the most commonly employed criteria (Bakan, 1973; Nebes, 1971b). Self-report is an equally common index (see, e.g., Fennell, Satz, Van Den Abell, Bowers, & Thomas, 1978; J. Levy, 1969; Nebes, 1971b) and is equally suspect. Neither criterion yields information on *consistency* of usage across a variety of tasks (some "sinistrals" may write with the left hand and use the right for practically everything else), and both generally correlate poorly with the other indices to be considered later (Benton, Meyers, & Polder, 1962; Satz, Achenbach, & Fennell, 1967). These criteria essentially dichotomize handedness, whereas it is perhaps better viewed as a continuously distributed function. Three other indices are typically employed:

1. Observation of a subject employing or manipulating asymmetrical tools or instruments (objects that cannot be easily operated by the nonpreferred hand) such as scissors, corkscrews, and golf clubs. Such implements are those that typically give sinistrals the most difficulty and that might therefore impose cultural pressures to conform. With prolonged practice the nonpreferred hand may even become functionally superior to the preferred hand.
2. Assessment by questionnaire (see, e.g., Annett, 1967; Briggs & Nebes, 1975; Crovitz & Zener, 1962; Oldfield, 1971) of a person's preferred hand for such activities as throwing a ball, dealing cards, using a comb, scissors, hammer, and screwdriver, brushing teeth, striking matches, and unscrewing lids from jars.
3. Measurement of performance (for speed and accuracy) when the person engages in certain standardized tasks involving manipulative dexterity, such as Annett's (1970a, b) pegboard task. In this task the subject is timed in moving a row of tightly fitting pegs from one row of holes to another. In another such task (Benton, 1962) subjects are timed in picking up pins with tweezers, placing them in holes, and fitting small metal collars to the pins with the tweezers. The nonpreferred hand typically has the less precise control (Peters, 1980) and sinistrals in general show greater variability and smaller performance differences between hands (Benton, 1962).

Questionnaire methods (which essentially measure consistency of hand *preference*) and performance tasks (which in contrast grade *performance* in terms of degree of relative superiority) are the two most commonly employed "rigorous" criteria, though they may well be measuring two only loosely related entities. Direct comparisons of these two techniques are reported by Annett (1976), Palmer (1974), and Provins and Cunliffe (1972). As Johnstone, Galin, and Herron (1979) point out, different handedness measures probably assess different aspects of a complex construct. They found that the best general "predictor" of handedness was the questionnaire: Speed (in tapping), strength (by dynamometer), and dextrality (pin-and-tweezer task) correlated better with the questionnaire than with each other. The questionnaire best discriminated subjects on EEG and dichotic measures, and writing hand was the poorest discriminator.

However, a number of problems arise with the use of questionnaires. How many items should be incorporated? Should we include highly correlated items (and run the risk of redundancy) or *unrelated* items (which might measure irrelevant attributes)? Should equal weight be given to all items? Does it matter that some objects are differentially used by the sexes (e.g., razors), that some questions are ambiguous (threading a needle can be done by moving the thread to the needle or vice versa)? Do we use a two-point (yes-no, left-right) scale or a many-point scale for graded responses? Is it meaningful simply to sum the results across items and scales, perhaps artificially giving the impression of a continuous distribution and quantitative value? How do we assess reliability and validity? These problems have yet to be resolved. Until such practical problems and techniques for assessing handedness are standardized, it looks as if we shall continue to be faced with a bewildering variety of idiosyncratic techniques and instruments.

The problems, however, are not simply practical. At the theoretical level, given that handedness appears to be (and possibly really is) continuously distributed from left to right, where do we draw the (apparently arbitrary) line between dextral and sinistral? Do we include an intermediate "ambilateral" or "ambidextrous" category? Is the distribution normal or J-shaped, unimodal or bimodal? These questions are discussed at length by McManus (1979), and some of the possible distributions are graphed in Figure 10-1. Thus some questionnaires generate a J-

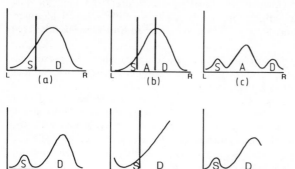

FIGURE 10-1 Possible handedness distributions resulting from questionnaire assessment: unimodal, bimodal, and J-shaped, with various divisions between dextrals and sinistrals.

S - sinistral   ordinate –number of subjects
D - dextral   abscissa –strength of preference
A - ambilateral
L - left
R - right

shaped distribution (e); others generate an almost bimodal distribution (f). Such a bimodal distribution may be asymmetrical, showing a surfeit of *weakly* left-handed subjects over strongly sinistral ones. We shall see later that there is other evidence that sinistrals may also be less strongly lateralized than dextrals, with more variability in their distribution.

Sex Differences and Developmental Aspects

It is often reported (e.g., Loo & Schneider, 1979; Oldfield, 1971) that sinistrality is more common in males than females. However, sinistrals tend to be less strongly lateralized (i.e., more ambidextrous; see, e.g., Carter-Saltzman, 1976; Hicks & Kinsbourne, 1976b; Newcombe, Ratcliff, Carrivick, Hiorns, Harrison, & Gibson, 1975; A. L. Thompson & Marsh, 1976). If so, and this appears to be a consistent finding, it is an interesting departure from the general rule in relation to *cerebral* laterality (see Chapter Eleven) that males are *more* strongly lateralized. As we shall see later, the greater liability to birth pathology in males, or a sex difference in either the way the sexes respond to extremes on a questionnaire or to environmental pressures (e.g., females may be more submissive) could possibly account in part for the greater tendency toward sinistrality in males.

As noted earlier Peters and Petrie (1979) found that the leading leg in the stepping reflex of infants born of dextral parents tends to be the right leg, even as early as the seventeenth day. Ramsay, Campos, and Fenson (1979) observed that infants start to demonstrate handedness in *bimanual* tasks shortly after the first year of life; they wondered whether this relates to the acquisition of language, since both bimanual manipulation and speech require a person to order constituent actions (manual and articulatory acts) into an integrated segmental sequence (cf. the view put forward in Chapter Nine, that the left hemisphere is specialized for analytic segmental processing). Ramsay (personal communication) found that *unimanual* handedness emerged around seven months. Before then, infants touched toys equally often with either hand; thereafter the right hand was preferred. As early as two months, infants typically hold toys longer with the right hand (Caplan & Kinsbourne, 1976; Hawn & Harris, 1979), and for the first few months after birth infants show an asymmetry in their hand position associated with the tonic neck reflex posture, an asymmetry that Coryell and Michel (1978) believe may lead to subsequent manual preferences.

Language Lateralization in Sinistrals

It has been suggested that lateralization in sinistrals may be either less complete or in certain circumstances qualitatively different from that in dextrals. In this section we shall systematically review evidence bearing on this issue.

Anatomical asymmetries of the cortex. Galaburda, LeMay, Kemper, and Geschwind (1978) review much of the work in the field of asymmetries of brain morphology and conclude that these asymmetries are less common in sinistrals, who are also more likely to show weaker or even reversed asymmetries. Witelson (1980) reaches a similar conclusion in her review. However, a recent study by Chui and Damasio (1980), who performed computed tomographic scans of fifty dextrals and twenty-five sinistrals (thirteen of whom were classified as ambidextrous) and who measured frontal and occipital lobe widths, petalia, and the direction of straight sinus deviation (see Chapters Three and Twelve), found that dextrals and nondextrals did not differ in any respect. Regardless of handedness, right frontal petalia was more common than left, left occipital petalia was more common than right, and straight sinus deviation was more common toward the right. Alone perhaps in specifically comparing cortical asymmetries of dextrals and sinistrals, Chui and Damasio conclude that there is no support for the concept of reverse asymmetry or cerebral *symmetry* associated with sinistrality or ambidextrality. Since their study was a comparatively large one, their findings must be recognized, but it is just possible that their technique of *in vivo* computed tomography is for some reason insensitive to such differences, though it was used successfully in this context by LeMay (1977).

Another technique that can inform us, albeit less directly, about brain asymmetries and that has demonstrated differences between dextrals and sinistrals was developed by Carmon and Gombos (1970; see also Chapter Three). They measured systolic blood pressure asymmetries in the ophthalmic artery, as an index of arterial blood pressure to one or the other cerebrum. Dextrals had a higher pressure on the right side; sinistrals showed smaller and less consistent differences. Carmon, Harishanu, Lowinger, and Lavy (1972) also directly measured hemispheric blood volume. Most dextrals showed a greater peak over the right hemisphere; most sinistrals showed the reverse. Using measures of electroencephalographic activity, Butler and Glass (1974b; the EEG asymmetry) and Kutas and Donchin (1974; the evoked potential response) found similar effects.

Clinical studies, the Wada test, and lateralized ECT. Rasmussen and Milner (1977) assessed speech dominance by intracarotid injection of sodium amytal; in 262 patients *without* clinical evidence of early damage to the left hemisphere, they found evidence of left hemisphere language dominance in 96 percent of dextrals and 70 percent of sinistrals; evidence of right hemisphere language in 4 percent of dextrals and 15 percent of sinistrals; and evidence of bilaterality in none of the dextrals and 15 percent of the sinistrals. (They also studied 134 patients with definite clinical evidence of early left hemisphere injury, and obtained similar results, with a shift towards the right hemisphere in all cases.)

Turning to lateralized ECT, McManus (1979) tabulates five studies (from 1970 to 1978) that determined the cerebral speech dominance of dextrals and sinistrals as assessed by unilateral electroconvulsive therapy. Of the 127 dextrals from all five studies, 91 percent had left hemisphere dominance, and of the 48 sinistrals,

71 percent had left hemisphere dominance, figures which are in remarkably and reassuringly close agreement with the Wada test results of Rasmussen and Milner. Since the subjects in these ECT studies were psychiatric patients with no evidence whatsoever of local or lateralized brain damage, they may be regarded as being representative of normal people with respect to language lateralization. In summary then, left hemisphere language dominance is more general than dextrality, and reversed dominance less frequent than sinistrality (Hécaen & Sauguet, 1971).

With respect to clinical records of aphasia, Satz (1979) finds that 70 percent of sinistrals are bilateral for language, 15 percent have right hemisphere language and 15 percent left hemisphere language. While, unfortunately, similar quantitative data obtained under exactly comparable circumstances for dextrals are not available, the general consensus of clinical opinion (see, e.g., Chapter Eight) is that damage to the left hemisphere in dextrals is far more likely to result in aphasia than with sinistrals.

Normal subjects: Dichotic and tachistoscopic studies. As Johnstone et al. (1979) point out, one problem of comparing handedness and cortical organization is that different measures of handedness and of cortical organization are used; for example, dichotic and tachistoscopic indices of cortical organization often correlate poorly (Bryden, 1975; E. B. Fennell, Bowers, & Satz, 1977), either because of noise in the measures or because different aspects of language (e.g., listening vs. reading) are being assessed. Visual and auditory language, and orthographic, phonological, lexical, semantic, and syntactic aspects of language may well be lateralized in different ways, perhaps more so in the case of sinistrals. The general concept of a language hemisphere may be more useful for describing typical dextral males, who show greater evidence of consistent language organization (see Chapter Eleven). A number of reviews (e.g., Hardyck, 1977a; Hicks & Kinsbourne, 1978) show that visual field and ear superiorities are larger with dextrals than with sinistrals. McManus (1979) tabulates ten large-scale studies from 1967 to 1978 that determined the cerebral speech dominance of dextrals and sinistrals as assessed by the dichotic listening task; subject numbers ranged from 22 to 144, with a mean of 70. Of 373 dextrals, an overall average of 81 percent had left hemisphere dominance, and of 328 sinistrals the number dropped to 62 percent. Obviously, these figures are not as extreme as those noted above in connection with the Wada test and lateralized ECT, but it should be noted that these two types of test primarily assess *expressive* speech, which we know (see Chapter Eight) to be more strongly lateralized than comprehension, which is what the dichotic task taps. Again, we cannot directly compare figures with clinical studies since what constitutes aphasia may be interpreted differently by different clinicians, since there has often been time for cerebral reorganization in clinical patients, and since control over the extent of damage is generally impossible to achieve.

Hicks and Kinsbourne (1978) and J. L. Bradshaw (1980a) review other aspects of cognitive and motor performance in normal subjects whereby sinistrals appear to be less, or more variably lateralized for language than dextrals. Tasks included the ability to balance dowels or tap with left or right hand while talking, gesture activity of either hand while talking, the perception of temporal order, and tactile sensitivity of the two hands. Hines, Fennell, Bowers, and Satz (1980) found that sinistrals were more variable in test-retest performance scores on dichotic and tachistoscopic laterality tasks than dextrals. Finally, Rubin and Rubin (1980) found that there were handedness differences in the asymmetry of posed facial expressions: Dextrals were more left-faced; sinistrals showed smaller differences between the two sides.

Generally, therefore, a right hemisphere language contribution is more likely in sinistrals than in dextrals. They have a better prognosis for aphasia after left hemisphere trauma (Hécaen & Sauguet, 1971; Zangwill, 1967) and an increased tendency toward dysphasia after right hemisphere insult, ECT, or amytal injection. However, there is an as yet unresolved debate as to whether all sinistrals are less lateralized (i.e., have more bilateral speech) than dextrals or, alternatively, are as strongly lateralized as dextrals but include a sizable number of individuals with reversed asymmetry. This dispute arises because studies fail to report *absolute* magnitudes of lateral asymmetries (of whatever type) *without* regard to direction. Satz (1980) believes that sinistrals are composed of several subgroups, those largely left hemisphere dominant for language, those largely right hemisphere dominant for language, and a sizable minority who are bilateral. Sex differences (females, see Chapter Eleven, being less lateralized than males) could account for some of the uncertainty (few studies into handedness have attempted adequately to control for sex differences). In three studies where magnitude of asymmetries was assessed, independently of direction, two (J. L. Bradshaw, Nettleton, & Taylor, 1981a; Geffen & Traub, 1979) found that sinistrals were no less lateralized than dextrals in terms of overall magnitude of asymmetries but merely contained more reversing subjects. One (J. L. Bradshaw & Taylor, 1979) did find overall weaker asymmetries in the sinistrals, irrespective of direction. It is perhaps possible that both factors may normally operate, as suggested by the clinical data mentioned earlier.

Other problems to be resolved are whether strength of handedness and sinistrality in the *immediate family* may interact with language lateralization. We shall discuss questions of handedness strength and familial sinistrality in the next section, but it can be concluded that to date no study has adequately controlled all of the variables. Until then (and that will be a major undertaking), the issue must remain largely unresolved.

Strength of Handedness in Dextrals and Sinistrals

Demarest and Demarest (1980) found that, when given dichotic tasks of a verbal nature, strongly sinistral subjects (as judged by magnitude and extent of hand preferences) showed a large LEA, strongly dextral subjects a large REA, and moderate or weak dextrals and sinistrals small or nonsignificant ear differences. As they observe, this finding contradicts that of Dee (1971), who claimed that both strongly dextral and strongly sinistral subjects give REAs, and weakly sinistral subjects give LEAs. Several other studies support the general position of Demarest and Demarest (1980), that the strongly sinistral rely less on the left hemisphere than the weakly sinistral (e.g., A. W. Knox & Boone, 1970; Lishman & McMeekan, 1977; Satz et al., 1967; and Searleman, 1980). On the other hand, two studies (Dee, 1971; Hécaen & Sauguet, 1971) found that the strongly sinistral were like dextrals in relying on left hemisphere language processes, and only the moderate sinistrals were atypical in cerebral organization.

If we can take the view of the majority in this contentious field, it would seem that *strength* of handedness is possibly a more important determinant than its *direction.* Indeed Silverman, Adevai, and McGough (1966) and Thomas and Campos (1978) both claimed that the degree of handedness, irrespective of its direction, determines overall differences in cognitive performance with tasks of a verbal and a visuospatial nature, even with nonlateralized presentations. Such a conclusion is comparable with the observation (see the following section) that genetic influences may determine the degree but not the direction of lateralization (Collins, 1977a; Coren & Porac, 1980b; M. Morgan, 1977). In conclusion, we wonder whether strong or weak lateralization should be associated with superior cognitive performance. On the one hand a high degree of hemispheric asymmetry should avoid some of the problems associated with "crowding" of cognitive functions, mutual interference, and competition, for example, for access to the articulators (see Chapter Nine); on the other hand, weaker lateralization and less asymmetry could possibly permit readier interhemispheric cooperation.

Sinistrality in the Immediate Family
of Dextrals and Sinistrals

Dextrals with sinistrality in the immediate family (i.e., who have a parent or sibling who is sinistral) are often said to have a better prognosis for recovery from aphasia resulting from left hemisphere trauma (Hécaen & Sauguet, 1971; Luria, 1970; Subirana, 1958, 1964) and to experience a relatively higher rate of crossed aphasia (i.e., aphasia in a dextral resulting from right hemisphere trauma: Ettlinger, Jackson, & Zangwill, 1956). In the normal population, reduced asymmetries are often reported in dextrals with familial sinistrality (Andrews, 1977; Gilbert, 1977; Hannay & Malone, 1976; Hines & Satz, 1971, 1974; Kellar & Bever, 1980; Ketterer & Smith, 1977; Lake & Bryden, 1976; McKeever & Gill, 1972b; McKeever, Gill, & Van Deventer, 1975; McKeever & Jackson, 1979; McKeever, Van Deventer, & Suberi, 1973; Springer & Searleman, 1978; Varney & Benton, 1975). A somewhat smaller number of studies (see Searleman, Tweedy, & Springer, 1979, for review) report no effect from the presence of sinistrality in the immediate family of dextrals (J. L. Bradshaw, Nettleton, & Taylor, 1981a; Briggs & Nebes, 1976; Hicks, 1975; Hines & Satz, 1974; McKeever & Van Deventer, 1977a).

However, as pointed out by J. L. Bradshaw et al. (1981a) it may be important to discriminate between sinistrality in the subjects' siblings and in the parents. Whether we are discussing the effect of sinistrality in the immediate family on either dextrals or sinistrals, the problem of family size has never been satisfactorily resolved: A subject with many siblings is inevitably more likely than an only child to have one or more sinistral brothers or sisters. One possible solution is to set a minimum criterial number of exclusively dextral first-degree relatives (e.g., Varney & Benton, 1975). McKeever and Van Deventer (1977a) suggest that second-degree relatives should be included and given suitable weightings, but there is then the increasing problem of validation (even first-degree relatives are usually unavailable for screening). Do we give parents and siblings equal weighting? If a recessive component is found to be important in determining handedness, it becomes necessary to treat two groups of close relatives differently. Moreover, there is the possibility of systematic error in that sinistrals may be more aware of their parents' (or siblings') left-handedness than "normal" dextrals, who conversely may tend to overestimate their parents' dextrality significantly (Porac & Coren, 1979b).

A similar debate has arisen over whether sinistrals with sinistral close relatives ("familial sinistrals") or those without such sinistrality in the immediate family ("nonfamilial sinistrals") are the less lateralized and therefore less like dextrals in their pattern of cerebral organization. Hécaen and Sauguet (1971) found familial left-handers were equally likely to suffer from dyslexia and dysphasia after left *or* right hemisphere damage; sinistrals without left-handed relatives were unlikely to suffer such problems after damage to the right hemisphere. Newcombe and Ratcliff (1973), however, found that among male sinistral patients with right hemisphere lesions the only ones to show symptoms of aphasia had *no* history of left-handedness in the family; sinistrals with right hemisphere lesions and sinistrality in the family were not aphasic. Thus, one clinical study (Hécaen & Sauguet, 1971) finds that the brains of nonfamilial sinistrals more closely resemble those of dextrals than do the brains of familial sinistrals (it should be noted that *strength* of handedness also interacted with their findings); another study (Newcombe & Ratcliff, 1973) found the opposite.

Studies with normal subjects are almost equally divided as to whether familial or nonfamilial sinistrals more closely resemble dextrals. Those showing that left-handers with sinistrality in the immediate family are the least lateralized or the most abnormally lateralized (i.e., the traditional viewpoint) include Gilbert (1977); R. E. Hicks (1975); Hines and Satz (1971); Lishman and McMeekan (1977); Schmuller and Goodman (1979, 1980); Zurif and Bryden (1969). Varney and Benton (1975) found that only familial sinistrals whose *parents* rather than *siblings* were also left-handed showed the pattern of reversed dominance. On the other hand studies showing that nonfamilial sinistrals (whose close relatives are exclusively dextral) are the ones who are abnormally lateralized include J. L. Bradshaw et al. (1981a); J. L. Bradshaw and Taylor (1979); Bryden (1965); Geffen and Traub (1979, 1980); Lake and Bryden (1976); McKeever and Van Deventer (1977a, b); Nilsson, Glencross, and Geffen (1980); Satz et al. (1967); and Warrington and Pratt (1973). Indeed both Bradshaw et al. (1981a) and Nilsson et al. (1980) found that normal lateralization in familial sinistrals occurred with subjects whose parents, rather than siblings, were also sinistral. Obviously, any firm conclusion is as yet premature, though we believe that the more recent studies, which have attempted to control as many of the variables as possible, indicate that *nonfamilial* sinistrals are the more deviant in their lateralization. We cannot simply conclude, as most authors do, that it is the presence of sinistrality in the immediate family that leads to or is associated with abnormal lateralization, whether in dextrals or sinistrals. If it is confirmed that parental sinistrality is a more important determinant of an individual's performance than sibling handedness, then the problem of family size ceases to be an issue, as the number and handedness of an individual's siblings is no longer important. Whether or not abnormal lateralization might stem from the effects of minimal brain pathology will be discussed in a subsequent section.

Determinants and Models of Human Handedness

A vast number of explanations have been proposed to account for patterns of human handedness, ranging from purely environmental factors (inclusive or exclusive of perinatal pathology) to a variety of genetic and nongenetic accounts where inheritance is at least partly implicated.

The environmental learning account. Perhaps the most extreme position was espoused by A. Blau (1946), who argued that sinistrality is learned, that it is a deviation in the learning process that normally leads to dextrality and results from faulty education and emotional negativeness. Collins (1977b) also believes that environmental factors are entirely responsible for swinging handedness one way or the other, but while his account perhaps works well enough for most other species of vertebrates, it cannot easily explain why a *majority* of us in *all* societies continue to be dextral. Few would deny that environmental influences can be very powerful in this context. Thus Provins (1967) acknowledges that *some* degree of inheritance seems to be operating in the transmission of family handedness patterns but since the *potential* skill of the nonpreferred hand can with training approximate or even surpass that of the preferred, he suggests that differential training underlies hand preferences. Such a viewpoint would predict that the incidence and degree of dextrality will change with age. Hicks and Kinsbourne (1976a) review eight studies that do not support such a prediction; however, a number of studies not noted by them do find life-span changes in the incidence and degree of sinistrality (e.g., Annett, 1973; Carter-Saltzman, 1976; Coren & Porac, 1979; Fleminger, Dalton, & Standage, 1977).

Apart from the effects of continued exposure to a right-handed world with all its asymmetrical implements and the possibility that older people may be less inclined to admit or even notice their sinistrality, it is also possible that younger people have been exposed to a less authoritarian and more permissive educational and socialization process. Certainly, authoritarian societies do appear to have fewer sinistrals (Dawson, 1977). This last explanation can also account for the finding (see above) that fewer females are sinistral if they are socially more submissive. Certainly, preferred handedness is markedly affected by such factors as family and cultural preferences, educational practices, and the prevalence of certain types of asymmetrical implements or tools, but it is very doubtful if we can regard this as the whole story. Teng, Lee, Yang, and Chang (1976) found that social pressure in a large Chinese population reduced sinistral writing and eating but had little effect on other activities. Carter-Saltzman (1980) and Hicks and Kinsbourne (1976a) found that handedness was determined biologically, not culturally, in that the hand preferences of offspring correlated significantly with the writing hands of biological but not of foster parents.

Genetic accounts.   It is clear from the two studies just mentioned that there is a heritable component in handedness. This is further demonstrated by the observations of Annett (1973), Chamberlain (1928), Merrell (1957), and Rife (1940), among others, that there are more dextral offspring if both parents are dextral than if one is sinistral, and fewest dextral offspring from two sinistral parents (though even here the frequency is very far from zero). However, the absence of any clear correlation between siblings or even between identical twins poses problems, as we shall see, for any simple genetic account. Although these facts suggest an extrachromosomal explanation, especially perhaps the observation that a child's handedness is determined more by the mother than the father (Corballis & Morgan, 1978), we should also note the observation of Liederman and Kinsbourne (1980a) that rightward head turning in neonates is found only if both parents are dextral and not if the father is sinistral. This instead suggests a genetic rather than an extrachromosomal mechanism. To complicate matters still further, Coren and Porac (1980b) examined hand, foot, eye, and ear preferences in 459 biologically related parent-offspring triads and 434 sibling pairs. On computing correlations for both strength and direction, they found no strong familial patterns for *direction* but did find positive correlations for *strength* of laterality. They conclude that inheritance is probably polygenic, thus accounting for the continuous nature of the various distributions, with no single causal mechanism for lateral preferences of limbs and senses.

Twin studies.   It might be thought that twin studies (a comparison of monozygotic and dizygotic twins) would help resolve some of the issues associated with the genetic inheritance of laterality. However, special factors may operate in twinning, such as an increased danger of pathology from intrauterine crowding and competition for blood supply, which might lead to pathological left-handedness and the reported tendency for monozygotic twins to experience mirror-imaging effects, in which structures derived from the ectoderm (the skin and nervous system) are reversed in one twin. For example, the shape of one twin's left ear may match that of the other's right ear, and mirror-imaging of brain function and handedness is not uncommon. This has led to suggestions that each embryo is derived from opposite lateral halves of an original "parent" embryo that split, each replacing its "missing half" from developmental potential not yet fully committed (see, e.g., Boklage, 1980; Springer & Searleman, 1980). However, according to the mirror-imaging hypothesis, at the very least a majority of monozygotic twins should show opposite handedness instead of the few that do. Second, a "left half" should replace a missing "right half" either with a *normal* right-sided structure, or with something more like the left side, or otherwise anomalous, depending on the remaining uncommitted developmental potential. The same argument should apply to the right half. The left-half embryo would still be left-sided on its left side, and the right half would still be right-sided on its right half. Therefore, we would not get mirror-image pairs; at the most we might find one twin anomolous on one side, and the other twin anomolous (in not necessarily a similar fashion) on the other side. Finally, if the mirror-imaging hypothesis were true, the distribution of handedness in dizygotic twins should be different from that of monozygotic twins, and that is not the case; the two distributions are similar.

Whether for reasons of pathology (fetal crowding, competition, etc.) or of mirror imaging, sinistrality is said to be more common in twins than in singletons (for reviews, see Boklage, 1980; Springer & Searleman, 1980). The general consensus is that the incidence of nondextrality is the same in both monozygotic and dizygotic twins and is twice that of singletons. According to Boklage (1980) even the *parents* of twins, of either zygosity, are twice as often nondextral as are their own same-sexed siblings, suggesting that both nondextrality *and* twinning are caused by the transmission of some kind of developmental instability. But even these conclusions are not universally accepted. McManus (1980) reports that the incidence of sinistrality is the same in twins of both zygosities and in singletons, so that twins are not subject to any special factors that might modify their handedness. The whole issue of twinning is as yet unresolved, though we can conclude that no simple genetic model for the inheritance of handedness can apply, since it would predict both concordance of handedness in monozygotic twins, which manifestly is not the case, and that such concordance would be lower in dizygotic twins, also contrary to the facts. We shall briefly review three genetic models and their associated problems in the following section.

Annett's first model. Annett (1964) proposed that handedness is genetically determined by a dominant (D) and a recessive (r) gene pattern. Dominant homozygotes (DD), who have inherited dominant handedness genes from both parents will be consistently right-handed with left hemisphere language. Recessive homozygotes (rr), who have inherited recessive handedness genes from both parents, will be consistently left-handed with language dominance in the right hemisphere. The heterozygotes (Dr), who have inherited a dominant gene from one parent and a recessive gene from the other will usually be dextral with left hemisphere language dominance, but under certain circumstances they may use either hand or hemisphere. Thus the distribution should be binomial; e.g., in every 100 people $[8^2 + (2 \times 8 \times 2) + 2^2]$ there could be 64 dominant homozygotes, 4 recessive homozygotes, and 32 heterozygotes. However, sinistrals, as we have seen, do *not* usually have right hemisphere language (though the incidence is admittedly higher than in dextrals). Moreover, an even more serious problem is that, according to the model, homozygosity should breed true, with only dextral offspring from fully dextral parents and only sinistral offspring from fully sinistral parents. Unfortunately, Annett's (1973) own data disprove this—84 percent of sinistrals have two dextral parents and 50 percent of children of two sinistral parents are dextrals.

Annett's second model. In this version Annett (1972) views handedness (in humans and other species) as a continuous variable, normally distributed as left, mixed, and right, with the mode *in humans* shifted towards the right hand. Only a small proportion of people at the one end are left-handed and many are mixed. The shift is at least partially genetically determined, with two phenotypes demonstrating the presence (RS+) and the absence (RS−) of the right shift factor. RS+ virtually ensures left hemisphere language, though right-handedness itself may also be partially determined by environmental factors. RS− subjects have no systematic intrinsic tendency to brain lateralization for either language or handedness; both are determined, probably independently of each other, by environmental factors. Half of them would be left lateralized and half would be right lateralized for either function. Annett appears to assume that RS+ acts like a dominant allele, and RS− as a recessive (Annett, 1978). This model would therefore make the following predictions: The products of matings involving the two dominant alleles (25 percent of the possible outcomes) would be perhaps very strongly dextral. The products of a dominant and a recessive (25 percent) or of a recessive and a dominant mating (again 25 percent) would be dextrals of normal strength and of course constitute 50 percent of the outcomes. The products of matings of the two recessive alleles (again 25 percent) would be split between half (12.5 percent) weakly dextral (by chance) and half (12.5 percent) weakly sinistral (by chance). A total of 87.5 percent of the population would be dextral, and 12.5 percent would be sinistral. These predicted figures (for handedness and language lateralization) at first glance fit the empirical values very nicely, and one can speculate whether there should be advantages or disadvantages in cognitive functioning (verbal and nonverbal) for the possession of the right shift factor in single or double dose. However, the model still does not easily cope with the twin data in particular or sibling handedness in general, since knowledge of a person's handedness tells us very little about that of his or her siblings (Corballis, 1980b). According to Corballis this seems to be a problem for any simple genetic theory.

The Levy-Nagylaki model. J. Levy and Nagylaki (1972) propose a two-gene, four-allele model, which as Hardyck and Petrinovich (1977) point out is undoubtedly the most detailed and comprehensive of the models. It attempts to account for the fact that a knowledge of a person's preferred hand does not, at least in sinistrals, allow us safely to predict his or her language hemisphere. According to the account, one gene locus determines the hemisphere that is dominant for language; the other determines whether the dominant hemisphere controls the ipsilateral or contralateral hand for writing and other fine, skilled, sequential movements via the uncrossed or crossed pyramidal motor tracts. (J. Levy & Reid, 1976, 1978, cite studies that found that there are individual differences in the pyramidal decussation pathways, and that maybe 5 percent of us have more fibers in the uncrossed than in the crossed tracts, and a few have no decussation at all. The pathway with the greater number of fibers would then be the more important with respect to hand preference.)

According to Corballis and Morgan (1978) the model accounts fairly well for the breeding ratios for handedness and for the distribution of people among the four categories of handedness and cerebral lateralization, and for the fact that only a very few dextrals have right hemisphere language. Hudson (1975), however, has critically evaluated the model and argues that it cannot satisfactorily account for all the handedness data (e.g., that parents are usually *less* left-handed than their offspring), and as Corballis and Morgan (1978) observe, there are still the problems associated with the twin and sibling concordances. For psychologists, perhaps the most controversial aspect of the model is its extension (J. Levy & Reid, 1976, 1978), which claims that we can predict the hemisphere that is dominant for language from a knowledge of which hand is employed for writing and how it is held (hooked and inverted or normal). In the normal hand posture (assumed to be controlled via the contralateral motor pathways), the hand is held below the line of writing, the pencil is slanted upward, and the tip points toward the top of the page. In the inverted posture (controlled via the ipsilateral motor route), either the hand or the paper is rotated to bring the hand above the line of writing; the tip of the pencil points towards the bottom of the page. (At this point it should be noted that people do not unambiguously adopt either position: It is often difficult to assign them to one or the other category, judges often disagree, and writers *can* and *do* change posture.) Left-handers writing with a normal (i.e., contralaterally controlled) posture should therefore have right hemisphere language dominance, and sinistrals writing with the inverted (ipsilaterally controlled) posture should have language in the left hemisphere. Most dextrals write with the normal (contralateral, left hemisphere) posture, and very few adopt the inverted (ipsilateral, right-hemisphere language) posture.

J. Levy and Reid (1978) gave two tachistoscopic tests, one verbal and one spatial, to assess the language lateralization of four groups of subjects (dextral and sinistral inverters and noninverters). They claimed that a knowledge of the hand used and its posture correctly predicted (in terms of the results of the tachistoscopic studies) the hemisphere dominant for language. This itself would be surprising, given the well-known inability of such tests to replicate exactly the findings of the Wada test and unilateral ECT studies. (We saw in Chapter Eight that this inability is ascribed to noise in such tools or to the fact that they are assessing the locus of *visual receptive* language functions rather than that of *expressive* speech, which may only loosely intercorrelate.) In any case a number of studies (see, e.g., J. L. Bradshaw, 1980a; Weber & Bradshaw, 1981) have failed to confirm either the theoretical rationale or the empirical predictions of the theory, and we can only conclude that Levy and Reid's conclusions are erroneous and are perhaps based on certain misapprehensions: The inverted posture is probably *not* determined entirely centrally but rather is under at least partial voluntary control and is subject to directional patterns of writing in a person's culture; writing with the hand ipsilateral to the language hemisphere may not necessarily depend on the ipsilateral pathways; the percentage of individuals with predominantly uncrossed ipsilateral pathways probably does *not* match the percentage of inverters; a number of relationships concerning partial agenesis of the corpus callosum and mirror-synkinetic movements postulated in inverters are probably unsupported; and the original Levy-Nagylaki model itself still fails to fully account for the empirical breeding ratios of parents to offspring and between siblings.

Corballis and Morgan's left–right maturational gradient account.   A pervasive idea frequently encountered in this chapter is that genes do not encode *direction* (they are "left–right agnosic"; Corballis & Morgan, 1978) but only the *degree* or *extent* of handedness. With this in mind, and in view of the problems that face any simple genetic account, Corballis and Morgan (1978) propose the idea of a cytoplasmic (i.e., nonnuclear, nongenetic) growth gradient of embryonic and subsequent development. They suggest that this gradient underlies handedness and other left–right asymmetries and is coded in the spatial structure of the oocyte (the precursor of the female germ cell). This growth gradient is therefore intrinsic, derived from the mother, and subject at most to only *indirect* genetic influences—though this point is hotly disputed. It is held to favor the development of the left side of the embryo before the developing embryo's own genes can take over and is said to account for all the recently observed asymmetries in the animal world (see Chapter Two). If the growth-enhanced, left-side member of a pair of structures is removed at an early age, the right side is released from inhibition and may develop almost normally. However, critics (see associated commentaries with the Corballis & Morgan, 1978, paper) claim that there are many exceptions to the left-side rule and condemn the tally-count approach across species. Indeed, there is at the moment really very little evidence for the idea and an embarrassingly large number of exceptions to the postulated left-side superiority in animal structures.

Sinistrality and Pathology

A disproportionate number of sinistrals are found among a number of clinical populations, including mental retardates, epileptics, stutterers, and sufferers from dysarthria, cerebral palsy, developmental aphasia, and dyslexia (for reviews, see Carter-Saltzman, 1979; Hicks & Kinsbourne, 1978; Satz, Baymur, & Van der Vlugt, 1979; Springer & Searleman, 1980). There are even said to be more nondextrals among smokers (Harburg, Feldstein, & Papsdorf, 1978) and criminals (Andrew,

1978)! Sinistrality is also said to be more common among the first- or late-born, those born of very young or old mothers, twins (though see our earlier discussion on this), males (who are larger at birth), and those known to be the products of complicated pregnancies. Consequently, the claim is sometimes made (Bakan, 1971, 1977; Bakan, Dibb, & Reed, 1973) that sinistrality stems largely or even entirely from birth stress. Bakan and his coworkers report an increased incidence of birth trauma (in terms of being born first or fourth or later, when complications are commoner) in sinistrals and also in their families. He suggests that sinistrality runs in families as a sequel to an increased risk of birth trauma, the latter being what is inherited. However, a considerable number of studies (Bakketeig & Hoffman, 1979; R. A. Hicks, Elliott, Garbesi, & Martin, 1979; Hicks, Pellegrini, & Evans, 1978; R. A. Hicks, Pellegrini, Evans, & Moore, 1979; Hubbard, 1971; Tan & Nettleton, 1980; Teng et al., 1976; M. Schwartz, 1977; see also Annett & Ockwell, 1980) have been quite unable to confirm the correlations between birth rank and sinistrality that Bakan claims to find, though the general question of some form of birthstress being a contributory cause of sinistrality must remain open.

Satz (1973) argues that there are two groups of sinistrals, natural sinistrals (who will tend to have sinistrality in the family) and pathological sinistrals (whose sinistrality is associated with a number of possible birth stressors and who come from a largely dextral family). For similar reasons, there should also be a small number of *pathological dextrals,* natural sinistrals who for reason of birth stress have become dextral. It is of course very difficult adequately to ascertain the occurrence of birth stress. One can place an ascending order of reliability on self-reports, reports of parents, reports of physicians, and hospital records, but even then the events are long past, different specialists will have different criteria for what constitutes birth stress, and a sinistral (or the parents or physician) may be sensitized to detect birth stress as a possible explanation for sinistrality where none really existed. There is some evidence (Coren & Porac, 1980a) that maternal age may predict nondextrality and also that there may be a higher incidence of Rh incompatibility between mother and child in the case of sinistrals (Kocel, 1977). McManus (1979) constructed perhaps the most ambitious of all questionnaires for assessing the risk from ante-, peri- and postnatal complications; he reported results from two moderately large retrospective studies and one very large prospective study of the possible relation between birth complications and subsequent left-handedness. None of his studies produced any substantial evidence for a relationship between birth stress and left-handedness. Annett and Ockwell (1980) also conclude from their study that pathology of the left hemisphere due to birth stress is not a major determinant of sinistrality. In addition, they found that the children of sinistral mothers were not more likely to report birth stress than children of dextral mothers. They even speculate whether increased experience of birth stress could possibly be a result rather than a cause of potential sinistrality. They cite evidence by Churchill, Igna, and Senf (1962) that fetuses that later turned out to be sinistral had adopted disadvantageous fetal positions.

Sinistrality and Cognitive Performance

We have seen that direct evidence linking sinistrality and birth stress is at best tenuous. Indirect support would be adduced if it could be shown that a population of otherwise apparently normal sinistrals was cognitively slightly inferior to dextrals, as a result of very mild, subclinical brain damage around birth. (A distinct hypothesis, which we shall discuss in a moment, is that due to simple differences in cerebral organization such as ambilaterality and crowding, dextrals and sinistrals would differ in their relative verbal and nonverbal processing capacities.) R. E. Hicks and Kinsbourne (1976a, 1978) review a number of studies that do demonstrate such a cognitive deficit in sinistrals, though at least as many (e.g., Hardyck, 1977b; Teng et al., 1979; McBride, Black, Brown, Dolby, Murray, & Thomas, 1979; Newcombe & Ratcliff, 1973) failed to find a deficit. A resolution to this issue is offered by Annett and Turner (1974), who showed that when a large random sample is classified for handedness, and the resultant groups compared, for example, on reading scores, no significant differences emerge. However, if one then looks only at those with very low scores, more sinistrals *do* emerge, a finding that is compatible with Satz's (1973) position that some, but not all, sinistrality is pathological. Confirmation is offered by Bishop (1980), who took an unselected group of preadolescents, tested them on intelligence, reading ability, and manual dexterity, then chose a target group *not* on the basis of sinistrality but on the basis of very poor performance by the nonpreferred hand (i.e., usually but not always the left hand). These subjects were impaired in intelligence and reading, and sinistrals in the target group had a lower incidence of familial sinistrality than other sinistrals, who were not as impaired in performance on the nonpreferred (right) hand. These target-group (nonfamilial) sinistrals were presumably pathological left-handers, perhaps with mild unilateral brain abnormality leading to a depression of contralateral performance, clumsiness, poor cognitive performance, and sinistrality. In two of our own studies (J. L. Bradshaw et al., 1981a; J. L. Bradshaw & Taylor, 1979), we found in a sample of university students that nonfamilial sinistrals performed significantly more poorly on tachistoscopically presented verbal tasks (naming and word–nonword decisions) than either familial sinistrals or dextrals. We must, however, conclude that across the whole population, excluding university students and clinical samples, which between them seem to have attracted an undue degree of research attention to date, there is comparatively little evidence of any obvious deficit in sinistral functioning.

Apart from the birth stress hypothesis per se, it is also possible that a language invasion into right hemisphere processing space (which, to judge by their possibly reduced asymmetries might seem to be more common among both sinistrals and females), might make sinistrals inferior to dextrals on nonverbal tasks and possibly superior on verbal abilities (J. Levy, 1969). (Such a double dose of language, apart from boosting that faculty, could also account for the reportedly higher incidence of stuttering among sinistrals because of hemispheric competition for the unpaired articulators.) Females *are* superior to males verbally, and inferior in nonverbal tasks (see Chapter Eleven). Some empirical support is claimed for the Levy hypothesis, though others have found no differences between handedness groups (for detailed reviews, see Carter-Saltzman, 1979; Swanson, Kinsbourne, & Horn, 1980). Since those reviews were published, O. Johnson & Harley (1980) found that strongly sinistral university students were better on verbal and worse on spatial tasks than strong dextrals. J. L. Bradshaw et al. (1981a) found evidence of a significant nonverbal intelligence deficit among sinistral university students, particularly *familial,* with parental handedness being a better predictor of performance than sibling handedness. Exactly comparable findings in a dichaptic shape discrimination task were reported by Nilsson et al. (1980): very poor performance by *familial* sinistrals, especially when the relationship was one of *parent* rather than *sibling* sinistrality. Such findings suggest that sinistrals have a somewhat different cognitive organization from dextrals, and that both environmental factors (inferior *nonfamilial* sinistral processing on speeded tasks) and genetic factors (inferior *familial* sinistral processing on unspeeded intelligence tests) may operate in sinistrality.

The other side of the coin, however, is the finding that in certain visuospatial or nonverbal auditory tasks sinistrals may be superior to dextrals (Beaumont, 1974; G. Cohen, 1972; Craig, 1980; Deutsch, 1978; Dimond & Beaumont, 1973; Herrman & Van Dyke, 1978; Provins & Jeeves, 1975). Moreover, it is possible that sinistrals are overrepresented in certain nonverbal occupations (art, architecture, music, engineering; see, e.g., Byrne & Sinclair, 1979; Mebert & Michel, 1980; J. M. Peterson, 1979; J. M. Peterson & Lansky, 1974). Some very nonverbal geniuses were sinistral (Leonardo, who also mirror-wrote; Einstein, who was a delayed reader; and Michelangelo). There may be more than one kind of sinistral (strongly or weakly sinistral, familial or nonfamilial, "natural" or pathological), or sinistrals may tend to choose those occupations or become interested in those skills where, in a largely verbal world, any deficit is less apparent or disabling.

In conclusion, though genetic factors are almost certainly important in determining handedness, as yet no satisfactory genetic model has been devised. A polygenic explanation will probably eventually emerge, involving a number of genes, each with relatively small effects on the whole. Many of these genes might influence various aspects of neurological lateralization, either in a strictly deterministic fashion or involving aspects of pathology. Polygenic inheritance would account for the variety of phenotypes observed in the direction and strength of both handedness and cerebral lateralization, and for cognitive and laterality differences between familial and nonfamilial sinistrals and dextrals. Polygenic inheritance is easily modifiable by environmental influences and produces quantitative and continuously distributable functions of the sort typically observed in laterality research, as compared with qualitatively and dichotomously different effects. It is probable that three major types of sinistral will emerge:

1. The environmental pathological
2. The genetic pathological
3. The genetic nonpathological

The first two types will tend to have indications of birth stress and the last two left-handed relatives.

Summary and Conclusions

There is a long historical tradition of denigrating sinistrals for clumsiness and incompetence. The observed preponderance of human dextrality, which is unique in the animal kingdom, has not changed since at least paleolithic days, to judge from an analysis of archeological artifacts.

Laterality effects are strongest and most manifest for handedness, descending through footedness, eye dominance, and ear dominance. However, leggedness and footedness should be distinguished, probably in terms of three possible aspects—posture, operant behavior, and locomotion. A large number of tests assess eye dominance, but all probably measure different aspects, which may reduce to three major factors—sighting dominance (a preference measure), sensory dominance (as in ocular rivalry), and acuity (refractive) dominance. The latter, which is uncorrelated with the others, has the lowest incidence of right-sided superiority.

Weak correlations emerge between hand, foot, eye, and ear dominance; correlations are strongest between the first two and weakest between the last two. No single causal mechanism can account for all of these manifestations of lateral preference, and all may be subject, in varying degrees, to both genetic and environmental influences.

A vast range of testing techniques have been used to assess handedness, which partly accounts for the range of estimates for population sinistrality, the mode being around 10 percent. Writing hand and self-report are two of the most popular techniques, but neither give information on the *consistency* of hand preference and usage, and individuals are often unaware of their own ambilaterality. These two measures may also give the false impression that handedness is dichotomously rather than continuously distributed. Other *preference* measures include observation of how people use tools and implements and questionnaires. *Performance* measures, on the other hand, assess speed and accuracy in tasks stressing manipulative dexterity. In such tasks sinistrals typically show greater variability and smaller performance differences between hands. Although questionnaires are generally thought to be reliable and valid instruments, there is disagreement as to the number, nature, and weighting of the items to be included, the nature of the response (dichotomous or graded), whether the resultant scores should simply be summed, and so on. Such factors can account for the different types of distribution that have been reported—J-shaped, bimodal, normal, asymmetrical, and so on.

Sinistrality is more common in males. Although sinistrals seem to be less lateralized than dextrals, males are generally more lateralized (at least with respect to language processes) than females. Possible explanations could invoke the fact that males are more likely to suffer from birth trauma (though it is disputed whether this is a major cause of sinistrality) as well as sex differences in responses to extremes on questionnaires and to environmental pressures.

Asymmetries in favor of the right leg's leading in stepping reflexes appear within the first three weeks after birth. Infants demonstrate consistent hand superiorities between six months and a year, earlier for bimanual tasks. Asymmetries in brain morphology (which are apparent in fetal life) are weaker, less common, or more likely to be reversed with sinistrals. The same holds true for asymmetries in arterial blood pressure, EEG, and evoked response indices. The Wada (amytal) test, unilateral ECT, and clinical records of the incidence of aphasia after unilateral trauma all give values of around 96 percent left hemisphere language dominance for dextrals, 70 percent for sinistrals. The remaining 4 percent of dextrals and 15 percent of sinistrals are right hemisphere dominant, with the balance (15 percent) of sinistrals appearing to have (*expressive*) language bilaterally distributed. With normal subjects, using dichotic or tachistoscopic measures, which assess the (probably less lateralized) *comprehensional* functions, 80 percent of dextrals and 60 percent of sinistrals are left-lateralized. Again, sinistrals generally show both weaker and more variable effects, and more reversals in dichotic, tachistoscopic, and tactile studies and in dowel-balancing and tapping tasks where concurrent verbal or nonverbal tasks are also presented.

Strength of handedness may possibly be a more important determinant of performance than direction, and genetic influences may determine the degree of lateralization more than its direction. The strongly sinistral may rely less on the left hemisphere for language processing than the weakly sinistral.

Familial sinistrality is an important determinant of performance, but often cannot be easily validated. There is some evidence, though it is disputed, that dextrals with sinistrality in the immediate family have a better prognosis for recovery after left hemisphere trauma, and that they have an increased incidence of crossed aphasia and reduced behavioral asymmetries. Some of the contradictory results may stem from whether the studies assess parents or siblings. Probably only parental influences are important; if so, the vexing problem of family size (there being a greater probability of familial sinistrality with increasing number of siblings) ceases to be an issue. With sinistrals there is also a dispute whether those with or without sinistrality in the immediate family are more likely to suffer from language-related problems after left hemisphere trauma. With the normal population, a majority of recent and well-controlled studies now indicate that *nonfamilial* sinistrals are the least lateralized or the most likely to demonstrate abnormalities of lateralization.

Environmental learning may influence certain aspects of handedness in human populations; it is, however, a critical determinant only in nonhuman vertebrates and certainly cannot explain why dextrality is more common in all human populations. The less authoritarian and more permissive societies have more sinistrals, though cultural pressures may be more important for determining hand usage for writing and eating than for other activities. The importance of biological rather than cultural determinants of handedness is shown by studies of the effects of biological and foster parenting. Other evidence of a heritable contribution comes from the fact that the incidence of dextrality is highest in the offspring of two dextral parents, lower where one parent is nondextral, and lowest where both

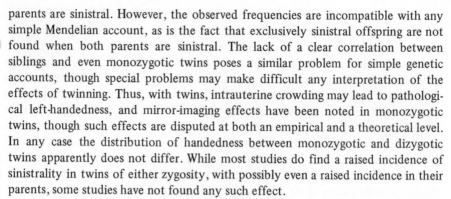

parents are sinistral. However, the observed frequencies are incompatible with any simple Mendelian account, as is the fact that exclusively sinistral offspring are not found when both parents are sinistral. The lack of a clear correlation between siblings and even monozygotic twins poses a similar problem for simple genetic accounts, though special problems may make difficult any interpretation of the effects of twinning. Thus, with twins, intrauterine crowding may lead to pathological left-handedness, and mirror-imaging effects have been noted in monozygotic twins, though such effects are disputed at both an empirical and a theoretical level. In any case the distribution of handedness between monozygotic and dizygotic twins apparently does not differ. While most studies do find a raised incidence of sinistrality in twins of either zygosity, with possibly even a raised incidence in their parents, some studies have not found any such effect.

Annett's first genetic model claimed that a person would be consistently dextral if he or she inherited two dominant genes, one from each parent. A recessive homozygote who inherited recessive handedness genes from both parents would be consistently left-handed with right hemisphere language. However, sinistrals do not usually have right hemisphere language, and homozygosity does not breed true. In her second model Annett argued that handedness is a continuous normally distributed variable with the mode in humans shifted to the right, this shift being genetically determined. The presence of the right-shift factor virtually ensures left hemisphere language, though right-handedness may also be partially determined by environmental factors. The absence of this factor will result in the absence of any systematic tendency to lateralization; chance and environmental factors alone will determine it. Although this model nicely predicts the observed frequencies of dextrality and sinistrality, it does not cope with the twin data or sibling handedness.

The two-gene, four-allele model of Levy and Nagylaki holds that one gene determines hemispheric language dominance, and the other determines whether the dominant hemisphere controls the ipsilateral or contralateral hand for writing or other skilled sequential movements—that is, whether the crossed or uncrossed pyramidal tracts predominate. While accounting well for breeding ratios, the distribution of handedness, and language dominance, this model still cannot cope with twin and sibling concordance, and contrary to the author's claim, a knowledge of writing-hand posture does not and cannot accurately predict language lateralization.

According to Corballis and Morgan's maturational gradient account, genes are left–right agnosic and do not encode the direction of handedness, only the degree and strength of it. A cytoplasmic growth gradient underlying left–right asymmetries is coded in the spatial structure of the oocyte and so is subject only indirectly to genetic influences. The left side of a developing embryo is favored before the latter's own genes can take over. There are, however, too many interspecific and intraspecific exceptions to the left-side rule.

A disproportionate number of sinistrals is found in clinical populations, and, it is said, among first-born or late-born children, children of very young or old mothers, twins, males, offspring of complicated pregnancies, and so on, suggesting an association between sinistrality and birth stress. On the other hand, sinistrality may run in families because of an inherited high risk of birth trauma. However, many have been unable to confirm the above correlations. It is possible that sinistrality may arise from at least two groups of causes, natural and pathological, that pathological dextrality may also occur, and that pathology of the left hemisphere due to birth stress is not a major determinant of left-handedness. Although there is some (disputed) evidence of a cognitive deficit in sinistrals, it may be most prominent at the bottom end of the ability distribution. In addition to the pathology explanation, sinistrals may have a cognitive deficit stemming from a language invasion of right hemisphere processing space. There is some evidence of a visuospatial inferiority in sinistrals, but there is also evidence of a sinistral superiority in certain nonverbal auditory tasks and a possible overrepresentation of sinistrals in certain artistic occupations, though this may be due to sinistrals' avoiding occupations where verbal skills are at a premium. If sinistrals do possess a "double dose" of language, the evidence generally points to its being to their *disadvantage.*

In conclusion, no satisfactory genetic explanation has been devised to account for the heritability of handedness. A polygenic explanation, with effects that are easily modifiable by environmental influences, is probably called for.

FURTHER READING

CORBALLIS, M. C., & MORGAN, M. J. On the biological basis of human laterality. *Behavioral and Brain Sciences,* 1978, *2,* 261–336.

HARDYCK, C. A model of individual differences in hemispheric functioning. In H. Whitaker & H. A. Whitaker (Eds.), *Studies in neurolinguistics* (Vol. 3). New York: Academic Press, 1977.

HARDYCK, C., & PETRINOVICH, L. F. Left handedness. *Psychological Bulletin,* 1977, *84,* 385–404.

HERRON, J. (Ed.). *Neuropsychology of left-handedness.* New York: Academic Press, 1980.

PORAC, C., & COREN, S. The dominant eye. *Psychological Bulletin,* 1976, *83,* 880–897.

CHAPTER ELEVEN
Sex Differences in Cognition and Lateralization

A Victorian physician once said, "The tendency to symmetry in the two halves of the cerebrum is stronger in women than in men" (Crighton-Browne, 1880, p. 65). It is perhaps a further reflection on the history of medical research in general and the study of sex and laterality differences in particular that the title of the prescient paper was "On the weight of the brain and its component parts in the insane." The main burden of this chapter will be the evidence for reduced asymmetries in females.

In a changing sociopolitical climate, it is probably no coincidence that in the last seven years at least seven major monographs have dealt, wholly or in part, with sex differences in information processing and cognitive performance (Maccoby & Jacklin, 1974; Hutt, 1975; Lloyd & Archer, 1976; J. A. Sherman, 1978; McGee, 1979; Nicholson, 1979; Wittig & Petersen, 1979). However, even earlier Porteus (1965, cited by McGee, 1980) in his review of fifty years' application of the Porteus Maze Test said:

> Someone rather whimsically has remarked that if a visitor from outer space, who was familiar with only asexual reproduction, were to survey the human scene, the subject of his greatest mystification would be the differentiation of the sexes. The obvious outward physical, physiological and mental differences would seem to him tremendous, but when confronted with the observation of temperament, disposition, habits, attitudes, strengths and weaknesses, predispositions or immunities in health, and records of literary, inventive, scientific, and artistic achievement, he would probably conclude that men and women belonged in two distinct species. And being devoid of sexual experience, only the fact that the two species interbred freely might possibly disturb his theory. (Porteus, p. 111)

It is sometimes said, only partly in jest, that the brain is a sex organ. In other vertebrate species, castrated animals given sex hormones appropriate to either their own or the opposite sex frequently display sexual behaviors appropriate to the hormone. Arnold (1980) reviews the evidence for permanent organization or change of neural circuits underlying sexual behaviors by hormones administered at critical developmental periods. Work on the anatomy and morphology of the brains of certain species of song birds shows sex-related differences that are partly amenable to hormonal influence (Nottebohm, 1979; Rogers, 1980), as we saw in Chapter Two. As yet there are very few analogous mammalian findings, perhaps partly because only very recently have either sex differences or left–right differences or an interaction between the two been demonstrated in the human brain. There is some evidence of male rats outperforming females in mazes (Ingle, 1980), of sex differences in asymmetrical turning movements in response to injections of amphetamine (Glick, Schonfeld, & Strumpf, 1980), but that is about all. We certainly cannot claim with McGlone (1980) that the human brain is sexually *dimorphic*, not just for the control of reproductive behavior but also for the mediation of cognitive functions, since, as M. J. Morgan (1980) points out, males and females cannot be discriminated in this way (in terms of either brain morphology or cognitive functioning) like they can by the possession of the appropriate genitalia. Differences in brain structure or cognitive function are merely the effects of sex influences on observed continuous variation; in height, for example, males *on average* tend to be taller than females, but in a given population many females will still be considerably taller than the average male.

Sex Differences in Verbal and Nonverbal Tasks

Although intelligence tests free of sex bias have been constructed, measures of general intelligence have been found by factor analysis to be made up of a constellation of specific abilities, and among these, sex differences have been observed. Specifically, girls tend to score higher on tests of verbal abilities; boys tend to score higher on measures of spatial abilities (Burstein, Bank, & Jarvik, 1980). Moreover, differences tend to be stronger after puberty (Burstein et al., 1980; McGlone, 1980). Tasks evincing male superiority include maze performance, picture assembly and block design tests, mechanical skills, alignment of a rod to the gravitational vertical in the presence of conflicting cues, disembedding figures, mental rotation, point localization, and even chess (see, e.g., Harris, 1978; McGee, 1979; Vandenberg & Kuse, 1979, for reviews). It might be observed that among a plethora of grand masters of chess, there has never been a single grandmistress! Nor, incidentally, in music have there been many or possibly even any women great composers, though there has been no shortage of great players. The same is said to be true of mathematicians (Benbow & Stanley, 1980). On the other hand, females outperform males on certain executive speech tasks such as speed of articulation, fluency, verbal production, and grammar, but possibly not in tests of verbal reasoning (see, e.g.,

Harris, 1977; McGee, 1980; McGlone, 1980). Moreover, females are in general far less susceptible to language-related learning disorders such as developmental dysphasia, developmental dyslexia, stuttering, and infantile autism (Benton, 1975; Hier & Kaplan, 1980; McGee, 1980). Compared to boys, girls speak earlier, develop larger vocabularies, can cope with more complex syntactic forms, articulate more quickly and more clearly, are more fluent, and are better readers (Harris, 1977, 1978).

For various reasons—not, one hopes, just sociopolitical ones—the nature of the male superiority in nonverbal and visuospatial functioning seems to have received more research attention. (For the sake of convenience in this and subsequent chapters we shall continue to employ the verbal–visuospatial dichotomy, which in any case has a long history in the literature of individual differences, rather than any other dichotomy such as the analytic–holistic that might possibly underlie it.) Male superiority in nonverbal and visuospatial functioning may have received greater attention because such superiorities are more diverse and less immediately easy to define, quantify, and observe, though as McGee (1979) notes, male superiority on tasks requiring spatial visualization and spatial orientation is among the most persistent of individual differences in the abilities literature. Although such differences really become manifest at or just before adolescence, right from the beginning boy infants are more inclined to explore; girls tend more to engage in choral activities, socialization, verbal behavior, and stasis. Such elementary differences in patterns of behavior could either be precursors of later-appearing cognitive differences between the sexes or could, possibly via feedback mechanisms, differentially expose and condition the developing children to environments of a predominantly spatial or verbal nature. The latter hypothesis will be considered further in the context of possible environmental explanations for observed sex differences.

On the basis of his review of a number of remarkably uniform factor analytic studies McGee (1979) divides male cognitive superiority into two factors: a spatial visualization factor and a spatial orientation factor (see also Burstein et al., 1980). Spatial visualization essentially involves the ability to manipulate parts of a stimulus configuration while maintaining a mental image of relationships among the parts, for example, the ability to imagine the rotation of a depicted object, the folding or unfolding of flat patterns, the relative changes of position of objects in space, the effects of movements of the internal parts of a configuration. All the various factorial studies agree that spatial visualization involves the ability to mentally manipulate, rotate, twist, or invert a pictorally presented stimulus and to recognize or recall a configuration where there is movement among the internal parts of a configuration or where the object is manipulated in three-dimensional space. Imagery and mathematical ability, especially geometry and algebra, seem to be related to this. (According to Benbow & Stanley, 1980, very substantial sex differences favor boys in mathematical reasoning ability, as opposed to computational competence, in which girls may excel. Their studies showed that this effect could not be ascribed to differential course taking, educational experiences, etc.)

The factor of spatial orientation, on the other hand, involves the perception of the position and configuration of objects in space, generally with the observer as a reference point. It measures the ability to determine relationships between stimuli that differ in their spatial arrangements, to comprehend the arrangement of elements in a stimulus pattern, to recognize an object seen from different angles or in different positions, to perceive spatial patterns accurately, and to remain unconfused by changes in orientation within which a spatial configuration may be presented. McGee (1979) claims that measures of field dependence–independence may be related to the spatial orientation factor as measured by the rod-and-frame and the embedded-figures tests. In the rod-and-frame test, the examinee adjusts a luminous rod to the gravitational vertical in the absence of visual clues other than a luminous frame that surrounds the rod. The frame, the examinee, or both may be tilted. Adult females are said to be more dependent on the field (i.e., influenced by the orientation of the otherwise irrelevant frame) in setting the rod than males. The embedded-figures test requires the examinee to view a simple geometric figure and then identify it within a more complex pattern. Similar tasks involve map reading, maze solving, pattern walking, and tests of sense of direction.

These two factors, the spatial visualization factor (the ability to mentally manipulate a stimulus configuration) and the spatial orientation factor (the perception of the position and configuration of objects in space from the viewpoint of the observer), though independently derived solely within the area of individual differences, are almost identical to the two factors encountered in Chapter Four. There we saw that brain damage produced two broadly distinguishable modes of visuospatial deficit, exactly comparable to those currently under discussion. Such parallelisms in otherwise independent disciplines can only strengthen our belief in the reality of such distinctions.

Heritability of a Spatial Superiority Factor

Familial correlations (between parents and children, between siblings, and between identical and nonidentical twins) suggest that both verbal and spatial abilities may have high levels of heritability, and that while verbal ability may also be influenced by cultural and educational variables, this may be less true of spatial abilities (Vandenberg, 1968; Vandenberg & Kuse, 1979). Prominent among genetic hypotheses on this issue is that of the sex-linked major recessive gene (O'Connor, 1943) on the X chromosome enhancing performance on visuospatial tasks. In all normal persons the twenty-third pair of chromosomes (the sex chromosomes) is designated either XX or XY. In XX the sex is female and in XY male. Because the mother (XX) can endow her child with only an X chromosome, it is the father (XY) who determines the offspring's sex, and a son receives an X chromosome only from his mother. A sex-linked recessive trait, therefore, can be expressed in females (XX) only if present on *both* X chromosomes (i.e., on the X from the father and the X from the mother). However, it can be expressed in *any* male (XY) because there is no dominant counterpart in the absence of a second X chromosome. Thus, if the mother carries the gene for spatial ability on *both* her X chromosomes, then *all* her sons will inevitably express the spatial ability trait. On the other hand, a daughter's second X chromosome, contributed by her father, may or may not bear the spatial ability gene. If it does not, the daughter will not express the spatial ability trait since the trait is recessive. Thus the model predicts that males will more often score highly on spatial tasks than females. On this basis the likely rank orders of correlations (r) in spatial abilities between parents (mother and father) and children (sons and daughters), and between the various sibling pairs can also be calculated. For parent-child correlations, one would expect:

$$r_{\text{father son}} < r_{\text{mother daughter}} < r_{\text{mother son}} = r_{\text{father daughter}}$$

For the sibling correlations, one would expect:

$$r_{\text{son daughter}} < r_{\text{son son}} < r_{\text{daughter daughter}}$$

When the expected and the empirical values were compared, despite some initial support (see Bock & Kolakowski, 1973), the hypothesis failed to be confirmed (DeFries, Johnson, Kuse, McClearn, Polovina, Vandenberg, & Wilson, 1979; Loehlin, Sharan, & Jacobs, 1978; see also Boles, 1980; Burstein et al., 1980; Harris, 1978; McGee, 1979; Vandenberg & Kuse, 1979, for critical reviews). Another problem for the model is Turner's syndrome, a chromosomal abnormality characterized by short stature in a person with the body morphology of a girl. Most of these individuals have a missing sex chromosome, the remaining one always being an X. Thus instead of XX (female) the Turner's syndrome karyotype is XO. If spatial ability is indeed a recessive ability carried on the X chromosome, individuals with Turner's syndrome (XO) should show superior spatial ability in equal proportion to normal males (XY)—that is, more frequently than in normal females (XX)—but they do not; they are usually considerably inferior in spatial performance (though they often have good to excellent verbal abilities). One possible resolution would be to posit a gene for spatial organization located on the Y chromosome; however, this would predict the highest correlation to be between father and son, which is manifestly not the case (Harris, 1978; McGee, 1979; Vandenberg & Kuse, 1979). Another possible resolution would be to invoke the role of sex hormones. Thus in Turner's syndrome, sex hormone levels are grossly disturbed, and if an optimum balance is required for setting into operation the spatial and verbal blueprints for the organization of brain function and the ultimate expression of spatial performance, then we might expect poor spatial performance in such individuals (Harris, 1978). There is indeed some evidence that females who are high and males who are low in the male sex hormone (androgen) score higher on spatial ability tests (see McGee, 1979). While this would support the idea of the need for an optimal (i.e., *intermediate*) level of hormones, the methods of estimating such hormone levels (e.g., gross observation of the body and of primary and secondary sexual characteristics) leave much to be desired, and a clear understanding of a hormonal role is yet to be achieved.

Environmental Influences

We have already seen that research on twins (identical and fraternal) indicates a strong heritable component perhaps particularly for spatial skills, which may be less subject to environmental influences than other skills (see McGee, 1979; Vandenberg & Kuse, 1979). Again, as we have seen, boy infants are more inclined to explore. While this may well be an innately determined factor, it will nevertheless tend to bring them into contact with novel objects, scenes, and experiences, a sort of environmental enrichment that could feed back on preexisting innate tendencies and magnify their effect. Boys may also tend to choose toys and games that sharpen their spatial skills, while girls opt for those activities that enhance their social and verbal skills. These tendencies may then be further strengthened by the expectations and pressures of parents, family, and society. To what extent, then, may we invoke the effects of differential socialization, sex roles, stereotypes, cultural pressures, and expectations in producing these sex differences in cognition? Consistent sex differences often tend to appear only in middle or late childhood, though this could be a maturational or even hormonal effect rather than the result of cumulative exposure to environmental pressures. There is also some evidence that spatial skills in girls may be improved by selective training and nonsexist education; some claim that improvement of this sort will occur, if at all, for both sexes if the opportunity is given, thus maintaining a constant differential (see, e.g., Benbow & Stanley, 1980). Cross-cultural studies (see reviews by Witkin, 1967; Kagan & Kogan, 1970; Vandenberg & Kuse, 1979) suggest that greater sex-related differences on spatial tasks may be found in authoritarian cultures with rigidly defined sex roles that force women to maintain a submissive position. We must conclude, however, that while social and experiential influences and their interaction with the developing nervous system may plausibly account for some sexual variation in overall cognitive performance, nevertheless no compelling environmental arguments have yet been advanced to account for sexual variation in the cerebral representation of verbal and spatial functions.

Sex Differences
in Degree of Cerebral Lateralization

Evidence discussed so far suggests that the sexes differ, probably innately, in verbal and spatial processing abilities: Females outperform males in certain verbal tests, and males outperform females in certain aspects of visuospatial processing. In effect, this double dissociation, which was originally made without reference to the theories and findings of human laterality research, can be regarded in statistical terms as an interaction (i.e., sex by task). We now come to another such interaction, sex by side, whereby the magnitude and possibly the direction of visual field or ear superiorities for verbal and spatial tasks may be found to differ between the sexes. We can ask two questions: To what extent are these two interactions related? Are males apparently more or less lateralized than females? We shall later argue that recently demonstrated sex differences in the nature and extent of cerebral lateralization almost certainly underlie the long-established findings of sex differences in verbal and spatial abilities. With respect to the second question, there are three possible positions, and all three have been proposed at one time or another. Buffery and Gray (1972) argued that females are more lateralized than males. At the height of the debate on sexism Fairweather (1976) claimed that there was no good evidence for sex differences in either degree of lateralization or level of performance in verbal and visuospatial tasks. Lately, data (reviewed by McGee, 1979; McGlone, 1980) have been accumulating that indicate females are less lateralized than males. Evidence for this last position comes from clinical findings that adult females suffer less incapacity and deterioration of language function than males after left hemisphere trauma, and that in children developmental dyslexia and dysphasia, stuttering, and infantile autism (all putatively involving lateralized functions to some extent) are less common in girls. Anatomical and behavioral studies also give evidence that cerebral lateralization is reduced in females.

The position of Buffery and Gray (1972) that females are more lateralized than males was based mainly on developmental data from children. Indeed, as Buffery and Gray themselves point out, sex differences in children are difficult to interpret when an advantage is in favor of girls, since it may always be due to their general maturational advantage over boys. Maturer subjects (girls mature earlier and are more cooperative and tractable than boys) will probably have higher motivation levels and longer attention spans; they will then tend to provide clearer and less noisy data and to give stronger effects. Thus children will tend, artifactually, to appear less lateralized than adults, and boys less than girls. Recent well-controlled developmental studies (see Chapter Twelve) do show that while children are no less lateralized than adults, girls are nevertheless less asymmetrical than boys in visual field and ear superiorities for both verbal and spatial tasks (C. Knox & Kimura, 1970; Witelson, 1976a).

Turning to adults, at the moment fairly undisputed evidence has accrued for the position that females are less lateralized than males in only three research areas: clinical studies, normal studies, and studies of brain anatomy and morphology. Until recently few studies have bothered to keep the sexes apart, or to have equal numbers of both sexes in their studies, or even to control for such factors as age and handedness, which are likely to contaminate any sex effect. Moreover, sex differences themselves tend to be very small and often "merely statistical"; the variability *within* a sex is often larger than the variability *between* the two sexes. Sex differences are often at most an even smaller difference superimposed on a preexisting small laterality difference, especially where visuospatial functions in normal subjects are involved. This is probably because, despite our earlier claim that male visuospatial superiority may possibly be less subject to environmental factors and more under genetic control than female verbal superiority, right hemisphere visuospatial superiorities are generally harder to demonstrate (and the corresponding tasks are harder to isolate in a pure form) than left hemisphere verbal superiorities.

Other problems in interpreting the data stem from the possibility that subjects differ in their attentional and information processing strategies. Thus Bryden (1979, 1980) argues that sex differences may be strongest when subjects are free to interpret attentional and other response aspects as they wish; they are weakest (but we would add by no means nonexistent) when the experimenter exerts stringent control over attentional and response strategies. However, sex effects in the predicted direction still appear in verbal, tachistoscopic reaction-time tasks where alternative (i.e., visuospatial) strategies could hardly occur and would in any case be maladaptive for females if they are indeed deficient in such skills; this argues against Bryden's position. Indeed, the general picture is one of more frequent reversal of asymmetries in females together with a greater tendency towards smaller asymmetries.

McGlone (1980) reviews the clinical studies and finds that while males show big differences in their verbal–nonverbal performance ratio scores, depending on whether they had experienced left or right hemisphere trauma, these differences are much smaller or even nonexistent in females. When the two functions (verbal and nonverbal performance) are examined separately, verbal functions in males appear to be much more exclusively mediated by the left hemisphere; thus left hemisphere lesions have much more serious consequences for language in males than in females, who recover quicker and more completely than males. Females are more likely to be affected in their speech than males after *right* hemisphere lesions. For nonverbal functions, again there is a relatively greater local representation in the right hemisphere for males, but the effects are not as striking as for nonverbal functions. As we noted earlier it is more difficult to demonstrate right hemisphere superiorities anyway, and, as McGlone observes, praxis (i.e., the initiation of overt motor responses) rather than performance at a more purely perceptual level may be important. We shall return to this issue later.

As early as 1880 studies of asymmetry of brain anatomy and morphology showed that differences in weight between the two hemispheres are smaller in females (McGlone, 1980). The shape of the Sylvian fissure is symmetrical in a greater percentage of females. The temporal planum (the superior surface of the temporal lobe posterior to Heschl's gyrus and a major speech area) is less often larger on the left in females (Wada, Clarke, & Hamm, 1975). Left–right asymmetries in the region of the first and second temporal gyri are more common in males than females (Kopp, Michel, Carrier, Biron, & Duvillard, 1977), and according to McGlone (1980) atypical asymmetries in vascular drainage patterns occur more often in females.

Turning to studies on normal subjects, findings on hand preferences are somewhat anomalous with respect to our general thesis that females are rather less later-alized than males, since sinistrality appears to be rather more common among *males,* and dextral females, at least from questionnaires, rate themselves as being more strongly right-handed than dextral males (see Chapter Ten). This, however, as McGlone observes, could be an artifact of females generally tending more than males to endorse extreme items on a questionnaire. In dichotic listening with verbal stimuli, where there are significant sex differences in either the magnitude or direc-tion of ear superiorities, REAs are more often apparent or greater for male than for female subjects. To date, there is no evidence of sex differences in ear effects for nonverbal stimuli. In the visual modality McGlone finds an apparent double disso-ciation: Male subjects show a greater RVF superiority for verbal materials and a greater LVF superiority for nonverbal and face stimuli. Such sex effects appear to be much weaker with nonverbal and face stimuli, just as the visual field effects themselves appear to be weaker with visuospatial than with verbal stimuli.

In more than twenty studies of our own (J. L. Bradshaw, 1980b) involving schematic faces, house fronts, bugs, and other patterns, we found no hint of an interaction with sex. However, these were perceptual tasks, and we wonder whether such an interaction might appear if manual praxis (see above) were somehow incor-porated in the experimental design. In the verbal mode, on the other hand, we have found consistent evidence of reduced or reversed asymmetries in females, usually *early* in an experimental series and only with *nonvocal* responses (i.e., where the subjects perform lexical—word–nonword—or semantic decisions) rather than where they name the stimulus aloud (J. L. Bradshaw & Gates, 1978). Later in the se-quence, or throughout the experiment with vocal responding, we found that fe-males gave RVF superiorities as large as males. To a limited extent, therefore, as a function of level of practice and mode of responding, dextral females resemble sinistral males in demonstrating a verbal contribution from the right hemisphere. We can ask whether the right hemisphere, normally reserved for visuospatial process-ing, has been invaded in females by secondary speech mechanisms acting in a sup-portive or auxiliary capacity for difficult or unfamiliar material where overt naming is not required. It might be the difficulty or unfamiliarity of the response, rather than the use of a vocal or a manual response *per se,* that is the more important factor (see, e.g., Goldberg & Costa, 1981). However, McGlone (1980) observes that females with *right* hemisphere damage showed depressed verbal IQ scores but no dysphasia, thus supporting our suggestion that the right hemisphere in females is involved more for the comprehensional lexical or semantic aspects of speech than for its expression. It is perhaps for this reason that sodium amytal (Wada) tests do not normally demonstrate sex effects; they are really only geared to demonstrate effects on expressive speech. This position contrasts with our earlier observations that a female verbal superiority is generally manifest more in executive (expressive) speech than in tasks involving verbal reasoning. The conflict can perhaps be at least partly resolved if it is determined whether with localized lesions the sexes differ more in one type of aphasia (fluent versus nonfluent) than in the other.

Rate of Maturation, Cerebral Asymmetry,
Developmental Dyslexia, and Language Functions

Waber (1976) argued that differences in verbal and spatial skills may not be due to sex differences *per se* but may instead be related to rate of maturation. Regardless of sex, early-maturing adolescents performed better on tests of verbal than of spatial abilities; late-maturing adolescents showed the opposite pattern and were more lateralized for speech than those who matured early. (This, incidentally, contradicts the claim of Buffery & Gray, 1972, discussed earlier.) Normally, of course, boys mature later than girls. Differences in mental abilities would thus reflect differences in the organization of cortical functions, which in turn would relate to different rates of physical maturation. Boys would establish hemispheric specialization later than girls, and if language normally develops before spatial skills, the delay in late-maturing adolescents in general and in boys in particular would benefit the development of spatial ability. This is said to be the case because in early maturers and girls, the first stages of language development may occur as both the left and then the right hemispheres traverse a critical stage of neural plasticity, leading to a possibly lasting involvement of both hemispheres in language processes, to the detriment of visuospatial processing and the advantage of language skills. Late-maturing adolescents, on the other hand, would have a protracted opportunity to establish language in the left hemisphere. Language would then be limited, remaining in the left hemisphere and not encroaching on the right, which would then be free to excel at nonverbal functioning. Consequently, the prolonged maturation typical of males would ultimately lead to greater lateralization, greater separation of function and spatial (but not verbal) superiority, and a greater opportunity for language malfunction to occur. This would account for the greater incidence in boys of speech-related disorders such as stuttering, developmental aphasia and dyslexia, and infantile autism (Benton, 1975).

In similar vein, Witelson (1976a) found that greater right hemisphere specialization in adolescent boys was associated with superior spatial processing; she also explains dyslexia in boys in terms of bilateral representation of *spatial* (not *verbal*) skills, with partial encroachment on the language hemisphere and an overemphasis (in *Western* scripts) on nonphonological spatial processing mechanisms of a right hemisphere nature (1977b). The earlier maturation and more bilateral representation of verbal and spatial skills in the two hemispheres of girls, resulting in relatively poorer spatial and superior verbal performance than boys, would reduce the opportunity for or risk of serious brain malfunction and, together with a reduced reliance on visuospatial functioning, would result in a reduced predisposition to developmental (and presumably late-acquired or traumatic) dyslexia. Such an explanation is, however, somewhat *ad hoc*. Denckla, Rudel, and Broman (1980) likewise find that strong visuospatial skills are often present in (predominantly male) developmental dyslexics, who are often left-handed and rely heavily on right hemisphere processing at all developmental stages. Other claims that the left hemisphere matures before the right in girls and the right before the left in boys have been made by J. Levy (1976), Harris (1978), and J. A. Sherman (1974). Again, it would be the boys' lag in expressive language development that would facilitate the development of spatial skills; the girls' earlier-developing left hemisphere verbal superiority would orient them toward the use of phonological mechanisms in reading and the use of verbal means of solving (even visuospatial) problems. Such an account would suggest that the exaggerated hemispheric dominance in the male brain would have evolved not to heighten language abilities but rather to protect spatial skills (in the male), which may normally develop later than language in ontogeny. However, the whole issue (of whether lateralization for language and, separately, for spatial functions appears earlier or later in boys or girls, is stronger or weaker, or more or less consistent) is in the last analysis highly confused and contradictory (see, e.g., Waber, 1979). The question of the possible development of lateralization will be dealt with in the next chapter; how this relates to developmental reading disorders will be considered in more detail in Chapter Thirteen. Perhaps the only safe conclusion is that the greater degree of hemispheric specialization in males puts them at greater risk at all ages for the development or occurrence of language disorders, because of the absence of alternative systems in the other hemisphere (see, e.g., Hier & Kaplan, 1980). It also accounts for male visuospatial superiority.

However, a number of empirical and theoretical issues remain to be settled. If an individual is strongly (or weakly) lateralized for one function, is he or she also strongly (or weakly) lateralized for the other? Are the effects constant across modalities (visual, auditory, and tactile) and across tasks (phonological, lexical, and semantic processing of verbal stimuli)? Are individuals superior in the task for which they have strongest (or weakest) asymmetries? If males show greater RVF superiorities than females in a verbal task, are males superior to females for stimuli presented to the RVF, are females superior to males in the LVF, or are both true? If, for example, members of the two sexes were equated for spatial ability, would sex differences in lateralization still appear? Are reduced *behavioral* asymmetries in normal females simply due to better interhemispheric communication in females? If there is a more fundamental processing dichotomy (e.g., analytic–holistic; see Chapter Nine), or a more fundamental left hemisphere specialization for motor sequencing, then might we expect stronger sex differences to appear when these aspects, rather than verbal–visuospatial stimuli, are addressed? Why is there such a difference between the sexes (we have already seen that it is inappropriate to call it a fully-fledged dimorphism)? Is it the remnants of specialized evolutionary adaptations, such as sharper visuospatial skills for males in hunting, territoriality, mate acquisition, tool making and using versus the contrasting requirements for females for food gathering, nurturing, and teaching communicatory skills to offspring (Kolakowski & Malina, 1974)? Many of these questions of course apply, with the appropriate changes, as much to the issue of handedness (Chapter Ten) as they do to sex.

Summary and Conclusions

In nonhuman species many sex-related differences in behavior, brain function, and performance depend on hormonal influences at critical ontogenetic stages. There is currently a resurgence of interest in sex differences in human cognitive and brain functioning. While many of these differences are fairly profound, they are not of the sort or the magnitude to warrant their being described as instances of sexual dimorphism.

Although intelligence tests have been constructed to be free, overall, of sex bias, girls consistently score higher on verbal tasks and lower on visuospatial tasks than boys, especially after puberty. These differences may also be reflected in the distribution of the sexes in certain occupations (e.g., music composition and professional chess), in clinical disorders (developmental dysphasia and dyslexia, stuttering, and autism), in developmental milestones (e.g., learning to speak), and in general behavior in infancy.

Two factors in male visuospatial superiority have been isolated: spatial visualization (the ability to mentally manipulate a stimulus configuration) and spatial orientation (the perception of the position and configuration of objects in space from the observer's viewpoint). These two factors are almost identical to those isolated in studies on the effects of localized brain damage on nonverbal cognitive performance.

According to one hypothesis there may be a sex-linked major recessive gene on the X chromosome whose presence will enhance visuospatial performance. Such enhanced performance will be expressed in females only if the gene is present on *both* X chromosomes; it will be expressed in *any* males since there is no dominant counterpart in the absence of a second X chromosome. However, the empirically obtained rank orders of correlations in spatial abilities between parents and children and between the various sibling pairs are not what the model would predict. Nevertheless, heritable influences are probably stronger for spatial skills and environmental influences for verbal ones.

Male infants tend to explore more, and female infants to socialize more. These effects could feed back into reinforcement from parents and society. Sex differences do appear to be greater in authoritarian cultures with rigidly defined sex roles. However, no compelling environmental arguments have yet been advanced to account for sexual variation in the cerebral representation of verbal and spatial functions.

The sexes differ not only in verbal and nonverbal processing abilities but also in the degree of lateralization. It was first thought, due perhaps to a confounding with the effects of differential rates of maturation in the two sexes, that females were more lateralized than males. It is now known that the reverse is true, though the effects are often small differences superimposed on fairly small baseline laterality effects. Smaller left–right differences in females appear in studies of asymmetries in brain morphology, clinical studies (females being less incapacitated than males after left hemisphere trauma), and studies with normal subjects. Although, paradoxically, males are more often and more strongly left-handed than females, RVF superiorities and REAs for verbal materials are stronger and more consistent with males. Indeed, sex differences are generally easier to demonstrate with verbal materials, just as verbal tasks generate stronger and more consistent asymmetries than nonverbal, visuospatial materials.

Females often show a LVF superiority for lexical decision tasks (but not where vocal naming latencies are measured) early in the task. They resemble sinistral males to some extent in that they demonstrate a verbal contribution from the right hemisphere, suggesting that in females right hemisphere processing areas normally reserved for visuospatial processing have been invaded by secondary speech mechanisms acting in an auxiliary capacity for the *comprehension* of difficult or unfamiliar material. Moreover, females with right hemisphere injury show depressed verbal intelligence scores but no dysphasia. Thus the right hemisphere in females appears to participate more in comprehensional than expressive speech, hence the absence of any apparent effects when it is suppressed by unilateral amytal injection.

It is possible that sex differences in verbal and spatial skills are due to differences in rates of maturation. Early-maturing adolescents (and females generally mature earlier than males) score better on verbal than on spatial tests and are less lateralized. Late maturers might establish hemispheric dominance later, to the advantage of spatial ability if language normally develops before spatial skills. Late maturers (such as boys) would have a protracted opportunity to develop language exclusively in the left hemisphere, without its encroaching on right hemisphere functions; the right would be free to excel at visuospatial capacities. The prolonged maturation typical of males, apart from leading to greater lateralization and separation of function, would also provide a greater opportunity and period of risk for malfunctions to occur in the establishment of verbal functions. Developmental dyslexia in boys could be due to overreliance on late-developing bilaterally represented spatial functions, from which girls are protected due to their earlier-maturing language capacities. However, such ideas, together with the suggestion that exaggerated cerebral asymmetry in the male brain has evolved so as to protect later-developing spatial skills essential for the male role as hunter, are at this stage largely speculative. Nor, as we shall see in the next chapter, is there much evidence for the *development* of lateralization. Nevertheless, the greater degree of hemispheric specialization in males probably does put them at greater risk with respect to disorders of language functions, given the absence of an alternative back-up system in the minor hemisphere, and could account for their visuospatial superiority over females. This perhaps is the only safe conclusion that can be drawn so far. Many issues in the general area of sex differences still await resolution.

FURTHER READING

BRYDEN, M. P. Evidence for sex-related differences in cerebral organization. In M. A. Wittig & A. C. Petersen (Eds.), *Sex-related differences in cognitive functioning: Developmental issues.* New York: Academic Press, 1979.

BURSTEIN, B., BANK, L., & JARVIK, L. F. Sex differences in cognitive functioning: Evidence, determinants, implications. *Human Development,* 1980, *23,* 289–313.

HARRIS, L. J. Sex differences in spatial ability: Possible environmental, genetic and neurological factors. In M. Kinsbourne (Ed.), *Asymmetrical function of the brain.* Cambridge: Cambridge University Press, 1978.

MACCOBY, E., & JACKLIN, C. *The psychology of sex differences.* Stanford, Calif.: Stanford University Press, 1974.

MCGEE, M. G. Human spatial abilities: Psychometric studies and environmental, genetic, hormonal and neurological influences. *Psychological Bulletin,* 1979, *86,* 889–918.

MCGLONE, J. Sex differences in human brain asymmetry: A critical survey. *Behavioral and Brain Sciences,* 1980, *3,* 215–263.

VANDENBERG, S. G., & KUSE, A. R. Spatial ability: A critical review of the sex-linked major gene hypothesis. In M. A. Wittig & A. C. Petersen (Eds.), *Sex-related differences in cognitive functioning: Developmental issues.* New York: Academic Press, 1979.

CHAPTER TWELVE
Developmental Aspects of Lateralization

Hemispheric asymmetry is still widely believed to develop slowly during childhood, with speech not fully lateralized to the left hemisphere until puberty. The two hemispheres are said to initially play an active and more or less equipotential role in verbal processes, at least until language is fully established, with the left gradually assuming functional prepotency, possibly by actively inhibiting the right. Once left hemisphere dominance is complete, the other hemisphere is said to be no longer capable of taking over language functions. These views were initially proposed by Lenneberg (1967) on the basis of studies by Basser (1962) and Zangwill (1960, 1964), among others, who claimed that early damage to either hemisphere was equally disruptive to the development of speech; in either case early damage permitted its ready reestablishment. Other findings compatible with this position were that acquired dysphasia after lesions to the right hemisphere is commoner in children than adults.

In recent years, however, a number of findings have emerged that are incompatible with a strong form of what we might call the equipotentiality theory. These findings can perhaps be grouped into three broad areas: evidence for consistent patterns of head turning in neonates; the onset and development of handedness patterns in infancy; and evidence for an early and more or less unchanging degree of left hemisphere specialization for language in infancy. The last is perhaps the most interesting and important and will be dealt with in the most detail.

Head Turning in Infancy

Turkewitz (1977a) reviews evidence for the assertion that the newborn child is asymmetrical in its response to auditory, tactile, and visual stimulation from the age of 24 hours or earlier. It has a lower right-ear threshold for auditory stimulation and turns more reliably to tactile stimulation on the right side of its face or body. This greater sensitivity does not appear to be due to asymmetrical head positioning (even though for unknown reasons neonates usually lie with heads turned to the right, thus differentially occluding receptors on that side). Nor is it likely to result from asymmetrical muscle tone or posture, since the psychophysical asymmetries persist even after the postural asymmetries have been eliminated. This seems to suggest an initial left hemisphere superiority in responsiveness to simple unimodal *stimuli* (Turkewitz, 1977a, b). This claim, however, is disputed by Liederman and Kinsbourne (1980b), who instead argue that an innate neural *response* asymmetry in the programming of movement is sufficient to account for the findings. Thus, rather than Turkewitz's account based on an asymmetrical sensitivity, these authors prefer a motor hypothesis, a tonic rightward motor bias. Whatever the cause of this asymmetrical head turning in neonates (and the issue as yet is far from resolved), it suggests that the hemispheres are not as completely equipotential at birth as once was thought.

The Onset of Handedness in Infancy

The study of the relative *skill* of the hands at different ages is probably of more direct relevance than studies of hand *preferences,* since skill differentiates better between the hands than preference (see Chapter Ten, and A. W. Young, 1981b). However, for obvious reasons only the latter can be assessed with infants.

G. Young (1977) and Witelson (1977c) review all the older literature on the development of hand preferences in early infancy (e.g., before one year) and conclude that a combination of poor methodology and differences in criteria (e.g., grasp strength, duration of hold, hand first or most often reaching for an object) accounts for the woeful contradictions in this area. Some studies find a right-handed preference in early infancy, and others find the opposite; still others find no difference between the hands. One possible resolution is that in these early months hand preference is subject to differential maturation of the two hemispheres, with first one then the other in ascendancy and with differing maturational rates among subjects. If it is possible to generalize across all the studies reviewed by Witelson (1977c) and G. Young (1977), the general trend seems to be that young infants grasp more with the right hand but reach more with the left hand, if indeed any consistent preferences are shown at all. Right-hand preference, however, does seem to be firmly established by five years of age (Witelson, 1977c) and possibly even by the end of the first year (Ramsay, 1980), when speech is unfolding and expressions with different consonant and vowel sounds across syllables are appearing.

Ramsay found in a *bi*manual manipulation task that the effects are strongest for girls and wondered whether these effects coincide with the period when speech might first depend on the presence of laterally specialized structures. He noted that both bimanual manipulation and speech itself require the ability to order consistent actions (manual and articulatory acts) into an integrated sequence. True *uni*manual handedness may emerge as early as seven months (Ramsay, personal communication), while according to Caplan and Kinsbourne (1976; see also Hawn & Harris, 1979), infants typically hold toys longer with the right hand as early as two months. Caplan and Kinsbourne queried whether this meant preferential attention by the left hemisphere (right hand) or, instead, that the left hand was quicker to "drop the rattle" to be free to undertake new initiatives (i.e., a hidden left-hand preference). Finally, for the first few months of life neonates show an asymmetry in their head position associated with the tonic neck reflex posture, an asymmetry that Coryell and Michel (1978) believe may lead to subsequent manual preferences. Thus there appears to be a correlation between the tendency of a prone neonate to adopt an exceptional left-facing posture (left arm extended and right flexed behind the head—the left tonic reflex posture) and left-handedness at ten years (Gesell & Ames, 1947).

In summary, while there is a suggestion that patterns of hand preference may change with age and may even be subject to developmental processes, this may simply reflect the different ways children learn to pick up and manipulate objects. Perhaps the more difficult the preference test, the less likely it is that any developmental effects will emerge (see, e.g., Annett, 1970b; Ramsay, Campos, & Fenson, 1979), since such tests tap *performance* effects rather than preference per se (A. W. Young, 1981b), and developmental changes in laterality measures are generally not found when performance is measured. Thus studies, where for example children are assessed in moving pegs rapidly on a pegboard or in rhythm tapping, have not generally found any developmental increases in asymmetry with subjects who ranged from three to sixteen years (Knights & Moule, 1967; Annett, 1970b; Denckla, 1973, 1974; Ingram, 1975; Finlayson, 1976; Wolff & Hurwitz, 1976).

Evidence for Left Hemisphere Specialization
for Speech in Early Infancy

The discrimination of speech sounds.   Molfese and Molfese (1979a, b) review a number of converging studies of theirs that demonstrate that children as young as one month can discriminate speech sounds in a manner similar to that shown by adults. In one study (1979a) they employed consonant-vowel syllables differing in the second formant transition, corresponding to /bae/ and /gae/, and they measured the auditory evoked response (AER). They found that in neonates (less than one day old) there are lateralized perceptual mechanisms in the left hemisphere that are sensitive to specific acoustic cues (see also A. E. Davis & Wada, 1977b). In another group of studies also using the AER Molfese and Molfese (1979b) examined the ability of infants from two and a half to five months old to discriminate between speech sounds varying in voice onset time (VOT; one of the cues utilized by adults to discriminate between various voiced and voiceless stop consonants, e.g., /b/ and /p/). They found that their subjects could perform these discriminations, even though they did not demonstrate categorical differentiation like adults, and that there were significant interhemispheric differences. Interestingly, it seems to be a *right* hemisphere mechanism that differentiates voiced from voiceless stop consonants (see also Molfese, 1980, and Chapter Nine), a mechanism that is also sensitive to such cues as steady-state onset asynchronies in nonspeech acoustic stimuli.

Molfese and Molfese also reviewed a number of other studies that demonstrate the ability of infants to discriminate speech sounds. These studies employed AER and other techniques such as high-amplitude sucking (HAS) and heart-rate habituation (HRH), which depend on the differential habituation of a response (nonnutritive sucking or heart rate) to graded stimuli. Thus, for example, Entus (1977) gave two-month-old infants dichotic stimuli contingent on their high-amplitude sucking on a blind nipple. Infants first showed an increase in the rate of sucking, then a decrease with habituation. With speech stimuli, there was a greater recovery (disinhibition) after a stimulus change at the right ear. With nonverbal sounds there was a greater effect after a change at the left ear. Turkewitz (1977b) reports similar results with infants twenty-four hours old, but Vargha-Khadem and Corballis (1979) in two experiments were quite unable to replicate the findings of Entus. Other studies showing the presence of asymmetries at or near birth include A. E. Davis and Wada (1977b; evoked potentials), Crowell, Jones, Kapuniai, and Nakagawa (1973; EEG), and Glanville, Best, and Levenson (1977; heart-rate deceleration in response to the introduction of a contrast stimulus with dichotic presentation of speech sounds).

Morphological asymmetries of the brain in early development. As we said in Chapter Three, there are a number of anatomical asymmetries in the human brain, some or all of which may be present at or even before birth (Chi, Dooling, & Gilles, 1977; LeMay & Geschwind, 1978; Teszner, Tzavaras, Gruner, & Hécaen, 1972; Wada, Clarke, & Hamm, 1975; Witelson & Pallie, 1973). As Witelson (1977c) observes, these left–right asymmetries are strictly only indicative of a preprogrammed bias in structure that may underlie subsequent functional asymmetries and of a potential for eventual language development in the left hemisphere. The presence of anatomical asymmetries at birth does not necessarily indicate asymmetrical neural *functioning* at birth. Similar points are made by Kinsbourne and Hiscock (1977; they argue that the brain is specialized for a function before it can perform such a function) and by Woods (1980), who seeks to distinguish between hemispheric potential for language acquisition and an actual hemispheric role in ongoing language functions. As he observes, the critical test for the potential of a given hemisphere would be the ultimate clinical outcome following loss of the speech areas of the *opposite* hemisphere, while the test for the actual role of a given hemisphere in ongoing speech would be the short-term effect of impairment of language areas in *that* hemisphere itself, always assuming (which, unfortunately, one cannot) that facilitatory and/or inhibitory interhemispheric influences can be discounted. We shall consider this point further in the next section.

Clinical studies: The effect of early brain damage on developing language functions and hemispheric asymmetry. In Chapter Eight we reviewed evidence for language mediation by the minor hemisphere in the event of damage to the speech areas of the dominant hemisphere. The critical aspect for our current discussion is what happens to the development of language and of cerebral asymmetry when such damage occurs prior to the onset of speech. Dennis and Whitaker (1977), Hécaen (1976), and Woods (1980) review their own work and the rest of the clinical literature, and all agree that the incidence of aphasia after damage to the right hemisphere in infancy is far lower than after damage to the left, even though such an incidence (after right hemisphere damage in infancy) might possibly be higher than when similar injuries are incurred in adulthood. Woods (1980), however, in a review of recent aphasia reports, claims that very few instances of aphasia in infancy result from right hemisphere injury. Moreover, Witelson (1977c) argues that the nature of infantile brain damage is likely in any case to be different from what happens to the adult: In the adult, lesions are more likely to be neat surgical ablations or to be discretely localized; in the infant, damage is more likely to be gross, may involve contracoup, and in any case will probably involve the other (left) hemisphere as well. Furthermore, any sort of brain damage in a very young child is likely to produce behavioral consequences in a child's most salient and complex capacity—speech—whether or not the speech mechanisms are themselves directly affected.

Another reason for an apparently raised incidence of expressive speech difficulties in infancy after right hemisphere damage is that comprehensional processes are affected. Comprehension, as we saw in Chapter Eight, may involve the right hemisphere even in adults. This further limitation on an already developmentally limited capacity for social interaction may artificially appear to be an instance of expressive aphasia.

Such arguments can account for apparent instances of temporary aphasia after right hemisphere trauma in infancy, a phenomenon that is rare with adults. However, according to Rasmussen and Milner (1977) an early (*left* hemisphere) lesion that does not modify hand preference is on the whole unlikely to change the side of speech representation (to the right). Rasmussen and Milner used the Wada amytal test on 134 patients with left hemisphere lesions incurred before the age of six (and in most cases perinatally). They found a strong tendency in most subjects, especially dextrals, for the left hemisphere to become and remain speech dominant wherever possible—that is, at least whenever there was still some residual parietotemporal and frontal cortex remaining. They believe that young children so successfully (compared with adults) reestablish speech after left hemisphere trauma not so much by the development of such functions in the minor hemisphere, but rather by *intra*hemispheric reorganization and the recruitment of neighboring cortex. They claim that there is an upward displacement of the posterior speech zone to include a larger area of the parietal cortex by way of compensation.

We can therefore conclude that left hemisphere injury is more likely, even in infancy, to result in (possibly temporary) aphasia and also that recovery therefrom, though "clinically complete" and a consequence of the greater plasticity of the infant brain, is very variable in the time required and usually is *not* in fact complete when sufficiently subtle testing is employed (Dennis, 1980a, b; Dennis & Whitaker, 1976; Woods, 1980). The critical-age concept of Lenneberg (1967) may therefore be an artifact of the methods employed to diagnose aphasia, and the strong form of his equipotentiality hypothesis should be rejected, though at *this* stage of the argument we cannot yet reject the possibility that some of the left-right differences found in infancy may become more pronounced or that new differences may emerge as the child matures and increases his or her cognitive repertoire (Moscovitch, 1977).

Gesture and tapping as indices of early lateralization. We saw in an earlier section that there is little evidence for a developmental increase in lateralization as measured in terms of hand preference or skill. There are, however, other indices involving use of the hands that are perhaps more directly related to cerebral lateralization and language functions. Thus Ingram (1975) found that even three-year-olds gesture more with the right hand than the left while speaking, just like adults with assessed left-hemisphere language dominance (Kimura, 1973b). Similarly, Piazza (1977) and Hiscock and Kinsbourne (1978), in studies of dual task performance where subjects were required to talk while carrying out independent manual tasks (e.g., tapping), found that talking interfered more with right- than with left-hand performance for children as young as three years. Moreover, there was no developmental increase in the laterality effect.

The REA as an index of early lateralization. There is now abundant evidence that under conditions of dichotic listening with verbal stimuli, the right ear is consistently superior to the left by four years of age or earlier. The numerous studies prior to 1978 that demonstrate this are listed and reviewed by Bryden (1979), Bryden and Allard (1978), Witelson (1977c), and A. W. Young (1981b). Does the REA increase or change in magnitude during subsequent development? There appears to be only one study (Grant, 1980) reporting a developmental *decrease* in the REA, though several studies report an increase (e.g., Bryden, 1973; Bryden & Allard, 1978; Satz, Bakker, Teunissen, Goebel, & Van Der Vlugt, 1975; Tomlinson-Keasey, Kelley, & Burton, 1978; Reynolds & Jeeves, 1978; Flanery & Balling, 1979; Galin, Johnstone, Nakell, & Herron, 1979; Yamamoto, 1980). Bryden and Allard (1978) argue that while the REAs may be present from an early age, they

may increase with development, possibly because the processing of stop consonants by the left hemisphere develops slowly, not reaching an adult level until at or
near puberty.

On the other hand even more studies claim the opposite, that there is *no*
developmental increase in magnitude of the REA. Kinsbourne and Hiscock (1977)
and A. W. Young (1981b) make a very strong case in favor of the latter position,
and we ourselves are aware of at least fourteen reports since 1978 that also find
no such developmental increase. Witelson (1976a) employed a nonverbal tactile
analogue to the dichotic listening paradigm; subjects palpated two hidden nonsense
shapes simultaneously and then chose (visually) the correct shape from an array of
alternatives. She found a left-hand superiority in boys from six to thirteen years
old, with no developmental increase in the effect. A. W. Young (1981b) reviews a
number of other tactile studies that have failed to demonstrate any developmental
increase in the laterality effect.

We believe that the evidence for a developmental increase in laterality effects
is very weak. Where it has been found, a number of artifacts in experimental procedures could have been responsible. These studies have used a huge range of techniques, items, lengths of list, intensities, signal-to-noise ratios, degree of channel
balance, rates of presentation, levels of required processing (phonemic or semantic
contrasts, perceptual target detection, or list memorization), and so on. Thus for
some subjects (e.g., older ones) a ceiling effect could have appeared because the
task was too easy; for other subjects (younger ones) a floor effect could have appeared because it was too difficult. Subjects may differ (other than just in age)
in terms of intelligence, education, or motivation. Attentional problems in younger
subjects could lead to greater variance in the results and spuriously nonsignificant
ear differences. Thus Geffen and her colleagues (Geffen, 1976, 1978; Geffen &
Sexton, 1978; Geffen & Wale, 1979; Sexton & Geffen, 1979) found that when
attentional strategies were controlled, there was no variation in the magnitude of
the REA, though the ability to deploy attentional strategies did vary with age, and
this caused apparent REA changes. In addition, the magnitude of the REA may
vary as a function of whether perceptual or memory factors are studied (see Chapter Seven), and perceptual measures, which are known to generate weaker REAs,
tend to be employed with younger children. These and other methodological problems are discussed further by Bryden and Allard (1978), Kinsbourne and Hiscock
(1977), Witelson (1977c), and A. W. Young (1981b).

On the other hand if no REA is apparent in younger subjects, it may not
necessarily mean that they are any less lateralized than older subjects; it may
merely indicate that we are testing for the lateralization of functions that are not
yet fully developed (Porter & Berlin, 1975; Witelson, 1977c). For this reason it
would be pointless to seek RVF superiorities with verbal stimuli in subjects who
have not yet learned to read, though such effects might well appear strong once
they learn to read. It would also be pointless to seek visual field asymmetries among
young subjects who cannot maintain central fixation. When such problems have
been adequately controlled, A. W. Young (1981b) in his comprehensive review finds

no good evidence of a developmental trend for the lateralization of either (visually presented) verbal or visuospatial tasks.

In the general context of the acquisition of new skills, it is interesting to note that, according to Silverberg, Gordon, Pollack, and Bentin (1980), when children first learn to read there is an initial LVF superiority (which possibly reflects a right hemisphere contribution to the preprocessing of difficult, unfamiliar material, cf. J. L. Bradshaw & Gates, 1978; Bryden & Allard, 1976), which later gives way to the "traditional" RVF superiority. Such effects (discussed in detail in Chapter Seven) could account for apparent increases in REAs with development, though this would not mean that lateralization *per se* is becoming more firmly established during ontogeny. One structure, however, that *is* thought to undergo further maturational development during the period in question and that could possibly serve to sharpen REAs through inhibitory influences, is the corpus callosum. According to Hewitt (1962) and Yakovlev and Lecours (1967) its myelination is not complete until puberty (see also Galin, Diamond, & Herron, 1977). During childhood the inferior parietal lobule itself does undergo further development in overall size (Blinkov & Glezer, 1968), dendrite formation, and myelination (Bailey & Von Bonin, 1951; Lecours, 1975).

Finally, we note that in terms of preferred usage, according to Porac, Coren, and Duncan (1980) hand, foot, and eye preferences become more right-sided and ear preferences more left-sided in adults throughout their life span. The authors claim that while this could be partly due to changing attitudes towards left-handedness, such an explanation can only account for a small part of the measured effect. They speculate whether it could be due to covert environmental pressures towards dextrality through continued exposure to right-sided tools, scissors, can openers, car controls, and so on, or due to physiological maturation processes. Although Borad and Goodglass (1980) found no effect of adult aging on the direction or magnitude of the REA, Riege, Mettler, and Williams (1980) did find that the left-hand superiority in tactile memory shows a decline with age.

The Development of Right Hemisphere Visuospatial Functions in the Young

It is not easy to devise tests to demonstrate asymmetries in nonverbal processing with the young. Clinical studies of the effects of right hemisphere lesions are usually performed long after the time of original injury. They can only tell us about right hemisphere performance at the *time of testing,* when normal maturational development, to say nothing of plastic reorganization of function, may have taken place. They cannot tell us much about right hemisphere capacities at the time of injury. Nevertheless, such studies do demonstrate very considerable deficits. With normal subjects, as we saw in Chapter Six, it is generally harder to demonstrate nonverbal LEAs and LVF superiorities than the REAs and RVF superiorities associated with verbal stimuli. This in itself could artifactually make young children appear less lateralized (for visuospatial or "right hemisphere" materials) than older subjects. However, from a review (Witelson, 1977c) of dichotic and tachistoscopic studies across the age range, there appears (just as with verbal materials) to be no real evidence for an increase in right hemisphere lateralization, at least after the age of five. Other experimenters, however, have appealed to differential rates of maturation of the two hemispheres (e.g., Goldman, 1972; Harris, 1978; J. Levy, 1976; J. A. Sherman, 1974), whether in the context of possible explanations of developmental dyslexia (Waber, 1976) or of the recognition of upright or inverted faces (Carey, 1978; Carey & Diamond, 1977). In many such cases the right hemisphere is said to be slower to mature and to be less specialized for a longer period (see Chapter Eleven). On the other hand there are also suggestions in the literature that gyri on the right temporal planum develop earlier (Chi, Dooling, & Gilles, 1977), that infant EEGs may develop earlier on the right side (Carmon, Harishanu, Lowinger, & Lavy, 1972), and that the right hemisphere matures more rapidly than the left on the basis of asymmetries in the site of epileptic disturbances in early childhood (Taylor, 1969). We believe that as yet there is no conclusive evidence one way or the other for a differential rate of hemispheric maturation.

General Conclusions on the Ontogeny of Asymmetry

The hemispheres are not equipotential from the beginning for language development. Nor do behavioral asymmetries increase with age, reaching a maximum at puberty, as Lenneberg (1967) believed, or even at an earlier age such as five or six years (Krashen, 1973b). Krashen reached this conclusion on the basis of his reanalysis of the clinical and the dichotic literature; it seemed to him that the percentage of speech disturbances in children older than five years is the same as in adults, and that only before the age of five did right hemisphere trauma affect speech. This, however, as we saw earlier, could be the result of a general cognitive deficit affecting the only readily available, observable, and measurable aspect of behavior in the repertoire of a child at that developmental stage—speech. A gradual decrease in neural plasticity almost certainly accounts for the fact that recovery of language processes after left hemisphere damage is faster and more complete the earlier the damage occurs (Moscovitch, 1977; Witelson, 1977c; Woods, 1980), though such recovery is never complete. Even in the adult there may be an inverse relationship between age of aphasia onset and extent of ultimate recovery, according to Kertesz and McCabe (1977). However, such a progressive reduction in youthful plasticity has nothing to do with the development of lateralization and probably involves otherwise uncommitted areas of the same hemisphere (Rasmussen & Milner, 1977) as much as takeover of function by the other hemisphere (Hécaen, 1976), though if one hemisphere does lag behind the other in maturation, such interhemispheric takeover may be facilitated.

The infantile hemispherectomy cases indicate that at birth both hemispheres can acquire language, and damage to either hemisphere does not prevent the development of apparently normal speech, though the right hemisphere is never quite as successful as the left. Thereafter, during the years of most rapid development, the left hemisphere plays the active role in speech production and comprehension, and the language potential of the right hemisphere gradually diminishes still further. The left hemisphere becomes firmly committed to speech, and these functions can no longer be crowded out by competing functions displaced from a damaged right hemisphere. On the other hand, the remaining language potential of the right hemisphere shows that it is not *irrevocably* committed to nonlanguage functions, though the transfer of language functions to the right will be at the expense of its non-linguistic capacities (Lansdell, 1969; Teuber, 1974).

By puberty, the potential of the right hemisphere for language acquisition will have diminished to the point where it is capable of mediating little or no propositional speech after left hemispherectomy. This ontogenetic reduction in neural plasticity may possibly be achieved by active suppression by the left hemisphere via the maturing corpus callosum. For this reason it is possible that congenital acallosals have bilateral language representation, in the absence of an inhibitory pathway (but see Chapter Five). One could even argue that lateralization would *decrease* with development in normal children, if it were not for the mutual inhibition of secondary capacities exerted by each hemisphere on the other via the developing commissures. The only way that left hemisphere specialization for language or any other functions may be said to increase is perhaps in the trivial sense that a child's repertoire of asymmetrically organized functions will probably increase during the early years. Conversely, for some skills the extent of asymmetric organization may even decrease as the skills become firmly established and integrated into a child's repertoire (A. W. Young, 1981b). It is even possible, as Witelson (1977c) observes, that environmental factors such as linguistic experience may influence the extent of left hemisphere control. She reviews the evidence for aphasia's being possibly less common in illiterates after left hemisphere damage, for weaker asymmetries among illiterates and the deaf (but see Chapter Eight), and for the idea that extreme language deprivation until puberty may result in subsequent mediation of language processes by the right hemisphere.

Such considerations do not necessarily reopen the question of whether asymmetries develop and increase with maturation. The findings are still compatible with the idea of decreasing neural plasticity, which may in turn be linked to both environmental experience and to the emergence of species-specific mental abilities at certain developmental milestones. Such milestones may include both Lenneberg's (1967) watershed at puberty, which presumably would be hormonally driven, and Krashen's (1973b) milestone at age five to six, when language is firmly established. Recent support for the reality of both these milestones comes from E. Zaidel's (1978b) findings with two selected commissurotomy patients and a third patient who had had a dominant hemispherectomy at the age of ten. With his technique (see Chapter Five) for presenting continuous lateralized visual stimuli to a single hemisphere, thus permitting free ocular scanning, he concluded that some language functions (e.g., syntax and phonology) of the right hemisphere are those of a five-year-old, and others (e.g., vocabulary) are those of someone at puberty. He therefore rejects the idea that the right hemisphere's linguistic competence is equivalent to that of a child of a certain developmental age, or that language development in the right hemisphere follows the sequence of stages of first-language acquisition by the left, in view of the great disparity in the right hemisphere between receptive and expressive speech. He concludes that until the first milestone both hemispheres may develop in parallel with respect to language competence in general and comprehension in particular. Thereafter, the left hemisphere surges ahead for fine motor programming and better control of the speech apparatus; the right progresses at a slower rate for some verbal functions (e.g., reading) and may even regress for others (e.g., expressive speech) as it continues to develop nonverbal functions. Such considerations, however, are still compatible with our own belief that these developmental milestones of E. Zaidel, Krashen, and Lenneberg are simply general *cognitive* developmental milestones and have little to do with the development of lateralization as such, or even with the gradual loss of neural plasticity.

We would therefore conclude that the two hemispheres are probably far from equipotential at birth. Although we cannot prove asymmetrical neural *functioning* at birth, there is plenty of evidence for its *potential.* Nor is there any strong evidence for an increase in lateralization during ontogeny (though this cannot be completely discounted), except perhaps in terms of the developmental unfolding and acquisition of new and more complex cognitive skills that will progressively "slot into" prespecialized asymmetrical structures. Instead, an account in terms of a gradually *decreasing plasticity* in neural functioning, both between and *within* the hemispheres, can account for the findings with clinical patients and normal subjects. This decrease in neural plasticity may possibly be related in some way to differential rates of maturation of the two hemispheres.

Summary and Conclusions

The traditional position on the question of whether lateralization develops was proposed by Lenneberg: Both hemispheres are initially equipotential for language, damage to either can be equally disruptive to the acquisition of speech in children, and lateral dominance develops slowly, reaching a peak at puberty. These views are all currently being questioned.

Morphological asymmetries of the brain are evident at or even before birth, though possibly they merely indicate a preprogrammed bias in structure that underlies subsequently developing functional asymmetries. Neonates show a pronounced asymmetry in their responsiveness to sensory stimulation, with a lower threshold on the right side and a greater tendency to turn to the right. These effects appear to be independent of prior asymmetrical head position. Whether the asymmetry is one of sensory sensitivity or a motor turning bias has not been resolved.

Studies of hand preferences—a weaker index than performance measures, which are inappropriate for testing the very young—have revealed many conflicting findings, often because of poor methodology and criteria. One suggestion is that there are different rates of hemispheric maturation, so that one hemisphere surpasses and then is surpassed by the other, with a wide range of individual differences. Right-handedness is firmly established by five years of age, possibly even within the first year, and may correlate with the unfolding of speech. Findings may depend on whether bimanual or unimanual activities are assessed. There is some evidence of very early asymmetries in holding, reaching, and dropping, though their interpretation and significance is unclear, and of a correlation between asymmetries in head position (associated with the tonic neck reflex posture) and later hand preferences. However, any developmental patterns in hand preference may largely reflect the way the child learns to pick up and manipulate objects. There is no evidence of developmental changes in measures of hand performance; however, such changes cannot be assessed before the age of about three.

There is evidence that at birth lateralized perceptual mechanisms are present for the discrimination of speech sounds, in terms of formant transitions and voice onset time. These have been measured using the auditory evoked response, high-amplitude sucking, and the heart-rate habituation technique.

The incidence of aphasia after right hemisphere damage in infancy is far lower than after damage to the left, contrary to the claims of Lenneberg. Moreover, many potential artifacts can increase the apparent incidence of right hemisphere aphasia in the very young, for example, the nature and extent of infantile brain damage, the limits on the way a child can be tested and can interact with its environment, and the fact that speech may be one of the very few available organized responses in its repertoire. Wada (amytal) tests indicate that early damage to the left hemisphere is unlikely to bring about a right hemisphere takeover of speech, Lenneberg's views to the contrary. The left hemisphere, unless totally removed, is likely to become and remain language dominant, despite often extensive damage. Thus, there is plastic reorganization at an *intra*hemispheric rather than an *inter*hemispheric level, wherever possible. Left hemisphere injury in infancy *does* usually result in some degree of aphasia, though it is usually much more transient than in the adult. Where the damaged left hemisphere cannot perform the plastic reorganization (which is the real key to such recovery), speech so mediated by the right hemisphere and tested years later in adulthood is never quite as complete as left hemisphere speech processes. The residual permanent deficit indicates the limits of early interhemispheric plastic reorganization.

Normal subjects even as young as three years old gesture more frequently with the right hand while speaking and show evidence of greater disruption of right-hand tapping performance than that of the left while engaged in a concurrent verbal task. There is a REA at least by four years of age. Although some studies indicate a developmental increase in this REA, far more fail to do so. There are many possible sources of artifact in such developmental studies; the nature of testing greatly varies between studies, as does the nature of required discriminations. Measures of memory rather than perceptual function are more likely to be used with older children, and perceptual measures have to be used for the younger, despite the possibility that laterality effects are weaker at the purely perceptual level. Ceiling and floor effects can obscure laterality differences. Above all, the ability to direct attention develops with age, and this factor is known to bring about increases in the REA; there is no such developmental REA increase when attentional aspects are controlled. In the visual modality, the very young may be unable or unwilling to maintain fixation on the fixation point. Some functions may not yet have developed in the young, and so may not be in their processing or response repertoire. When novel, unfamiliar, or difficult letters or words are read for the first time, a LVF (right hemisphere) superiority may initially emerge even with adults as a consequence of that hemisphere's involvement in preprocessing and novelty, and the act of reading for the very young is an intrinsically novel, unfamiliar, and difficult task.

It is difficult to devise suitable tests for nonverbal right hemisphere processing in the young. Moreover, even in adults it is normally harder to demonstrate nonverbal right hemisphere superiorities. But even in this area there is no evidence of developmental effects in lateralization. Some claim that the right hemisphere matures more slowly than the left on the basis of behavioral evidence, though other evidence (e.g., anatomical) goes against this. However, there is good anatomical evidence for the continued developmental myelination of the corpus callosum and possibly also the inferior parietal lobule up to puberty.

The hemispheres are therefore not equipotential at birth, and there is no real evidence that asymmetries develop and reach a peak at puberty or even at five years of age. Evidence supporting either position is likely to be artifactual. A developmental decrease in plasticity accounts for better recovery from early aphasia, but this phenomenon is unconnected with the development of lateralization. Later, by puberty, the left hemisphere becomes firmly committed to language, largely as a consequence of loss of neural plasticity. The only sense in which hemispheric specialization may be said to increase is in that a child's repertoire of asymmetrically organized functions will increase as it grows older. These functions may well tend to emerge at certain developmental milestones, such as puberty (which is hormonally driven) and possibly around five years (when language is firmly established). There may well be differential hemispheric development around these (and possibly other) milestones, which may also interact with a general decrease in neural plasticity.

FURTHER READING

BRYDEN, M. P. Evidence for sex differences in cerebral organization. In M. A. Wittig & A. C. Petersen (Eds.), *Sex-related differences in cognitive functioning: Developmental issues*. New York: Academic Press, 1979.

KINSBOURNE, M., & HISCOCK, M. Does cerebral dominance develop? In S. J. Segalowitz & F. A. Gruber (Eds.), *Language development and neurological theory*. New York: Academic Press, 1977.

MOLFESE, D. L., & MOLFESE, V. J. VOT distinctions in infants: Learned or innate? In H. Whitaker & H. A. Whitaker (Eds.), *Studies in neurolinguistics* (Vol. 4). New York: Academic Press, 1979.

MOSCOVITCH, M. The development of lateralization of language functions and its relation to cognitive and linguistic development: A review and some theoretical speculations. In S. J. Segalowitz & F. A. Gruber (Eds.), *Language development and neurological theory.* New York: Academic Press, 1977.

TURKEWITZ, G. The development of lateral differentiation of the human infant. *Annals of the New York Academy of Sciences,* 1977, *299,* 309–317.

WITELSON, S. F. Early hemispheric specialization and interhemispheric plasticity: An empirical and theoretical review. In S. J. Segalowitz & F. A. Gruber (Eds.), *Language development and neurological theory.* New York: Academic Press, 1977.

WOODS, B. T. Observations on the neurological basis for initial language acquisition. In D. Caplan (Ed.), *Biological studies of mental processes.* Cambridge, Mass.: MIT Press, 1980.

YOUNG, A. W. Asymmetry of cerebral hemispheric function during development. In J. W. T. Dickerson & H. McGurk (Eds.), *Brain and behaviour: A developmental perspective.* Glasgow: Blackie, in press.

CHAPTER THIRTEEN
Developmental Dyslexia, Schizophrenia, and Left Hemisphere Dysfunction

There is a reading disability in children that is known by a variety of titles, from word blindness, strephosymbolia, congenital alexia, specific learning disability, specific reading disability, and specific reading retardation to dyslexia, or congenital, specific, or developmental dyslexia (see, e.g., Critchley & Critchley, 1978; Pirozzolo, 1979). It is still not known whether it is a single syndrome or a loose collection of vaguely related disabilities. Few agree on either the condition's definition or on the criteria for distinguishing good and poor readers, with the consequence that there is often a considerable degree of nonhomogeneity in the groups given a particular label. Some (see, e.g., Pirozzolo, 1979) regard the condition as one aspect of the minimal brain dysfunction syndrome, a catch-all term for apparently normal children (without confirmed or obvious neurological, sensory, motivational, or sociocultural deficits) who fail to learn or to progress through the same developmental stages as their agemates. Some of these children may also be hyperkinetic, with or without associated learning disabilities. Benton (1975) reviews in detail the specific condition of reading disability in children (which for convenience we shall now refer to as developmental dyslexia). It is often associated with other developmental deficiencies, "soft" neurological signs, and such difficulties as telling time, naming months and seasons of the year, telling left from right, and so on (see Vellutino, 1978). Recently Ahn, Prichep, John, Baird, Trepetin, and Kay (1980) constructed a set of developmental equations that predict the distribution of the relative power in the delta, theta, alpha, and beta bands of the resting EEG from various scalp locations as a function of children's ages. They found that dyslexic children and those "at risk" for a number of similar dysfunctions demonstrated significant deviations from the normal values for these neurometric equations; in particular, they exhibited an excess of slow waves (delta and theta). However, apart from such findings, the evidence remains at best circumstantial that the syndrome is associated with demonstrable signs of "hard" neurological impairment, and many would stress the normality of developmental dyslexics in other aspects, how they are usually of average or even superior general intelligence (Gaddes, 1980). They are characterized not as being generally dull children, but as being specifically inferior in reading achievements, below what would reasonably be predicted of them on the basis of other information (intelligence, sociocultural background, achievement in other academic areas, and so on). In other words there is a significant disparity between what is expected of them and their actual performance in reading and writing. Such considerations led to the following definition of developmental dyslexia by the World Federation of Neurology in 1968:

> "A disorder manifested by difficulty in learning to read despite conventional instruction, adequate intelligence, and socio-cultural opportunity. It is dependent on fundamental cognitive disabilities which are frequently of constitutional origin." (Critchley, 1970, p. 11)

A problem with such a definition, of course, is that it is essentially *negative*: A child can only be correctly diagnosed as dyslexic if the *negative* conditions are fully satisfied, and this is notoriously difficult.

The Incidence of Developmental Dyslexia

There is disagreement not only on how to characterize the condition but even about its actual incidence. Estimates range from one in five hundred to one in three (Pirozzolo, 1979), and many believe that it affects up to 15 percent of American school children (Naylor, 1980). It is generally far commoner in boys than girls, perhaps in the ratio of four to one (Pirozzolo, 1979; Vellutino, 1978). Witelson (1976a) argues that the bilateral representation of language in females (see Chapter Eleven) may protect them from dyslexia. This is only one of the many possible associations between developmental dyslexia and cerebral asymmetry that we shall discuss, and Witelson's views on this matter will be covered more fully in a later section.

Not only is the incidence of the condition higher in boys, but there is also a strong familial or genetic predisposition to it (Critchley & Critchley, 1978; Gaddes, 1980; Vellutino, 1978). The exact nature of the hereditary influence remains unclear (Pirozzolo, 1979), but there appears to be a higher concordance rate for developmental dyslexia in monozygotic than in dizygotic twins (Bakwin, 1973; Hallgren, 1950; Hermann, 1959), and it may repeatedly crop up in family pedigrees (Finucci, Guthrie, Childs, Abbey, & Childs, 1976).

The Etiology of Developmental Dyslexia

There is still very little known about the likely causes of developmental dyslexia, except that there are probably several. It frequently resolves with maturity (Critchley & Critchley, 1978; Rourke, 1976) though it is uncertain whether this is because the dyslexic has learned to compensate for the condition by employing alternative strategies or even brain areas to mediate the process of reading and writing. Or the condition may resolve because some areas of the brain that are perhaps particularly slow to mature in dyslexics have now reached an adequate level of maturation. This "late maturation" or "physiological immaturity" hypothesis dates from W. P. Morgan (1896) and S. T. Orton (1925, 1937) and still has a wide currency (Bouma & Legein, 1980; Critchley & Critchley, 1978; Pirozzolo, 1979; and Satz, Taylor, Friel, & Fletcher, 1978). From the beginning it was suggested that in dyslexics the angular gyrus and the phylogenetically recent association area interconnecting and integrating visual, auditory, tactile, kinesthetic, and motor regions concerned with language may be undeveloped. This proposal, recently revived by Geschwind (1965), is supported by anatomical findings in that these regions develop slowly in cortical size (Blinkov & Glezer, 1968), dendrite formation (Von Bonin & Bailey, 1961, cited by Jorm, 1979), and myelination (Bailey & Von Bonin, 1951; Lecours, 1975; Selnes, 1974; Yakovlev, 1962; Yakovlev & Lecours, 1967) well into adolescence. Such late maturation could explain why around puberty the condition often suddenly resolves (Pirozzolo, 1979). Other evidence for the involvement of such regions (i.e., in the inferior parietal lobule) comes from the findings (reviewed by Jorm, 1979) of abnormal visual evoked responses from this region with developmental dyslexics.

The Orton Hypothesis

S. T. Orton (1928) made a number of observations on dyslexics: They typically have difficulty discriminating between letters that have a different value when left–right mirror-reversed, for example, b and d, p and q. They tend to confuse reversible words like *was* and *saw,* yet often display unusual ability in reading from a mirror and in producing mirror writing. They are often left-handed males. All this, Orton said, was due to a maturational lag resulting in poorly established cerebral dominance, which caused confusion between the representation of the visual stimulus in the normally dominant hemisphere and a mirror-image (antitropic) engram in the other. The latter would normally be suppressed or "elided" (S. T. Orton, 1925, 1937). According to Orton (1937, 1966) this incomplete cerebral dominance is also apparent as incomplete, mixed, or "crossed" handedness (whereby a person is, for example, right-handed and left-eye dominant); the person also has a tendency to left–right mirror confusion and a poor directional sense.

The essence of Orton's theory is that because the brain is symmetrical, its two halves should record events with opposite left–right orientations; the dominant hemisphere would normally record events in the correct orientation and the minor hemisphere in the reverse. It is not clear, however, why the dominant hemisphere should arbitrarily be credited with recording events in the correct orientation. Nor does it follow, as Corballis and Beale (1976) point out, that the two halves of a symmetrical brain would respond to any given stimulus pattern in mirror-opposite ways, as long as both eyes and both visual fields received and transmitted the perceptual information to the brain. The only circumstance in which the situation envisaged by Orton could arise is where for any reason only one hemisphere receives perceptual information. If that perceptual information is topographically represented in its single hemisphere, and if the interconnecting commissures homotopically join mirror-image points in the two hemispheres, then a *memory* representation of the topographically represented information in the trained hemisphere could, in theory, be mirror-reversed in its transcommissural transfer to the naive hemisphere. While corresponding points in the two cortices may be homotopically interconnected at a level appropriate for the transfer of memory functions, as Corballis and Beale (1976) observe, all the evidence suggests that at the *perceptual* level the commissures linking the visual areas cannot be homotopic but must instead maintain left–right equivalence, so that the individual can maintain continuity of visual processing across the retinal meridian. (According to Starr, 1979, paradoxical or mirror-image-preferred transfer in optic chiasm sectioned monkeys is a consequence of visual field neglect, and not of mirror-image topography in the two cerebral hemispheres.) We can therefore conclude that interhemispheric mirror reversal can occur only, if indeed at all, at the level of memory transfer, and this is the only sense in which Orton's theory can possibly be supported.

We shall see that certain aspects of Orton's theory are sometimes said to receive further weak support from the possible association of dyslexia with anomalies of hand or eye dominance and left–right directional confusion (Ginsburg & Hartwick, 1971; Sparrow & Satz, 1970). Of course as Corballis and Beale (1970a) observe, a perfectly bilateral machine or organism could not perform left–right discriminations, which must include scanning in a preferred (e.g., left-to-right) direction and distinguishing between such letters as *d* and *b, p* and *q* and such words as *saw* and *was*. Such an organism could only make mirror-image responses to mirror-image stimuli.

Mirror Writing and Mirror Confusions

The evidence for mirror writing among dyslexics is highly controversial (Benton, 1975). Even that attributed to Leonardo may possibly have represented a deliberately chosen private code. As Corballis and Beale (1976) observe, it is sometimes a symptom of left hemisphere damage and may also accompany a switch from the preferred to the nonpreferred hand. It is more easily performed with the nonpreferred hand if you simultaneously write forward with the preferred hand, but it can also be easily achieved with the preferred hand alone if you write on your own forehead or on the underside of a board. This observation might suggest that mirror writing involves a spatial skill (imagining a writing surface from various personal standpoints) rather than a motor skill. Indeed, it can be considered in a number of possible contexts—of two writing centers, one in each hemisphere; of two visual or memory images, one in each hemisphere; or of mirrored motor patterns from the two hands. We would add to this list the possibility that when writing with the nonpreferred hand we still read the engram out from the dominant hemisphere, and this motor trace is reversed during transcommissural transfer to the minor hemisphere for control of the nonpreferred hand.

It is disputable whether mirror-image confusion and a tendency toward left-right reversals is in fact any more common among developmental dyslexics than among beginning readers (see Corballis & Beale, 1976; D. J. Johnson & Myklebust, 1967). Kershner (1979) in a mental rotation task found no evidence that developmental dyslexics suffered from spatial confusion, mirror-image reversals, or inability (or abnormal ability) to transform mental images. Lyle and Goyen (1968) and Goyen and Lyle (1973) found that developmental dyslexics were no more likely than normals to wrongly choose a mirror version of a flashed letter. On the other hand, Belmont and Birch (1965) found that poor readers were inferior at differentiating left from right. From their clinical experience Critchley and Critchley (1978) claimed that dyslexics often mirror write and make nonverbal spatial confusions (left–right, and, perhaps significantly, up–down, which would *not* be predicted by the left–right mirror confusion hypothesis). Conversely, Newland (1972) reported that while dyslexics made more left–right perceptual errors, they did not differ from normals for up–down errors. Fischer, Liberman, and Shankweiler (1978) found (as did Lyle & Goyen, 1968; Goyen & Lyle, 1973) that *overall* dyslexics were no more likely to make reversal errors (of *all* types) than nondyslexic poor readers; however, the two groups did differ in that dyslexics, in misreading reversible letters, made more than twice as many reversals in the horizontal plane (e.g., *b* for *d* or *p* for *q*) as in the vertical plane (e.g., *b* for *p*, *d* for *q*), and much more often made a right-to-left (sinistrad) transformation (i.e., wrongly reading *b* as *d*) than a left-to-right (dextrad) transformation (i.e., wrongly reading *d* as *b*). Thus Fischer et al. concluded that there is, with a *fine grain analysis,* some support for Orton's (1925, 1937) view that developmental dyslexics may be distinguished by a sinistrad directional bias in their reversals.

Is There a Raised Incidence of Crossed Lateralization and/or Oculomotor Irregularities?

The claim that developmental dyslexics evince a raised incidence of crossed lateralization (i.e., right-handedness with left eye dominance or vice versa) is highly controversial. It is invoked by Bryden (1970) and Critchley and Critchley (1978) but is dismissed by Rourke (1978) and Rutter (1978). Dunlop, Dunlop, and Fenelon

(1973) studied ocular convergence, fusion, and dominance and found developmental dyslexics to have a higher incidence of ocular conditions, most notably convergence defects, defective stereopsis, and crossed hand-eye dominance. Both Pavlidis (1981) and Stein and Fowler (1981) found that erratic eye movements (e.g., esophoria, convergence insufficiency, and inability to make smooth pursuits or to maintain steady fixation) occur with dyslexics even when they are engaged in nonverbal visual tasks, and they speculate on whether this is the cause of dyslexia. Stein and Fowler believe that oculomotor insufficiencies lie at the root of the problem and argue that dyslexics fail to develop *stable* ocular dominance—rather than that their problem is one of *crossed* dominance. They believe that this may account for the apocryphal tales that dyslexics find it helpful to occlude one eye while trying to read and in fact confirmed this hypothesis in a clinical trial. They argue that such procedures effectively stabilize ocular dominance and so lead to better oculomotor control. Certainly, the idea of oculomotor and scanning irregularities in dyslexia has a long tradition (see, e.g., Zangwill & Blakemore, 1972), though according to Pirozzolo (1979) these phenomena characterize only one of his subgroups of dyslexics (to be discussed later in the chapter), the visual-spatial dyslexics.

Is There a Raised Incidence of Sinistrality in Developmental Dyslexics?

S. T. Orton (1925) was the first to suggest that there might be a raised incidence of sinistrality in developmental dyslexics, and it is still accepted by Critchley and Critchley (1978). Rutter (1978), however, rejects such an association. The issue is further reviewed by Hicks and Kinsbourne (1976a), who cite five studies in the last twenty-five years that find such a correlation (Vernon, 1957; Wold, 1968; Wussler & Barclay, 1970; Zangwill, 1962; Zurif & Carson, 1970) and three that do not (Applebee, 1971; Chakrabarti & Barker, 1966; Hartlage & Green, 1971). In addition to these studies, Dean (1978) finds that poor readers are more bilateral in their handedness preferences, are more ambidextrous, and are more apt to have non-dextral *fathers* (but not *mothers*) than would normally be expected; however, Richardson and Firlej (1979) find no difference in manual preference between normal subjects and dyslexics. There are a number of possible explanations for the inconsistencies in the findings of studies of the relationship between handedness and reading disability. Early studies relied heavily on clinical populations, and their results were not supported by large-scale studies of "normal" populations. Various methods of assessing handedness (see Chapter Ten) have been used (some simply rely on the subject's stated hand preference). The age group studied also seems to be important; while the incidence of reading disability and indeterminate handedness both decrease with age, this does not necessarily imply a causal relationship between them.

Is There Reduced or Reversed Cerebral Asymmetry in Developmental Dyslexics?

S. T. Orton again was the first to suggest that developmental dyslexia is a consequence of incomplete language dominance. Although Naylor (1980) concludes that the evidence is inconclusive in view of the lack of adequate controls, there are frequent reports that support Orton's position (e.g., Kershner, 1977, 1979; Leisman & Ashkenazi, 1980; McKeever & Van Deventer, 1975; Marcel, Katz, & Smith, 1974; Marcel & Rajan, 1975; Olson, 1973; Sparrow & Satz, 1970; M. E. Thomson, 1976; Tomlinson-Keasey & Kelly, 1979; Witelson & Rabinovitch, 1972; and Zurif & Carson, 1970). According to Hier, LeMay, Rosenberger, and Perlo (1978) the usual morphological asymmetries of the brain are reversed (see Chapter Three). However, in the behavioral studies the dyslexics' generally poorer performance could have resulted in reduced asymmetries as a consequence of floor effects. Moreover, incompetence in or unfamiliarity with reading could cause a reliance on right hemisphere visuospatial or preprocessing mechanisms (see Chapter Seven). Thus, there is some evidence that normal children initially show a LVF superiority with verbal material when learning to read; with developing expertise they shift to the normal RVF superiority (Carmon, Nachshon, & Starinsky, 1976; Silverberg, Gordon, Pollack, & Bentin, 1980). That this is not an age-maturation effect is evident from the finding that a similar shift occurs for Hebrew adolescents learning English while a RVF superiority for their native Hebrew persists throughout (Silverberg, Bentin, Gaziel, Obler, & Albert, 1979). The early LVF superiority presumably reflects visuospatial preprocessing with unfamiliar patterns. We can then explain persistent LVF superiorities with dyslexics as reflecting their continuing inability to get beyond this initial stage (cf. Bakker, 1973; Bakker, Smink, & Reitsma, 1973). We would thus view any behavioral evidence for cerebral bilaterality in dyslexics as probably an *effect* rather than a *cause* of their condition, as bilaterality for language functions in females is an advantage rather than a hindrance (see Chapter Eleven).

A. W. Young and Ellis (1981) argue that reduced or absent RVF superiorities in dyslexics could stem from a number of other possible artifacts. The dyslexics may simply have poor fixational control (as we saw earlier in the context of oculomotor irregularities), with the result that stimuli do not fall in the peripheral visual fields as intended. Poor readers may recognize only high-frequency, concrete, or imageable words, for which there is some evidence of extensive right hemisphere involvement anyway (see Chapter Eight). Young and Ellis also allude to the possibility, discussed above, that dyslexics, because of their lack of expertise, are forced to rely on right hemisphere mechanisms of visuospatial preprocessing or physical categorization.

However, very many studies (see Naylor, 1980, for review) fail to find any difference between developmental dyslexics and normal subjects in degree of visual or auditory laterality effects, a conclusion also reached by Hynd, Obrzut, Weed, and Hynd (1979); McKeever and Van Deventer (1975); Obrzut, Hynd, Obrzut, and

Leitgeb (1980); and Richardson and Firlej (1979). Keefe and Swinney (1979) found that while both dyslexic and control groups gave a REA and a RVF superiority on average, the distribution of the laterality scores for dyslexics was bimodal (that for the control group was unimodal) in that one subgroup showed a left and the other a right hemisphere deficit. These two subgroups may well correspond to those proposed by Boder (1971) and Pirozzolo (1979), which we shall shortly discuss, and their differential presence in the other studies may account for the contradictory findings. Moreover, just as the occurrence of possible artifacts was found to account in part for the absence of asymmetries with developmental dyslexics, so too the presence of asymmetries, equal in extent to those of normal readers, could be artifactual. Thus, as Naylor (1980) observes, not all of the target groups were in fact true dyslexics (many were just poor readers), and not all of the studies matched the target and the control subjects on IQ or on stimulus exposure duration.

Another possibility is that the presence or absence of dichotic ear asymmetries with dyslexics is a function of attentional demands. Thus Obrzut, Hynd, Obrzut, and Pirozzolo (1981) found no evidence of a developmental increase in the REA in either normal readers or dyslexics and found a normal REA with both groups when attention was not directed to either ear. With directed attention, normal readers continued to evince a REA; dyslexics showed a LEA when attention was directed to the left ear. They argue that this indicates an inability to simultaneously process competing verbal information and to suppress the nondominant ear, possibly due, they say, to relatively independent functioning of the two hemispheres, perhaps as a consequence of a callosal defect. As we have already seen, there is independent evidence that the corpus callosum is normally slow to myelinate.

Witelson (1977b), in addition to employing conventional, lateralized tachistoscopic presentation of letter stimuli, also employed dichaptic stimulation, whereby two different shapes (or letters) were simultaneously presented, one to either hand, for identification. The dyslexics showed no intermanual difference in accuracy scores in the shapes task, being equally accurate with either hand; the normal children, in contrast, showed a left-hand (right hemisphere) superiority. For the language tasks, the dyslexics showed the normal left hemisphere superiority, though at a deficient level of performance. She suggests that this indicates bilateral representation of the spatial, holistic (normally right hemisphere) mode of processing in dyslexics, with consequent "crowding" and deficient utilization by the left hemisphere of verbal modes of processing. This, she suggests, may lead to an inefficient and limited strategy for the reading of phonetically coded orthographies.

The question that Witelson fails to answer satisfactorily, of course, is why girls, with a normally bilateral representation of spatial functions, do not exhibit reading difficulty. However, support for Witelson's general viewpoint comes from several sources. Gordon (1980b) found that dyslexic children consistently scored better on the *Cognitive Laterality Battery* tests of right hemisphere function than on tests of left hemisphere function. Moreover, he found that most (90 percent) of the first-degree relatives of dyslexics also had this same right-dominant profile, even though they were not themselves dyslexic, further supporting the idea of a genetic component. In addition, Kershner (1979) found that while dyslexics and normal subjects did not differ in overall number of errors in an (unlateralized) mental rotation task, the dyslexics nevertheless preferred to employ a holistic and a context-bound strategy, whereas the fluent readers coded the visuospatial stimuli analytically. This leads to the suggestion (cf. Witelson, 1977b) that dyslexics are deficient in language processes because they wrongly rely on holistic mechanisms. When the condition eventually resolves and the dyslexics after much practice learn to read more or less satisfactorily, they may have belatedly acquired the appropriate analytic strategy, perhaps as a consequence of the eventual myelination of the requisite neural tracts, or they may, like deep phonemic (acquired) dyslexics, have learned how to cope by using a right hemisphere type of strategy. If so, we would predict that adults who were dyslexic as children should have a tendency to manifest paralexic errors. In this context we find it most interesting that Critchley and Critchley (1978), who seem to be quite unaware of the existence and nature of semantic paralexia in deep dyslexia as acquired in adulthood, nevertheless report examples of developmentally dyslexic children who have difficulty with grammatical and function words and make classic errors of paralexia. In fact, Jorm (1979) suggests that the symptoms of developmental dyslexia are similar to those of deep dyslexia, a claim that is criticized by A. W. Ellis (1979). If, however, there are two or more types of developmental dyslexia, then we feel that Ellis's objections lose some of their cogency.

Witelson's (1977b) account of an overrepresentation of and overreliance on (bilaterally represented) holistic processing mechanisms in developmental dyslexia would also predict that such individuals should possibly be superior in nonverbal, visuospatial, and perhaps mathematical (geometric rather than computational) skills. As we shall see in the next section, there does appear to be some evidence in support of such a proposition.

Ability of Developmental Dyslexics to Perform Nonverbal Functions

A recurring suggestion in the clinical literature is that developmental dyslexics are good or even superior at nonverbal, visuospatial, mechanical skills of the sort normally ascribed to the right hemisphere (Critchley & Critchley, 1978) and that high mathematical ability may be associated with dyslexia (Pirozzolo, 1979). L. J. Thompson (1969, 1971) suggested that many eminent men, including Leonardo, Edison, Einstein, the sculptor Rodin, and bacteriologist Paul Ehrlich, were dyslexic. Symmes and Rapoport (1972) found that healthy, well-adjusted, intelligent dyslexics were superior on WISC measures of spatial visualization. Denckla, Rudel, and

Broman (1980) found that dyslexics were poor at a spatial task (route walking) while very young, but by age ten years or older they were superior to normals. The authors developed a model involving differential maturation of the two hemispheres to account for their findings; this differential maturation itself differed between normal readers and dyslexics.

It is interesting to note that in one of her reports Witelson (1976b) also claims that among very young dyslexics the pattern of verbal and spatial asymmetries is similar to that of normal readers, only becoming aberrant around the age of ten. These findings are compatible with some sort of a delayed-maturation account, or even one involving maturation failure, perhaps involving regions in the vicinity of the angular gyrus, such as were originally proposed nearly a century ago and later taken up in modified form by Orton. Perhaps they also partly account for those studies (see next paragraph) that claim that in some perceptual respects dyslexics may be inferior to normal readers. Alternatively, these findings may also be perhaps better accounted for by the repeated, independent claims in the literature that there are two (or possibly more) major types of dyslexic with contrasting patterns of deficit.

Whether or not dyslexics are superior at certain nonverbal perceptual functions, it is common to deny any inferiority (Clifton-Everest, 1974; Jorm, 1979; Kershner, 1979; Vellutino, Pruzek, Steger, & Meshoulam, 1973; Vellutino, Steger, DeSetto, & Phillips, 1975; Vellutino, Steger, & Kandel, 1972). However, according to Lyle and Goyen (1968), Goyen and Lyle (1973), and Sabatino and Ysseldyke (1972), they are inferior at such tasks. Lovegrove, Heddle, and Slaghuis (1980) found that dyslexics have longer-lasting iconic storage than normal subjects at *low* spatial frequencies (for which receptors abound in the visual periphery and which are important for shape perception and holistic processing, faculties in which dyslexics are said to be superior). Conversely dyslexics have shorter-lasting iconic storage at high spatial frequencies (where foveal vision is involved, for example, for fine, detailed analytic processing of letters and words, at which dyslexics typically are inferior). Parenthetically, neither this paper nor the one we discussed by Kershner (1979) employed lateralized stimuli, but both concluded that dyslexics process visuospatial stimuli in a holistic mode. In a subsequent paper, Lovegrove, Bowling, Badcock, and Blackwood (1980) confirmed that dyslexics and controls differ in their pattern of sensitivity across the spatial frequencies, and that this difference depends on stimulus duration. At short stimulus durations both groups showed a monotonic decrement in sensitivity with increasing spatial frequency; with longer durations, especially those approximating reading fixation durations, normal readers were most sensitive at four cycles per degree, while dyslexics continued to show a decrease in sensitivity. Such findings, if confirmed, may account for some of the discrepancies reported in the literature; they might also suggest that, depending on appropriate conditions of stimulation (in terms of the frequency components in the stimulus and its duration), at least *some* dyslexics may be superior to normal readers in visuospatial tasks that can best be processed in a holistic mode.

One, Two, or Several Subtypes
of Developmental Dyslexia

We have already suggested that some of the inconsistencies in the literature could be resolved if it were found that dyslexics did not constitute a single homogeneous group (as many experimentalists seem to have believed) but instead comprised a number of possibly very different subtypes (as clinicians have long held, e.g., Critchley & Critchley, 1978; Satz & Morris, 1980). Vernon (1979) argues for at least two major types: those with predominantly auditory-linguistic deficiencies (difficulties in, e.g., performing grapheme-to-phoneme conversion, of the sort in fact exhibited by deep *acquired* dyslexics), and those with predominantly visuo-spatial problems. Such a distinction (characterized as dysphonetic versus dysei-detic) was made by Boder (1971) and is implicit or explicit in a number of other studies reviewed by Vernon (1979) (e.g., Doehring & Hoshko, 1977; D. J. Johnson & Myklebust, 1967; Kinsbourne & Warrington, 1963; Naidoo, 1972; and Vernon, 1971). In addition to these studies, Aaron (1978) found that there were two types of dyslexic, those with an analytic and those with a holistic type of deficit. Keefe and Swinney (1979), as we have already seen, found that the distribution of lateral-ity scores (dichotic and tachistoscopic) was bimodal for dyslexics and unimodal for normal readers and that the dyslexics fell into two subtypes, those with a left hemi-sphere deficit and those with a right hemisphere deficit. Fried, Tanguay, Boder, Doubleday, and Greensite (1981) have recently reported electrophysiological evidence that discriminates between two subgroups of dyslexics, those with a phonological and those with a visuospatial deficit.

Pirozzolo (1979) has perhaps taken the issue furthest, both empirically and theoretically. He claims that one subgroup (a majority) has problems with phonol-ogy; they read words as visual gestalts and are unable to decode them into phonetic units or to use grapheme-to-phoneme correspondence rules (like deep dyslexics). Another subgroup (a minority) cannot process words as visual gestalts but has to sound out the constituent letters of each word. He designates the two subgroups respectively as auditory-linguistic dyslexics and as visual-spatial dyslexics. Only the latter, according to his findings, typically show a normal RVF superiority together with deficits in visual, spatial, and oculomotor skills (with abnormal or regressive eye movement patterns) as well as tendencies toward directional and topographical disorientation, spatial dysgraphia and dyscalculia, and finger agnosia. Conversely, the auditory-linguistic dyslexics show no field asymmetries for verbal materials and exhibit impaired expression, lower verbal IQ, agrammatism, and faulty grapheme-to-phoneme matching in reading.

We believe that some such typology of dyslexia could eventually account rather well for much of the confusion and many of the positive empirical findings in the field of developmental dyslexia. At some time, however, a discrepancy be-tween the findings of Witelson and Pirozzolo will need to be resolved, in that Witel-son finds normal verbal asymmetries and reduced visuospatial asymmetries in her (unsubdivided) group of dyslexics, while Pirozzolo reports reduced verbal asymmetries in his larger subgroup of dyslexics, the auditory-linguistic subgroup, which has an apparent phonological deficit. Moreover, as we have earlier seen, two brain areas, the angular gyrus and the corpus callosum, are believed to be subject to late or even delayed maturation or myelination. It is quite possible, though speculative, that late development of these two areas is differentially involved in the two subtypes of developmental dyslexia. We can also speculate as to whether with essentially ideographic, nonphonological scripts (e.g., Chinese and the *kanji* form of Japanese) there is a reversal in the incidences of the two proposed types of dyslexia relative to the Western figures.

Dyslexia As a Deficit
in Serial Memory, Sequencing, and Segmentation

Jorm (1979) is adamant that there is only one type of dyslexia, which involves deficiencies in phonological coding in general and difficulties in coping with rapidly presented sequences of stimuli in particular. He reviews a number of studies dealing with the latter issue. Likewise, he reviews, as do Naylor (1980), Rourke (1978), Vernon (1979), and Vellutino (1978), twenty or more studies that bear on the idea that dyslexics have short-term memory problems with auditory and visual sequencing tasks, whether verbal or nonverbal, particularly where temporal rather than spatial order or analysis is concerned (and see also Gordon, 1980b). Such findings further support the concept (see Chapter Nine) that analytic, serial, segmental processing underlies the left hemisphere's superiority in mediating language functions. Since, as Pirozzolo (1979) observed, dyslexics who are unable to perform grapheme-to-phoneme conversions form the largest subgroup, most empirical studies that employed undifferentiated dyslexics would be expected to show deficits in serial or segmental processing.

Schizophrenia and Left Hemisphere Dysfunction

We have seen that the question of the etiology of developmental dyslexia is far from being resolved, but at least one form is likely to involve dysfunction of the left hemisphere, whether for grapheme-to-phoneme conversion or at the probably more fundamental level of serial, sequential processing. Another quite unrelated syndrome, schizophrenia, is the subject of no less controversy as to its nature and causation, which in any case are beyond the scope of this book. However, as a disorder it has one thing in common with developmental dyslexia—a postulated dysfunction of the left hemisphere.

The pioneering work of Flor-Henry (1969) initially suggested the link between schizophrenia and left hemisphere dysfunction. Since then a number of studies (for review, see Gruzelier & Flor-Henry, 1979) have indicated that the kinds of functional deficit manifested in schizophrenia are those that would normally be ascribed to lesions of the dominant or language hemisphere: impaired ability to conceptualize, use abstractions, draw logical inferences, and so on (R. E. Gur, 1979). Gruzelier and Hammond (1979) reviewed their own work and that of others, which indicated a left-sided deficit, probably resulting from left-sided temporal-limbic disturbances. This deficit was manifested in characteristic asymmetries of electrodermal responses to stimuli varying in emotional significance and in asymmetries of auditory thresholds and discriminations, with impaired performance on verbal subtests of the WAIS. Tomer, Mintz, Levi, and Myslobodsky (1979) and Gur (1979) also reviewed the evidence for abnormal EEG activity in the left hemisphere and the tendency of schizophrenics to give predominantly rightward lateral eye movements in response to *spatial* as well as verbal questioning. Gur (1979) also discussed the finding of abnormalities in schizophrenics' left hemisphere blood supply, as measured by the [133]Xenon inhalation technique.

According to T. H. Blau (1977) these phenomena can all be subsumed under a general disturbance in brain asymmetry, which he found to be manifest in a tendency for vulnerable children to draw circles in a clockwise rather than the far more "natural" counterclockwise fashion. Counterclockwise drawing of circles is natural for dextrals (see Chapter One), and though Blau did not comment on the handedness of his "at risk" children, we note that Krynicki and Nahas (1979), who found evidence in schizophrenics of increased incidence of crossed hand-eye dominance, poor right-hand tactile sensitivity, and right–left confusion, also reviewed evidence that left-handedness and ambidextrality occurred in schizophrenics more often than would normally be expected. Perhaps the most convincing evidence of asymmetrical cerebral involvement of this sort, and a possible relationship with handedness, comes from the findings of Naeser, Levine, Benson, Stuss, and Weir (1981) of significant differences in hemispheric asymmetries (by computerized tomographic brain scans) between schizophrenics and normals. Only half of the schizophrenics had the expected increased left-occipital width, and half had the unexpected equivalent, or increased, right-occipital widths.

Schizophrenia, therefore, like developmental dyslexia, would appear to be characterized by certain abnormalities of left hemisphere functioning. In both syndromes the exact nature of these abnormalities is yet to be elucidated; they may turn out to have little in common with each other, apart from left hemisphere involvement, and both syndromes may eventually be shown to consist of little more than collections of loosely interrelated symptoms going under a common label.

Summary and Conclusions

The issue of developmental dyslexia is surrounded by controversy and unanswered questions: Is there one or several distinct syndromes? How should the condition be defined and what are the criteria for its diagnosis? What is its relationship to other learning disabilities? Is it associated with hard as well as soft neurological signs? What is its incidence (though most agree that it runs in families and is more common in males), its likely etiologies, and so on? Many, however, stress the apparent normality of developmental dyslexics in most other respects, and the fact that the condition may involve a specific deficit limited more or less exclusively to levels of reading attainment.

Over fifty years ago Orton suggested that the condition was associated with left-right mirror reversals of letters and words, and with sinistrality, weak or mixed handedness, and crossed hand-eye dominance. He also suggested it was due to poorly established cerebral dominance. The latter effect, possibly a consequence of delayed maturation of regions in the vicinity of the angular gyrus (which is known to be involved in reading functions), was thought to lead to confusions between left and right hemisphere representations of visual stimuli, whereas normally the representation in the nondominant hemisphere would be suppressed. There is, however, no good evidence for mirror-symmetrical left-right coding in the two sides of the brain, certainly not at the level of perception, given the complete absence of appropriate homotopic interconnections, though it is just possible that such an effect could occur at the level of memory representations. Weak support for certain aspects of Orton's theory derives from the observation that developmental dyslexia does seem to be associated with anomalies of hand or eye dominance and with left-right confusion. Certainly, a perfectly bilateral machine could not perform left-right discriminations, which in one form or another are essential for reading our directionally coded Western script. Moreover, though the issue is not yet settled, it does seem likely that developmental dyslexics have a greater tendency towards mirror-image confusions and left-right reversals.

Also disputed is whether there is a greater incidence of crossed (hand-eye) lateralization among developmental dyslexics, though it is difficult to see exactly how the mechanics of such a "condition" would affect reading. However, it does seem indisputable that developmental dyslexics suffer more than would be expected from oculomotor problems, convergence defects, defective stereopsis, and erratic eye movements. Inability to develop *stable* ocular dominance (rather than crossed dominance) may be the critical factor, though possibly only for one subgroup, the visual-spatial dyslexics.

Also unresolved is the question of whether sinistrality, weak or mixed handedness, and reduced or reversed cerebral asymmetry is overrepresented among developmental dyslexics. Where anomalies of cerebral lateralization are apparent, they could possibly be a consequence of such artifacts as floor effects in testing procedures; poor fixational ability because of oculomotor irregularities; unfamiliarity or incompetence in reading, resulting in a reliance on right-hemisphere visuospatial strategies and preprocessing mechanisms; a relative overfamiliarity with only one class of words—high frequency, concrete, or imageable words—which may preferentially contact right hemisphere or bilateral mechanisms. Many recent studies have failed to show reduced or reversed cerebral asymmetry in developmental dyslexics, but again artifacts may be operating: Target groups may merely be poor readers rather than true dyslexics; dyslexics may fall into two subgroups, those showing a left and those showing a right hemisphere deficit; dyslexics may have an attentional deficit characterized by an inability to suppress the nondominant ear, possibly as a consequence of relatively independent functioning of the two hemispheres due to callosal insufficiency. (The corpus callosum is known to myelinate relatively late *normally,* and this maturation may be particularly late among developmental dyslexics.)

It is also possible that some or all developmental dyslexics overemploy a spatial, holistic mode of processing and that this mode may be represented *bilaterally* rather than just in the right hemisphere. This processing mode is of course inappropriate for Western phonologically based scripts. There is independent evidence that dyslexics prefer to use a holistic processing strategy and may perform at a high level in nonverbal tasks where such a strategy is advantageous. They also may tend to make errors of a paralexic nature and to perform at a good or superior level in mathematical or visuospatial tasks, unless they require resolution of high spatial frequencies or fine, detailed, analytic processing.

Such considerations lead to the possibility that there are at least two subgroups of developmental dyslexics. Those in the first (the majority) demonstrate auditory-linguistic deficits and problems in phonologically recoding the visual representation; they read words as visual gestalts. The second subgroup displays visual-spatial deficits and can only read words by sounding them out. These two subgroups may also differ in the extent and direction of any field or ear asymmetries. Probably because of the imbalance of representation in the two subgroups, some would argue that *all* developmental dyslexics also have difficulties with analytic, sequential, segmental processing in addition to their phonological incapacities and that these latter deficits are perhaps a consequence of the former.

Debate also continues on the etiology and typology of schizophrenia. Like developmental dyslexia, schizophrenia may possibly comprise several subgroups, though again, in some or all cases a left hemisphere dysfunction may be implicated. Deficits in logic and the capacity to use abstractions are evident. Further evidence of a left hemisphere involvement comes from a number of sources, which, though not all free of controversy themselves, add up to a fairly consistent picture. Perhaps the strongest evidence of a left hemisphere involvement in the condition comes from computerized tomographic brain scans and a raised incidence of anomalies of handedness.

FURTHER READING

BENTON, A. L., & PEARL, D. *Dyslexia: An appraisal of current knowledge.* Oxford: Oxford University Press, 1978.

CRITCHLEY, M., & CRITCHLEY, E. A. *Dyslexia defined.* London: Heinemann, 1978.

JORM, A. F. The cognitive and neurological basis of developmental dyslexia: A theoretical framework and review. *Cognition,* 1979, *7,* 19–33.

NAYLOR, H. Reading disability and lateral asymmetry: An information processing analysis. *Psychological Bulletin,* 1980, *87,* 531–545.

PIROZZOLO, F. J. *The neuropsychology of reading disorders.* New York: Holt, Rinehart & Winston, 1979.

VERNON, M. D. Variability in reading retardation. *British Journal of Psychology,* 1979, *70,* 7-16.

YOUNG, A. W., & ELLIS, A. W. Asymmetry of cerebral hemispheric function in normal and poor readers. *Psychological Bulletin,* 1981, *89,* 183-190.

CHAPTER FOURTEEN
General Conclusions and Clinical and Educational Implications of Human Cerebral Asymmetry

Before discussing the clinical and educational implications of our current knowledge of human cerebral asymmetry, it may be useful to summarize the earlier chapters. No specific references are given since these can be found in the main text.

Biological and Morphological Aspects of Cerebral Asymmetry

The apparent left–right symmetry of vertebrates is incomplete and often largely superficial, despite the advantages of symmetry for movement in a left–right unbiased world. Humans also exhibit many small departures from perfect symmetry, and this is perhaps partly responsible for their (imperfect) ability to perform mirror-image discriminations, together with their long fascination with the phenomenon of left and right and its relationship with other dichotomies.

Only humans (and possibly certain parrot species) show consistent patterns of asymmetry (i.e., their preponderant dextrality) at a population level. In other species paw preferences are idiosyncratic and not subject to the effects of selective breeding. However, several brain structures in nonhuman vertebrates—particularly some species of songbird—may be systematically asymmetrical. In the higher primates there is increasingly consistent evidence for morphological asymmetries in the cortex, in areas which in humans would mediate speech.

Such left–right asymmetries in the human peri-Sylvian cortex are present in human fossil remains and neonates; they are weakest and least consistent in nondextrals. Overall, the brain may be said to have a counterclockwise torque. These asymmetries appear to be related to the neurological substrate of language, though their full and exact significance is not yet completely clear.

Evidence from Clinical,
Split-Brain, and Normal Subjects

There are three sources of evidence of behavioral asymmetries in humans: clinical, split-brain, and normal studies. Evidence from the first of these sources, however, is often difficult to interpret. Aphasia may be induced, and studied, in a reversible form with unilateral barbiturate anesthesia, unilateral ECT, and electrostimulation of the brain at the levels of the cortex and thalamus. Traumatic aphasia may be divided into Broca's anterior expressive aphasia, Wernicke's posterior aphasia (which largely affects comprehension), and conduction aphasia (which involves the disconnection of the above two affected areas). Connectionist theory has proved very fruitful in explaining existing and in predicting hitherto undescribed syndromes, but some believe that it fails to capture the rich complexity of psycholinguistic organization and the dynamic processes of speech mediation.

As with the aphasias, there are at least two types of alexia, as would be expected on the basis of the known two routes to word recognition—direct access and the phonological route. Studies with the two unique forms of Japanese script confirm this division. The left hemisphere may mediate the analysis of figures into component elements, while the right is more concerned with the holistic global apprehension of the entire configuration, and of the interrelationships *between* the component elements rather than the actual elements themselves. Face recognition is largely but not exclusively a right hemisphere phenomenon, depending on whether discriminations or recognition involve familiar or unfamiliar faces. It is still unknown whether there is something special about face recognition, compared to other complex meaningful patterns, just as it is still debated whether there is something special about perceiving in the speech mode. Music also has a bilateral as well as a right hemisphere component.

Despite speculation for over a hundred years on the likely consequences of the commissurotomy operation, its psychological consequences have only been known for twenty years, and subtle testing procedures are usually required to demonstrate them. The most dramatic observation is that the hemispheres may be split into two largely independent cognitive systems, the left mainly subserving verbal and analytic processes and the right nonverbal, visuospatial, gestalt, or holistic aspects. Although the right hemisphere can comprehend much spoken speech and even read fairly simple text, its powers of expression are extremely limited—and practically nonexistent for propositional speech. Cross cueing between the two hemispheres may develop, and the naive hemisphere is likely to confabulate when questioned about something presented to the other. Certain aspects of vision, notably "ambient" vision as mediated by the undivided retinotectal system, may be unaffected by the commissurotomy operation. Other techniques that have been employed with commissurotomized patients include chimeric stimulation and prolonged lateralized viewing via a scleral contact lens. Such techniques have demonstrated the phenomenon of metacontrol, whereby a hemisphere may come to predominate on the basis of expectancies, and the seepage of mental "auras," probably through subcortical connecting systems. The scleral contact lens system has enabled the very considerable comprehensional powers of the right hemisphere to be mapped in detail and its "personality" and corpus of knowledge to be interrogated.

The question of whether the commissurotomy operation leaves two separate wills, consciousnesses, and volitions is not easily answered. While such a proposition would appear to be true in certain respects, it may also be partly true of a normal person. Only under very special and limiting circumstances can it be said that the operation leads to an increase in processing capacity. Normally, powerful factors for unification are present, such as a unilateral allocation of attention, even in the divided brain.

In cases of callosal agenesis there is surprisingly little evidence of the disconnection syndrome, possibly due to compensation in other areas and by other commissures. Apart from some slight deficits in bimanual coordination, the poor spatial functioning found in these cases may possibly be a consequence of bilateral language representation, though this is disputed.

In studies using normal subjects there is of course an absence of morbidity, but independent operation of the hemispheres cannot be observed. Lateralization of stimuli, moreover, forces the adoption of frequently unnatural and restrictive testing procedures. For these reasons, and because a great diversity of techniques has been adopted, many of the findings have often been difficult to replicate. The studies have generally found, however, that a RVF superiority occurs with visually presented verbal materials except perhaps when they require processing only at a physical or visuospatial level, or when the materials are briefly exposed, perceptually degraded, or require preprocessing. Semantic processing also fails to make big demands on left hemisphere mechanisms, the latter being preeminent when phonological or overt articulatory aspects are emphasized. These phenomena, however, are independent of the effects of directional reading processes or scanning. A LVF superiority typically appears with simple nonverbal stimulus dimensions, patterns, and face-processing tasks, especially when deeper levels of processing are required, though it is uncertain whether the right hemisphere's mediation of faces is completely independent of both the general visuospatial aspects and the emotional connotations. A RVF superiority in judging faces may be found when they are very difficult to discriminate (thus requiring the analytic mechanisms of the left hemisphere) and possibly when they are highly familiar or have to be categorized.

Bilateral visual presentations may generate larger field asymmetries, as a consequence of the competitive nature of the stimulation, but to avoid noncentral fixation under these circumstances a central fixation stimulus may be required.

Care must then be taken to avoid biasing the nature of the processing of the lateralized stimuli with the fixation stimulus.

Dichotic (and under certain circumstances, monaural) presentations demonstrate a REA for verbal and a LEA for nonverbal (intonational, environmental, melodic) stimuli. The REA is stronger for the more encoded stop consonants than for steady-state and unencoded vowels and stronger at a memory level than at a purely perceptual level. It is, however, more a correlate than an index of cerebral dominance, reflecting the lateralization of speech perception rather than production. A number of methodological problems can be avoided if reaction time in a target detection paradigm is measured. Another such technique is that of lateralized DAF, which shows that speech performance is more disrupted when the delayed signal is channeled to the right ear, although the opposite effects occur when simple music pieces are played.

Tactile analogues of the dichotic technique, employing dichaptic stimulation, also generate a double dissociation between directional asymmetries and the verbal-nonverbal nature of the stimulation. The left side of the body is generally superior in perceiving a number of spatial configurations, including Braille.

A double dissociation and material-specific effects may also appear with EEG measures, alpha activity, evoked potential responses, and the CNV. Similar effects are reported with measures of rCBF and CLEMs, though interpretation of the latter is disputed. However, such activation measures receive general support from the findings that asymmetries are modified by the subject's sex and handedness. An overflow of cognitive activity to motor areas of the same hemisphere, which may underlie the disputed CLEMs, does seem to trigger spontaneous hand activity or to interfere with it when it is generated as part of a concurrent task, such as rhythmic tapping or dowel balancing.

The fact that ear asymmetries may be demonstrated under certain circumstances with monaural stimulation, and that the nature of the competing materials may be at least as important as the presence of peripheral competition, argues against the need for a strong form of Kimura's model (of suppression of ipsilateral by contralateral pathways) to generate ear asymmetries. The Kimura model also holds that laterality differences reflect privileged access to uniquely specialized hemispheres, with the differences manifested in terms of either transcommissural transmission times or signal degradation during transmission. However, simultaneously presented information may sometimes be better processed when projected to different hemispheres than to the same, perhaps particularly with commissurotomy patients, but only as long as the tasks are simple and compatible. This interhemispheric superiority even occurs with normal subjects when the two streams must be integrated or compared, suggesting that interhemispheric communication does not involve any substantial delay or degradation. In any case reaction-time studies where the subject has to respond with a left or right limb to laterally presented light flashes demonstrate that transcommissural transmission times are of the order of only a few milliseconds (longer values with certain choice reaction-time paradigms reflect attentional effects with respect to sensory and motor hemispace). Most cognitive studies, however, find laterality differences to be of the order of tens of milliseconds, and so we can conclude that such differences do not reflect transcommissural transmission time and that the hemispheres differ quantitatively and relatively rather than qualitatively and absolutely.

According to Kinsbourne's attentional account, laterality differences reflect differential hemispheric activation. However, laterality effects still occur even when the subject cannot predict the verbal or nonverbal nature of the stimulus and when the subject knows in advance which visual field or ear will be stimulated. A variant of this account continues to emphasize the importance of apparent spatial origin of stimulation but disclaims the activational aspects of Kinsbourne's model. Nevertheless, laterality effects are generally stronger when memory rather than perceptual processes are tapped, when subjects have had practice and are familiar with the materials, and when deeper levels of cognitive processing are involved. Load and activation may eventually prove to be important determinants of the extent and direction of laterality effects, the direction possibly reversing when a processing hemisphere is overloaded. When the nature of hemispheric asymmetry is eventually resolved, it is likely that aspects of both Kimura's and Kinsbourne's accounts will be incorporated in a model that also recognizes the importance of processing load and strategy effects, together with at least some component of structural asymmetry, and of lateralized attention and activation. Indeed, the right hemisphere's own involvement in activational processes is revealed in the contexts of emotionality, unilateral hemineglect, arousal, vigilance, and novelty. Although there is some evidence that the right hemisphere may prove preeminent when processing novel, unfamiliar materials that do not readily lend themselves to encoding according to a preordained descriptive system, the evidence as yet is inconclusive, and the phenomenon could stem from right hemisphere holistic strategies. The only safe conclusion so far is that stable laterality effects are more likely to emerge with reasonably familiar materials and subjects who have had practice.

Language and the Nondominant Hemisphere

Stable laterality effects with verbal materials are more likely to emerge with adult, dextral, male subjects in the context of the expressive rather than the comprehensional aspects of speech. Left hemisphere anesthesia almost entirely suppresses speech production in these subjects, but it has very much less of an effect on comprehension. In split-brain patients, the right hemisphere is largely mute, though far from uncomprehending; it may even possess some limited writing capacity. It has limited phonological powers and a reduced lexicon, it may comprehend the written word directly rather than via phonological recoding, and it perhaps acts in an essentially supportive role in language mediation.

Early lesions that do not modify hand preferences do not seem to affect the lateralization of speech production, though comprehensional processes may become more bilateral. However, left hemispherectomies performed in infancy will result in the right hemisphere's taking over all language functions, though careful testing in adulthood may reveal subtle deficiencies at a syntactic and phonological level. When such an operation is performed on adults, there is usually little substantial recovery of expressive speech. Phonological access and aspects of the left hemisphere's normal reading mechanisms may be lost in the syndrome of deep or phonemic dyslexia. The ability to comprehend semantic aspects, possibly via right hemisphere mechanisms, and to read high-frequency, concrete, or imageable nouns, often with semantic paralexia, may be retained, while the capacity to read low-frequency, abstract, or nonimageable words and grammatical function words may be selectively lost. Attempts to demonstrate analogous phenomena with normal subjects have not always been successful.

There is, however, evidence of a double dissociation with normal subjects when Japanese *kana* and *kanji* are studied and when ear differences for processing encoded stop consonants and unencoded steady-state vowels are measured. A LVF superiority may also appear for the preprocessing of difficult, unfamiliar, or degraded letters or words or when the physical aspects of verbal stimuli are preeminent. A right hemisphere contribution may possibly occur with arithmetical tasks and second languages, but again these effects may depend more on visuospatial processes in the former and the relative unfamiliarity of the latter. Similar explanations may apply to reported anomalous asymmetries in processing signs in the congenitally deaf and in Braille reading in the blind, since there is no evidence that cerebral lateralization is otherwise any different in the deaf or blind. With respect to stutterers, however, the issue is not resolved.

The Nature of Human Hemispheric Asymmetry

The fact that the right hemisphere, though mute, is far from uncomprehending and may even play a role in reading is evidence against strict interpretation of a verbal-nonverbal dichotomy. Other evidence is the fact that unilateral lesions differentially affect space perception, drawing, and block design. Analogous findings are revealed by commissurotomy studies and experiments with normal subjects, with the left hemisphere generally superior at analytic modes of processing and the right at global, gestalt apprehension of the interrelationships between components. Ear asymmetries in listening to music are similar: A LEA appears for simple judgments of elementary acoustic properties, and a REA for the more complex, rhythmic, and time-dependent aspects. Listening strategies and variables such as musical expertise, competence, and talent also may determine the direction of ear superiorities in melodic recognition, again in terms of an analytic-holistic dichotomy. The underlying left hemisphere capacity, which may determine all other aspects of cerebral asymmetry, may be for discriminating between rapidly changing acoustic signals at the sensory level and for controlling fine, sequential, manipulative movements of the limbs, hands, fingers, and articulators at the motor level. This motor capacity may be the more fundamental: It may determine the mediation of language functions by the left hemisphere, and in consequence the superiorities of the right hemisphere may be simpler, less specialized, more primitive, and gained by default. Nevertheless, such interhemispheric differences appear more to be a matter of degree than a difference in kind. It is not yet resolved whether verbal REAs and RVF superiorities stem directly from the operation of such analytic segmental mechanisms in the left hemisphere or from that hemisphere's mediation of language in consequence of its prior analytic and segmental specializations. Nor is it yet clear whether there is something special about "perceiving in a speech mode."

A number of other issues also await resolution, such as the reason for cognitive and motor asymmetry in humans, why it is weak and incomplete, why a majority of us are lateralized in the same direction while a minority are sinistral, and whether it stems from shared tool use and the consequent need for "standardization," whether hand gestures gave way to facial gestures and then true speech, and so on. However, the incidence of sinistrality appears to have changed little from the days of the paleolithic when language perhaps first appeared.

Handedness and Sex Differences

Laterality effects are strongest and most consistent for handedness, and there is a fairly high correlation between handedness and foot dominance. Eye dominance may be a composite of a number of other loosely related factors. Of the general population, around 90 percent (perhaps more in the case of females) are dextral, depending on the measures used. Preference and performance measures need to be distinguished, but both indicate a continuum rather than a dichotomy between dextrality and sinistrality. While asymmetries in stepping reflexes (in favor of the right leg) may appear in neonates as early as the first few weeks, hand superiorities may not appear much before six months.

Asymmetries in brain morphology, in language lateralization as determined by clinical methods, and in electroencephalographic and behavioral indices are weaker and more variable with sinistrals. However, strength of handedness may possibly be a more important determinant of performance than direction, and genetic influences may determine the degree of lateralization more than its direction, a view that has recently been incorporated into a model invoking cytoplasmic growth gradients.

Familial sinistrality, and especially *parental* handedness, is an important determinant of performance. *Nonfamilial* sinistrals appear to be the least lateralized or the most likely to demonstrate abnormal lateralization. Although cultural factors undoubtedly play a role, handedness is subject to strong biological determinants, though its heritability does not appear to be compatible with any simple Mendelian account, as family, twin, and sibling studies have shown. A number of genetic models have been proposed, but all so far have foundered on the twin and sibling data. Nor does a knowledge of the writing hand and its posture accurately predict language lateralization, as has been claimed.

A disproportionate number of sinistrals are found in clinical populations. A relationship of any sort between sinistrality and birth trauma, however, is not universally accepted, whether or not an increased risk of birth trauma is itself heritable. Apart from the birth trauma explanation, there may be another reason for the reported existence of a cognitive deficit in sinistrals: cognitive crowding if language is bilaterally represented. Although sinistrals show some evidence of a visuospatial inferiority, they may be superior for certain nonverbal auditory tasks and, if they do possess a "double dose" of language, it appears that it may act to their *disadvantage* rather than their benefit.

The sexes also differ in their cognitive capacities: Girls score higher than boys on verbal and lower than them on visuospatial abilities. These differences also appear in choice of occupations and in the distribution of clinical disorders such as developmental dyslexia, stuttering, and autism. Male superiority in visuospatial processing has been ascribed to a sex-linked recessive gene on the X chromosome; despite some initial support, familial correlations have not borne out the hypothesis, though heredity does seem to play a part. Moreover, while environmental factors must inevitably also play a role, as shown by the effects of different cultures, they cannot account exclusively for the findings.

In addition to cognitive abilities, the sexes differ in the extent of lateralization; though the differences are small, females are generally found to be less lateralized than males, whether the studies examine asymmetries in brain morphology, the effects of brain damage, or visual field and ear asymmetries in normal subjects. In some respects females resemble sinistral males, leading to suggestions that in females, areas in the right hemisphere normally reserved for visuospatial processing have been invaded by secondary speech mechanisms that act in an auxiliary capacity for the comprehension of difficult or unfamiliar material.

Some of these sex differences could possibly be due to differences in rates of maturation, since early maturing adolescents (like females) generally score better on verbal than on spatial tasks and are less lateralized. Late maturers (like males) might establish hemispheric dominance later, to the advantage of spatial ability if language normally develops before spatial skills; language would thus have a protracted opportunity to develop exclusively in the left hemisphere without encroaching on right hemisphere functions, though it would also have a greater period of risk during which malfunctions could occur. Dyslexic boys might place more reliance, in attempting to read, on late-developing, bilaterally represented spatial functions. However, there is little evidence for the maturational development of lateralization, and the safest conclusion might simply be that the more pronounced hemispheric specialization in males deprives them of alternative backup systems in the other hemisphere.

Developmental Aspects of Lateralization

There is very little evidence for a general developmental increase in lateralization with normal children. Morphological asymmetries of the brain are evident in fetuses, and neonates show a pronounced (head turning) asymmetry in their responsiveness to sensory stimulation. Hand preferences are firmly established by the age of five, and possibly even one; any further developmental effects probably reflect the unfolding of manipulative skills. Lateralized perceptual mechanisms for the discrimination of speech sounds are found in the neonate.

Earlier claims (e.g., by Lenneberg) to the contrary, the incidence of aphasia after right hemisphere damage is far lower than after left hemisphere damage, in infants and adults. Many potential artifacts can increase the apparent incidence of right hemisphere aphasia in the very young. Unless the left hemisphere is completely removed, it is likely to become and remain language-dominant. The greater ability of the infant or child to recover language after left hemisphere trauma is due to *intra*hemispheric reorganization or plasticity. When the right hemisphere is forced to take over language (e.g., because of early left hemispherectomy), careful testing in adulthood reveals that it never acquires quite the degree of language competence that is characteristic of the left.

Asymmetries of gesture and of interference in tapping performance during concurrent verbal tasks are apparent at the earliest age at which testing is possible. There is a verbal REA at least by four years, and no real evidence for a developmental increase when performance levels and attentional aspects are controlled, though plenty of potential sources of artifact do give the appearance of such an increase. An early LVF superiority with verbal materials, when it occurs, can be put down to the employment of right hemisphere preprocessing mechanisms for difficult or unfamiliar visual material, which appears even with adults. The only senses in which developmental changes in asymmetry can be said to occur are in the unfolding of cognitive and manipulative skills, the continued myelination of certain cerebral structures related to language, and a general developmental decrease in neural plasticity.

Developmental Dyslexia

Some otherwise normal children fail to develop normal reading skills, and there have been repeated claims that this syndrome is associated with anomalies of handedness, eyedness, and cerebral asymmetry. There is no good evidence for mirror-symmetrical, left–right perceptual coding in brains lacking normal asymmetries, though such brains certainly might have difficulty discriminating between mirror-image stimuli or consistently scanning in a given direction. Developmental dyslexics do seem to have a greater tendency toward mirror-image confusions and oculomotor irregularities. However, as yet unresolved is the question of whether or not sinistrality, weak or mixed handedness, and reduced or reversed cerebral asymmetry is overrepresented among developmental dyslexics; numerous artifacts can account for both the presence or the absence of such findings. Some or all developmental dyslexics may overemploy a spatial, holistic mode of processing, which is inappropriate for Western phonologies. In dyslexics this mode possibly is bilaterally represented rather than mediated just by the right hemisphere. They certainly seem to prefer to use holistic processing strategies, and they perform at a high level in nonverbal tasks where such a strategy is advantageous.

There are in all probability at least two groups of developmental dyslexics, which accounts for many of the conflicting findings. The larger subgroup apparently suffers from auditory-linguistic (phonological) deficits, reads words as visual gestalts (like adult deep or phonemic dyslexics), and may display little or no field or ear asymmetries. This subgroup may also display difficulties in analytic segmental processing, which is perhaps the primary disability. The second (smaller) subgroup displays visual-spatial deficits, can only read words by sounding them out, and possesses normal asymmetries. Schizophrenics may share with the first group a subtle deficit in left hemisphere functioning.

Some Clinical and Educational Implications

While much is known about the nature of hemispheric asymmetry, our ability to apply this knowledge to the treatment of brain-damaged patients or to educational techniques and practices is, as yet, fairly limited. Unfortunately, a little knowledge has in some cases led to rather wild speculation and to some very dubious remediation procedures.

The treatment of language disorders. According to Benson (1979b) most current aphasia therapy consists of efforts to overcome expressive disturbances, particularly problems of articulation, phonation, and speech initiation. He points out that while problems of auditory language comprehension are the most difficult aspects of aphasia to treat, this is fortunately the area most likely to improve spontaneously (Vignolo, 1964).

Kertesz (1979) summarizes eleven current methods of language therapy. Early methods emphasized stimulation, facilitation (by repeated practice), and motivation (Wepman, 1951); these approaches still form an important part of current traditional techniques. Some therapists have used different language modalities for facilitation—for example, spelling aloud to assist writing (Schuell, Jenkins, & Jiménez-Pabón, 1964)—or have used a more intact language channel to eliminate or reduce a block in understanding or expression caused by a damaged channel (e.g., by presenting printed and spoken words simultaneously; Weigl, 1968). A logical extension of these facilitation and deblocking methods is to use right hemisphere mechanisms in a similar way. Benson describes the melodic intonation therapy (MIT) technique introduced by Sparks, Helm, and Albert (1974) as the "most successful innovation to date" (Benson, 1979b, p. 183). The patients first learn to tap out the rhythm of a phrase intoned by the therapist and then attempt to intone it themselves as they tap. As the patient progresses, the melodic aspect of the program is faded out. It is unclear whether the successful results are simply an example of interhemispheric facilitation or whether, as Sparks et al. (1974) suggest, by attaching melodic intonation to propositional language, the deleterious influence of the damaged left hemisphere is reduced. Benson (1979b) reports that this method has rapidly gained worldwide use but is useful only with a limited group of aphasics (those with severe output limitations and relatively intact comprehension).

The undamaged right hemisphere of aphasic patients may be better able to communicate via a symbolic system. Glass, Gazzaniga, and Premack (1973) and H. Gardner, Zurif, Berry, and Baker (1976) have used symbolic communication systems with aphasics based on the ones used to teach chimpanzees to "read" and "write" (R. A. Gardner & Gardner, 1969; Premack, 1971). Even if the global aphasics with whom either this system or one involving hand signals is used (Eagleson, Vaughn & Knudson, 1970; Chen, 1971) never regain normal language, they do have a means of communication (albeit a limited one), which is a tremendous psychological factor in their rehabilitation.

Alexia, an acquired inability to comprehend written language (Albert, 1979), agraphia, an acquired disorder of expression of written language (Marcie & Hécaen, 1979), and acalculia, acquired disorders of calculation (Levin, 1979), may occur independently, but they are more commonly associated with aphasia. Furthermore, there are several forms of these conditions, each with its own symptomatology (see Chapter Four). Many different cueing, deblocking, and facilitating techniques have been developed to assist the alexic, but Albert (1979) feels that little has changed since the publication of Benson and Geschwind's (1969) pessimistic views on treatment and prognosis. He suggests that since the right hemisphere has considerable language capacity, efforts should be made to retrain the alexic's language skills by emphasizing "right hemisphere" strategies. With agraphia and acalculia, as with other language disorders, far more seems to be written about symptoms and the type of lesions that may account for them than about treatment procedures. Levin states that "innovative methodologies are needed to investigate hemispheric dominance for calculation in normal persons" (1979, p. 139). This is also true for alexia and agraphia, and the effort may result in new and successful methods of remediation.

Benson concludes:

> Rehabilitation of the aphasic is a relatively new pursuit, a frontier situation both crude and exciting, which already offers valuable assistance to many aphasic patients. The future promises innovative advances in therapy and far greater appreciation of the appropriate technique for a given type of language disturbance. (1979b, p. 191)

It seems very likely that new knowledge of the language skills and processes of *each* hemisphere will contribute to these "innovative advances."

Treatment of right hemisphere disorders. Our earlier claim, that far more is written about symptoms and the type of lesions that may account for language disorders than about treatment procedures, is even more applicable to right hemisphere disorders (e.g., see Benton's, 1979, chapter on visuoperceptive, visuospatial, and visuoconstructive disorders). This may suggest that remediation of right hemisphere disorders is extremely difficult, but it is also probably true that such disorders are not considered to be as important in a highly literate society as left hemisphere language problems. Most individuals, unless they are artists, architects, or musicians can probably accept or tolerate right hemisphere disabilities. For example, Nash was able to revise his textbook, *Developmental Psychology: A Psychobiological Approach,* after suffering a right hemisphere stroke (see preface to Nash, 1978).

Possible implications of cerebral asymmetry for psychiatry. In Chapter Five we discussed whether the work with commissurotomy patients indicates simultaneous presence of two streams of consciousness or two wills within a single head. We saw that each disconnected hemisphere has independent perceptual, memory, and cognitive capacities and that even without subtle testing (Dimond, 1980) personality changes are apparent. However, powerful unifying factors appear to be present even in the divided brain, so that only under exceptional testing procedures can anything approximating a true duality of consciousness be demonstrated, and even then it may be little different from what obtains with normal subjects under equally artificial conditions of hypnosis and training to perform more than one task at a time. Thus the question as to whether there are two simultaneous, coexisting streams of consciousness in the divided brain remains as yet unresolved (but see Puccetti, 1981).

However, there have been speculations that an increased knowledge of left and right cerebral specialization may help us understand and manage at least some psychiatric problems. Galin sees "a compelling formal similarity between these dissociation phenomena seen in the commissurotomy patients and some phenomena of interest to clinical psychiatry" (1974, p. 574). He also likens certain aspects of right hemisphere functioning to "the mode of cognition psychoanalysts have termed primary process, the form of thought that Freud originally assigned to the system Ucs" (1974, p. 574); that is, he compares right hemisphere language with the sort of language that appears in dreams and slips of the tongue. Ornstein suggests that both the structure and function of our left and right hemispheres "underlie in some part the two modes of consciousness that coexist within each one of us" (1977, p. 20). He too sees Freud's "conscious" mind as related to the left hemisphere and accessible to language and to rational discourse and the "unconscious" mind as related to the right hemisphere and much less accessible to reason or verbal analysis.

As Galin himself admitted (1977), much of this work is still in the realm of speculation. It is therefore difficult to see what the practical outcomes may be.

Perhaps its greatest potential lies in bringing the disciplines of neuropsychology and psychiatry closer together.

"Patterning" and "neurological organization." The knowledge that most people have left hemisphere dominance for language almost inevitably led to the conclusion that this pattern of lateralization must therefore be advantageous and should be achieved by whatever means possible. This fallacious argument has led to many bizarre treatment procedures, which are still widely practiced at least in the United States (Kinsbourne & Hiscock, 1977) and in Australia (Sasse, 1977). For some twenty years Glen Doman, a physical therapist, and Carl Delacato, an educational psychologist, have been promoting a system of therapy for retarded and handicapped children. In it they place considerable emphasis on the need for a child to develop a dominant hemisphere (Delacato, 1959, 1963, 1966, 1970). An important aspect of their theory is that a basic difference exists between humans and lower animals because "man has achieved cortical dominance wherein one side of the cortex controls the skills in which man outdistances lower forms of animals" (Delacato, 1959, p. 21). This latter claim is not in itself in dispute since human use of tools and speech are both usually controlled by the left hemisphere (see Chapter Nine), but Delacato assumes that this "cortical dominance" is subject to maturational development and claims that if there is some obstruction to this development, communication and language problems result. To prevent these problems Doman and Delacato have developed a method of treatment known as "patterning." As summarized by H. J. Cohen, Birch, and Taft (1970) this method

> has purportedly been useful for (1) achieving greater "mobility" in patients with brain damage than has been achieved by classical therapy; (2) treating communicative disorders, including visual, speech, and reading disabilities; (3) enhancing intelligence and elevating I.Q. levels; (4) preventing communicative disorders, altering aberrant behavior, and improving coordination in normal infants, together with; (5) having other universal applications. (p. 302)

The wide range of conditions for which this treatment is recommended is exemplified by the title of Doman's (1974) book, *What to do about Your Brain-injured Child, or Your Brain-damaged, Mentally Retarded, Mentally Deficient, Cerebral-palsied, Emotionally Disturbed, Spastic, Flaccid, Rigid, Epileptic, Autistic, Athetoid, Hyperactive Child.*

Doman and Delacato believe that ontogeny recapitulates phylogeny (that is, that the development of the individual repeats the evolutionary pattern of the species). Treatment depends on determining what point children have reached without skipping any of the developmental stages—their "level of neurological organization"—and provides an opportunity for working through the higher levels in the correct phylogenetic sequence. If they are at a very low level and not yet walking, they are required to spend most of their waking hours on the floor and crawling and creeping are encouraged. Children who are unable to carry out the necessary movements for themselves are "patterned" by a team of three to five adults (therapists, parents, and volunteers) who manipulate the child's head and limbs through the necessary movements. Children who can walk but who have not learned to crawl in the prone position or to creep on their hands and knees—which are claimed to be absolutely essential to normal development—must go back and learn and practice at these levels. This may involve as little as an hour a day for a child who has only a mild reading problem, but more typically would involve eight hours a day and could even extend up to thirteen or more hours per day, seven days a week. Sleeping posture is also thought to be important and may be restricted.

Other techniques employed by Doman and Delacato with the more severely brain-damaged children include rebreathing through a mask (with the mistaken idea that retaining carbon dioxide dilates blood vessels in the brain and promotes healing of brain cells) and spinning the child upside down to supposedly increase cerebral blood flow (National Health & Medical Research Council, 1976).

In order to achieve hemispheric dominance, in which one side of the brain will control not only language but also the dominant hand, eye, and foot, it may be deemed necessary to restrict the use of one arm, occlude one eye, and prohibit singing and listening to music. Bimanual activity may be prohibited and one arm (normally the left) may be put in a sling. Music, particularly primitive folk-type melodies, is believed to be beneficial for children supposedly at the midbrain level of development (Delacato, 1963), but for children at the cortical level who have not established unilateral dominance, all tonal activity, both sensory and expressive, must be deleted (Delacato, 1959).

In their excellent critique H. J. Cohen, Birch, and Taft (1970) conclude that there is no substantial support in work on the development and organization of the nervous system for the theoretical bases of the Doman-Delacato method. Some ten years later this is still the position. We have already seen (Chapter Twelve) that hemispheric asymmetry does not develop but rather is almost certainly innate, and that in most individuals the left hemisphere, unless removed *in toto*, is likely to become and remain language-dominant, despite often extensive damage. Plastic reorganization, when it occurs, is more likely at an *intra*hemispheric rather than an *inter*hemispheric level.

Delacato's basic premise that hemispheric asymmetry is unique to humans has also been refuted (see Chapter Two). We will consider just two further points, which are each the basis of Delacato's remediation techniques. First, Delacato seems to assume that the dominant eye (or sighting eye) is directly connected to the dominant hemisphere (Delacato, 1970, p. 161). Anatomically, this is just not possible (see Figure 5-2). The optic nerves divide at the optic chiasm so that some fibers from each eye go to each hemisphere, the nasal fibers projecting contralaterally and the temporal ipsilaterally. It is therefore impossible to develop one hemisphere by restricting vision to one eye, and while it may possibly help some (visual-spatial) dyslexics develop stable *ocular* dominance (see Stein & Fowler, 1981), this practice may even be harmful unless prescribed and monitored by a qualified ophthalmologist.

Second, in his concept of a dominant hemisphere, Delacato appears to assume that the other hemisphere must be kept subdominant. Thus, in order to complete neurological organization, every effort is made to suppress the nondominant hemisphere, even if this means putting restrictions on enjoyable, beneficial, and relaxing activities involving music, which, as we have seen in Chapter Nine, is in any case not lateralized *per se* to the right hemisphere. This practice has absolutely no foundation in what we know about hemispheric organization. The relationship between the two sides of the brain is not one of dominance by one side and suppression of the other; rather, each side has differing abilities or processing capacities. Indeed, as we saw in Chapter Eight, the nondominant right hemisphere plays a not-inconsiderable role in mediating language-related behavior.

Delacato's techniques are frequently used with children with reading disabilities (Delacato, 1970), particularly children with mixed laterality and/or mirror-reversal problems. However, as we have seen in Chapter Thirteen, there is no good evidence for mirror-symmetrical, left–right coding in the two sides of the brain, certainly not at the level of perception, and there is considerable dispute as to whether there is a greater incidence of crossed lateralization among developmental dyslexics. There are only weak correlations between measures of hand, foot, eye, and ear dominance, and it is unlikely that any single causal mechanism can account for all these manifestations of lateral preference (see Chapter Ten). Crossed laterality does not necessarily indicate atypical hemispheric asymmetry, and no useful purpose is served by continually screening children for signs of it.

Although the theoretical foundations of the Doman-Delacato methods appear to be completely unsound, one should still ask whether the methods work. There have been numerous unsubstantiated claims of success, particularly in the popular press. Several attempts have been made to validate the claims made for these methods, but they have not shown that Doman and Delacato's techniques are significantly more effective than conventional methods of treatment and remediation (H. J. Cohen, Birch, & Taft, 1970; Robbins, 1966; Robbins & Glass, 1969; Neman, Roos, Menolascino, McCann, & Heal, 1975). Neman et al. did find some specific improvements, but the validity of their findings has been seriously questioned by Zigler and Seitz (1975; see also Hirsch & Anderson, 1976).

Official concern has also been expressed about the Doman-Delacato methods. In 1968 the American Academy of Pediatrics published a statement by seven professional organizations in the United States and Canada that are concerned with the care and rehabilitation of disabled and retarded children and adults, expressing their concern about the Doman-Delacato methods. The reasons for their concern included:

1. Promotional methods . . . appear to put parents in a position where they cannot refuse such treatment without calling into question their adequacy and motives as parents.
2. The regimens prescribed are so demanding and inflexible . . . that they may lead to neglect of other family members' needs. . . .

3. It is asserted that if therapy is not carried out as rigidly prescribed, the child's potential will be damaged, and that anything less than 100 per cent effort is useless. . . .

4. Restrictions are often placed upon age-appropriate activities of which the child is capable, such as walking or listening to music . . . though unwarranted by any supportive data and knowledge of long-term results published to date.

5. Claims are made for rapid and conclusive diagnosis according to a "Developmental Profile" . . . of no known validity. No data on which construction of the Profile has been based have ever been published, nor do we know of any attempt to cross-validate it against any accepted methods.

6. Undocumented claims are made for cures in a substantial number of cases . . . extending even beyond disease states to making normal children superior, . . . easing world tensions . . . and possibly "hastening the evolutionary process" . . .

7. Without supporting data, Doman and Delacato have indicated many typical child-rearing practices as limiting a child's potential, increasing thereby the anxiety of already burdened and confused parents.[1]

In October 1976 the National Health and Medical Research Council (Australia) released a report on methods used by the Institute for the Achievement of Human Potential (I.A.H.P.), which was established by Doman and Delacato in 1963. They found no scientific evidence to support either the theory of neurological organization or the treatment techniques used by the I.A.H.P. (National Health & Medical Research Council, 1976).

This is not to deny categorically that there may be some residual benefits from programs such as Doman-Delacato's, which make the child the focus of sustained attention, but since "close supervision, repeated testing, structured environment, and a favourable atmosphere all may produce substantial benefits in I.Q. and social functioning, there is ample reason to question the claim that the types of improvement reported by Doman and Delacato are the direct result of 'patterning treatment'" (H. J. Cohen et al., 1970, p. 308). H. J. Cohen et al. (1970) review several studies to support these claims and suggest that a similar analysis can be applied to other claims advanced by the advocates of "patterning"—for example, improvements in motor function, perception, speech, language, and reading. The enthusiastic judgment of parents and friends (and even of the media) under those circumstances in which a treatment appears to be helpful, while readily understood, is unlikely to reflect the scientific validity of the treatment.

Educational possibilities. Bogen, a neurosurgeon, is one of the few researchers to have written specifically on "educational aspects of hemispheric specialization" (Bogen, 1975, 1977). He writes that "the notion of two largely lateralized

---

[1]From the official statement on "The Doman-Delacato Treatment of Neurologically Handicapped Children" published in the *Journal of Pediatrics,* 1968, *72,* 750. Courtesy of the publishers, C. V. Mosby Company.

modes of thought [appositional and propositional] suggests that teaching by either precept or percept affects primarily one or other hemisphere" (1975, p. 27). He suggests that in emphasizing the three Rs our society has tended to educate mainly one hemisphere—the left. This may have not only caused difficulties for individual students but could mean "that an entire student body is being educated lopsidedly" (Bogen, 1975, p. 29).

Throughout the previous chapters we have frequently emphasized that hemispheric differences are quantitative, not qualitative, and that the hemispheres are relatively rather than absolutely specialized (except perhaps for expressive speech). Hence care should be taken before classifying any task as absolutely left or right, or any individuals or group as left or right hemisphere thinkers. With this caution in mind it is still possible to endorse Bogen's suggestions that we should give greater recognition to those who excel at "so-called" right hemisphere tasks, and should encourage greater right hemisphere participation in the educational process. Wheatley (1977), for example, suggests that right hemisphere involvement in mathematics is increased by the use of puzzles, particularly of a spatial nature, and problem-solving activities with tessellations, pentominoes, tangrams, and soma cubes. In other subjects, too, Bogen suggests that "greater right hemisphere participation would involve more laboratory and field experience at the expense of lectures and seminars" (1975, p. 30). Perhaps the new methods of tomographic mapping of human cerebral metabolism being used by Mazziotta and his colleagues (Mazziotta, Phelps, Miller, & Kuhl, 1981; Phelps, Mazziotta, Kuhl, Nuwer, Packwood, Metter, & Engel, 1981) will in due course enable determination of the relative involvement of different cortical areas in different problem-solving and learning tasks. Until then teachers should select a variety of techniques in order to assist as many different students as possible.

Gaddes presents "two cases with evidence of clearly defined regional cerebral dysfunction, one with left-hemisphere dysfunction and one with right-hemisphere impairment" (1980, p. 140). These case studies are good examples of the role of the teacher and the psychologist in attempting to integrate neurological information and behavioral data. The emphasis in both cases seems to be on highlighting the child's strengths. In a school system, which Gaddes suggests "tends to discriminate unfairly against the child with unilateral left-hemisphere dysfunction and to favour the right-hemisphere lesion child, because he usually has a better chance to satisfy the demands of the system" (p. 147), it is important to draw attention to a child's left and right hemisphere skills and to emphasize the importance of both. In this way teachers may come to give greater recognition to the poor reader with a performance IQ in excess of 130.

While little is known about the interaction between cognitive styles and instructional designs, teaching techniques, and modes of presentation, Ausburn and Ausburn (1978) see the real importance of cognitive styles lying in this area. They suggest that it is not only difficult but also unwise to try to alter a person's cognitive style, because the existing style may in fact be beneficial in some tasks or situations. Learning problems should instead be viewed as instruction-based, and appropriate instruction should be designed to help learners cope with the tasks that are causing them difficulty. This solution should be applied to children who are having difficulty learning to read. If Witelson is correct and dyslexics do use a spatial, holistic cognitive strategy in reading rather than a phonetic-analytic one (see Chapter Thirteen), then we should be trying to develop an approach to the teaching of reading that strikes a balance between linguistic processing ("phonetic" approach) and spatial processing ("look-and-say" method). While in "phonic" or "phonetic" methods children are taught to analyze words into their phonic components and then to synthesize these components into a spoken word, the "look-and-say," or "whole-word," approach teaches children to respond to the whole word as a total visual image, using various visual cues such as the word's shape, size, and initial grapheme (for review, see Southgate & Roberts, 1970). The balance might have to be adjusted either way, depending on the level of each cognitive mode a given child is capable of achieving. In some cases of acquired dyslexia resulting from severe left hemisphere damage, a "look-and-say" method may be the most appropriate approach because it would allow the nondamaged right hemisphere to take over the reading task via a visual holistic strategy (e.g., see Carmon, Gordon, Bental, & Harness, 1977).

As our understanding of the specialized roles of each hemisphere develops, and as our techniques for investigating individual differences in this specialization improve, we should be able to tailor our teaching methods to meet the needs not only of dyslexic and disabled persons but of all individuals. Whether they achieve their "human potential" will depend not on how they are "patterned" but on how well clinicians and educationalists apply our expanding knowledge of hemispheric processing.

References

Aaron, P. G. Dyslexia, an imbalance in cerebral information-processing strategies. *Perceptual and Motor Skills*, 1978, *47*, 699–706.

Abbs, J. H., & Smith, K. U. Laterality differences in the auditory feedback control of speech. *Journal of Speech and Hearing Research*, 1970, *13*, 298–303.

Ahn, H., Prichep, L., John, E. R., Baird, H., Trepetin, M., & Kay, H. Developmental equations reflect brain dysfunction. *Science*, 1980, *210*, 1259–1262.

Aitkin, L. M., & Webster, W. R. Medical geniculate body of the cat: Organization and responses to tonal stimuli of neurons in ventral division. *Journal of Neurophysiology*, 1972, *35*, 365–380.

Albert, M. L. Alexia. In K. M. Heilman & E. Valenstein (Eds.), *Clinical neuropsychology*. New York: Oxford University Press, 1979.

Allard, F., & Bryden, M. P. The effect of concurrent activity on hemispheric asymmetries. *Cortex*, 1979, *15*, 5–17.

Allard, F., & Scott, B. L. Burst cues, transition cues and hemispheric specialization with real speech sounds. *Quarterly Journal of Experimental Psychology*, 1975, *27*, 487–497.

American Academy of Pediatrics. The Doman-Delacato treatment of neurologically handicapped children. *Journal of Pediatrics*, 1968, *72*, 750–752.

Anderson, J. R. Arguments concerning representations for mental imagery. *Psychological Review*, 1978, *85*, 249–277.

Anderson, R. E. Short term retention of the where and when of pictures and words. *Journal of Experimental Psychology: General*, 1976, *105*, 378–402.

Andreewsky, E., Deloche, G., & Kossanyi, P. Analogies between speed-reading and deep dyslexia: Towards a procedural understanding of reading. In M. Coltheart, K. Patterson, & J. C. Marshall (Eds.), *Deep dyslexia*. London: Routledge & Kegan Paul, 1980.

Andrew, J. Laterality on the tapping test among legal offenders. *Journal of Clinical Child Psychology*, 1978, *7*, 149–150.

Andrews, R. J. Aspects of language lateralization correlated with familial handedness. *Neuropsychologia*, 1977, *15*, 769–778.

Annett, M. A model of the inheritance of handedness and cerebral dominance. *Nature*, 1964, *204*, 59–60.

Annett, M. The binomial distribution of right, mixed and left handedness. *Quarterly Journal of Experimental Psychology*, 1967, *19*, 327–333.

Annett, M. A classification of hand preference by association analysis. *British Journal of Psychology*, 1970, *61*, 303-321. (a)

Annett, M. The growth of manual preference and speed. *British Journal of Psychology*, 1970, *61*, 545-558. (b)

Annett, M. The distribution of manual asymmetry. *British Journal of Psychology*, 1972, *63*, 343-358.

Annett, M. Handedness in families. *Annals of Human Genetics*, 1973, *37*, 93-105.

Annett, M. A coordination of hand preference and skill replicated. *British Journal of Psychology*, 1976, *67*, 587-592.

Annett, M. A single gene explanation of right and left handedness and brainedness. Unpublished paper, 1978.

Annett, M., & Annett, J. Individual differences in right and left reaction time. *British Journal of Psychology*, 1979, *70*, 393-404.

Annett, M., Hudson, P. T. W., & Turner, A. Effects of right and left unilateral ECT on naming and visual discrimination analysed in relation to handedness. *British Journal of Psychiatry*, 1974, *124*, 260-264.

Annett, M., & Ockwell, A. Birth order, birth stress and handedness. *Cortex*, 1980, *16*, 181-188.

Annett, M., & Turner, A. Laterality and the growth of intellectual abilities. *British Journal of Educational Psychology*, 1974, *44*, 37-46.

Anzola, G. P., Bertoloni, G., Buchtel, H. A., & Rizzolatti, G. Spatial compatibility and anatomical factors in simple and choice reaction time. *Neuropsychologia*, 1977, *15*, 295-302.

Applebee, A. N. Research in reading retardation: Two critical problems. *Journal of Child Psychology and Psychiatry*, 1971, *12*, 91-113.

Arndt, S., & Berger, D. F. Cognitive mode and asymmetry in cerebral functioning. *Cortex*, 1978, *14*, 78-86.

Arnold, A. P. Sexual differences in the brain. *American Scientist*, 1980, *68*, 165-173.

Atkinson, J., & Egeth, H. Right hemisphere superiority in visual orientation matching. *Canadian Journal of Psychology*, 1973, *27*, 152-158.

Ausburn, L. J., & Ausburn, F. Cognitive styles: Some information and implications for instructional design. *Educational Communication and Technology*, 1978, *26*, 337-354.

Babkoff, H., Ben-Uriah, Y., & Eliashar, S. Grammatical decision time and visual hemifield stimulation. *Cortex*, 1980, *16*, 575-586.

Bailey, P., & Von Bonin, G. *The isocortex of man*. Urbana: University of Illinois Press, 1951.

Bakan, P. Handedness and birth order, *Nature*, 1971, *229*, 195.

Bakan, P. Left-handedness and alcoholism. *Perceptual and Motor Skills*, 1973, *36*, 514.

Bakan, P. Left handedness and birth order revisited. *Neuropsychologia*, 1977, *15*, 837-839.

Bakan, P., Dibb, G., & Reed, P. Handedness and birth stress. *Neuropsychologia*, 1973, *11*, 363-366.

Bakker, D. J. Ear-asymmetry with monaural stimulation: Relations to lateral dominance and lateral awareness. *Neuropsychologia*, 1970, *8*, 103-117.

Bakker, D. J. Hemispheric specialization and stages in the learning-to-read process. *Bulletin of the Orton Society*, 1973, *23*, 15-27.

Bakker, D. J., Smink, T., & Reitsma, P. Ear dominance and reading ability. *Cortex*, 1973, *9*, 301-312.

Bakker, D. J., & Van de Kleij, P. C. M. Development of lateral asymmetry in the perception of sequentially touched fingers. *Acta Psychologica*, 1978, *42*, 357-365.

Bakketeig, L. S., & Hoffman, H. J. Perinatal mortality by birth order within cohorts based on sibship size. *British Medical Journal*, 1979, *2*, 693-696.

Bakwin, H. Reading disability in twins. *Developmental Medicine and Child Neurology*, 1973, *15*, 184-187.

Bamber, D. Reaction times and error rates for same-different judgements of multi-dimensional stimuli. *Perception and Psychophysics*, 1969, *6*, 169-174.

Bartholomeus, B. Effects of task requirements on ear superiority for sung speech. *Cortex*, 1974, *10*, 215-223.

Barton, M., Goodglass, H., & Shai, A. Differential recognition of tachistoscopically presented English and Hebrew words in right and left visual fields. *Perceptual and Motor Skills*, 1965, *21*, 431-437.

Basser, L. S. Hemiplegia of early onset and the faculty of speech with special reference to the effects of hemispherectomy. *Brain*, 1962, *85*, 427-460.

Beaumont, J. G. Handedness and hemisphere function. In S. J. Dimond & J. G. Beaumont (Eds.), *Hemisphere function in the human brain.* London: Elek Science, 1974.

Beck, B. B. *Animal tool behavior: The use and manufacture of tools by animals.* New York: Garland, 1980.

Beller, H. K. Parallel and serial stages in matching. *Journal of Experimental Psychology,* 1970, *84,* 213–219.

Belmont, L., & Birch, H. G. Lateral dominance, lateral awareness, and reading disability. *Child Development,* 1965, *36,* 57–71.

Benbow, C. P., & Stanley, J. C. Sex differences in mathematical ability: Fact or artifact? *Science,* 1980, *210,* 1262–1264.

Benson, D. F. Aphasia. In K. M. Heilman & E. Valenstein (Eds.), *Clinical neuropsychology.* Oxford: Oxford University Press, 1979. (a)

Benson, D. F. *Aphasia, alexia, and agraphia.* New York: Churchill Livingstone, 1979. (b)

Benson, D. F., & Geschwind, N. The alexias. In P. J. Vinken & G. W. Bruyn (Eds.), *Handbook of clinical neurology: Disorders of speech, perception, and symbolic behavior* (Vol. 4). Amsterdam: North Holland, 1969.

Benton, A. L. Clinical symptomatology in right and left hemisphere lesions. In V. B. Mountcastle (Ed.), *Interhemispheric relations and cerebral dominance.* Baltimore: Johns Hopkins University Press, 1962.

Benton, A. L. Contributions to aphasia before Broca. *Cortex,* 1964, *1,* 314–327.

Benton, A. L. Differential behavioral effects of frontal lobe disease. *Neuropsychologia,* 1968, *6,* 53–60.

Benton, A. L. Developmental dyslexia: Neurological aspects. In W. J. Friedlander (Ed.), *Advances in neurology. Vol. 7: Current reviews of higher nervous system dysfunction.* New York: Raven Press, 1975.

Benton, A. L. The amusias. In M. Critchley & R. A. Henson (Eds.), *Music and the brain.* London: Heinemann, 1977.

Benton, A. L. The cognitive functioning of children with developmental dysphasia. In M. A. Wyke (Ed.), *Developmental dysphasia.* New York: Academic Press, 1978.

Benton, A. Visuoperceptive, visuospatial and visuoconstructive disorders. In K. M. Heilman & E. Valenstein (Eds.), *Clinical neuropsychology.* Oxford: Oxford University Press, 1979.

Benton, A. L. The neuropsychology of facial recognition. *American Psychologist,* 1980, *35,* 176–186.

Benton, A. L., Levin, H., & Varney, N. Tactile perception of direction in normal subjects: Implications for hemispheric cerebral dominance. *Neurology,* 1973, *23,* 1248–1250.

Benton, A. L., Meyers, R., & Polder, G. J. Some aspects of handedness. *Psychiatria et Neurologia* (Basel), 1962, *144,* 321–337.

Benton, A. L., Varney, N. R., & Hamsher, K. de S. Lateral differences in tactile directional perception. *Neuropsychologia,* 1978, *16,* 109–114.

Berlin, C. I. Hemispheric asymmetry in auditory tasks. In S. Harnad, R. W. Doty, L. Goldstein, J. Jaynes, & G. Krauthamer (Eds.), *Lateralization in the nervous system.* New York: Academic Press, 1977.

Berlin, C. I., Cullen, J. K., Lowe-Bell, S. S., & Berlin, H. L. Speech perception after hemispherectomy and temporal lobectomy. Paper presented at the Speech Communication Seminar, Stockholm, Aug. 1–4, 1974.

Berlin, C. I., Hughes, L. F., Lowe-Bell, S. S., & Berlin, H. L. Dichotic right ear advantage in children 5 to 13. *Cortex,* 1973, *9,* 393–402.

Berlucchi, G. Interhemispheric integration of simple visuomotor responses. In P. A. Buser & A. Rougeul-Buser (Eds.), *Cerebral correlates of conscious experience: Inserm symposium No. 6.* Amsterdam: Elsevier/North-Holland Biomedical Press, 1978.

Berlucchi, G., Brizzolara, D., Marzi, C. A., Rizzolatti, G., & Umiltà, C. Can lateral asymmetries in attention explain interfield differences in visual perception? *Cortex,* 1974, *10,* 177–185.

Berlucchi, G., Brizzolara, D., Marzi, C. A., Rizzolatti, G., & Umiltà, C. The role of stimulus discrimination and verbal codability in hemispheric specialization for visuospatial tasks. *Neuropsychologia,* 1979, *17,* 195–202.

Berlucchi, G., Crea, F., Di Stefano, M., & Tassinari, G. Influence of spatial stimulus-response compatibility on reaction time of ipsilateral and contralateral hand to lateralized light stimuli.

Journal of Experimental Psychology: Human Perception and Performance, 1977, *3,* 505–517.

Bertelson, P., Vanhaelen, H., & Morais, J. Left hemifield superiority and the extraction of physiognomic information. In I. Steele Russell, M. W. Hof, & G. Berlucchi (Eds.), *Structure and function of cerebral commissures.* London: Macmillan, 1979.

Bever, T. G. The nature of cerebral dominance in speech behavior of the child and adult. In R. Huxley & E. Ingram (Eds.), *Language acquisition, models and methods.* New York: Academic Press, 1971.

Bever, T. G. Broca and Lashley were right: Cerebral dominance is an accident of growth. In D. Caplan (Ed.), *Biological studies of mental processes.* Cambridge, Mass.: MIT Press, 1980.

Bever, T. G., & Chiarello, R. J. Cerebral dominance in musicians and nonmusicians. *Science,* 1974, *185,* 137–139.

Bever, T. G., Hurtig, R. R., & Handel, A. B. Analytic processing elicits right ear superiority in monaurally presented speech. *Neuropsychologia,* 1976, *14,* 175–181.

Bindra, D., Donderi, D. C., & Nishisato, S. Decision latencies of "same" and "different" judgments. *Perception and Psychophysics,* 1968, *3,* 121–130.

Birch, H. G., & Belmont, L. Auditory-visual integration in normal and retarded readers. *American Journal of Orthopsychiatry,* 1964, *34,* 852–861.

Birkett, P. Measures of laterality and theories of hemispheric processes. *Neuropsychologia,* 1977, *15,* 693–696.

Birkett, P. Relationships among handedness, familial handedness, sex and ocular sighting-dominance. *Neuropsychologia,* 1979, *17,* 533–537.

Birkett, P., & Wilson, I. Theory and practice in the measurement of laterality. *Cortex,* 1979, *15,* 507–513.

Bishop, D. V. M. Handedness, clumsiness and cognitive ability. *Developmental Medicine and Child Neurology,* 1980, *22,* 569–579.

Black, D., Young, C. C., Pei, W. C., & de Chardin, T. Fossil man in China. *Memoirs of the Geological Survey of China, Series A, No. 11,* 1933.

Blau, A. *The master hand: A study of the origin and meaning of right and left sidedness and its relation to personality and language.* Research Monograph No. 5. New York: American Orthopsychiatric Association, 1946.

Blau, T. H. Torque and schizophrenic vulnerability. As the world turns. *American Psychologist,* 1977, *32,* 997–1005.

Blinkov, S. M., & Glezer, I. I. *The human brain in figures and tables.* New York: Basic Books, 1968.

Blount, P., Holmes, J., Rodger, J., Coltheart, M., & McManus, C. On the ability to discriminate original from mirror-image reproductions of works of art. *Perception,* 1975, *4,* 385–389.

Blumstein, S., & Cooper, W. E. Hemispheric processing of intonation contours. *Cortex,* 1974, *10,* 146–158.

Bock, R. D., & Kolakowski, D. Further evidence of sex-linked major-gene influence on human spatial visualizing ability. *American Journal of Human Genetics,* 1973, *25,* 1–14.

Boder, E. Developmental dyslexia: Prevailing diagnostic concepts and a new diagnostic approach. In H. R. Myklebust (Ed.), *Progress in learning disabilities,* Vol. 2. New York: Grune & Stratton, 1971.

Bogen, J. E. The other side of the brain I. Dysgraphia and dyscopia following cerebral commissurotomy. *Bulletin of the Los Angeles Neurological Society,* 1969, *34,* 73–105. (a)

Bogen, J. E. The other side of the brain II. An appositional mind. *Bulletin of the Los Angeles Neurological Society,* 1969, *34,* 135–162. (b)

Bogen, J. E. Some educational aspects of hemispheric specialization. *UCLA Educator,* 1975, *17,* 24–32.

Bogen, J. E. Some educational implications of hemispheric specialization. In M. C. Wittrock (Ed.), *The human brain.* Englewood Cliffs, N.J.: Prentice-Hall, 1977.

Bogen, J. E. The callosal syndrome. In K. M. Heilman & E. Valenstein (Eds.), *Clinical neuropsychology.* Oxford: Oxford University Press, 1979.

Bogen, J. E., & Bogen, G. M. Wernicke's region—where is it? *Annals of the New York Academy of Sciences,* 1976, *280,* 834–843.

Bogen, J. E., & Gordon, H. W. Musical tests for functional lateralization with intracarotid amobarbital. *Nature,* 1971, *230,* 524–525.

Boklage, C. E. The sinistral blastocyst: An embryologic perspective on the development of brain-function asymmetries. In J. Herron (Ed.), *Neuropsychology of left-handedness*. New York: Academic Press, 1980.

Boles, D. B. Laterally biased attention with concurrent verbal load: Multiple failures to replicate. *Neuropsychologia*, 1979, *17*, 353-361.

Boles, D. B. X-linkage of spatial ability: A critical review. *Child Development*, 1980, *51*, 625-635.

Borad, J. C., & Goodglass, H. Lateralization of linguistic and melodic processing with age. *Neuropsychologia*, 1980, *18*, 79-83.

Borkowski, J. G., Spreen, O., & Stutz, J. Z. Ear preference and abstractness in dichotic listening. *Psychonomic Science*, 1965, *3*, 547-548.

Botkin, A. L., Schmaltz, L. W., & Lamb, D. H. "Overloading" the left hemisphere in right-handed subjects with verbal and motor tasks. *Neuropsychologia*, 1977, *15*, 591-596.

Bouma, H., & Legein, Ch. P. Dyslexia: A specific recoding deficit? An analysis of response latencies for letters and words in dyslectics and in average readers. *Neuropsychologia*, 1980, *18*, 285-298.

Bowers, D., & Heilman, K. M. Pseudoneglect: Effects of hemispace on a tactile line bisection task. *Neuropsychologia*, 1980, *18*, 491-498.

Bowers, D., Heilman, K. M., Satz, P., & Altman, A. Simultaneous performance on verbal, non-verbal and motor tasks by right-handed adults. *Cortex*, 1978, *14*, 540-556.

Bradley, L., & Bryant, P. E. Difficulties in auditory organization as a possible cause of reading backwardness. *Nature*, 1978, *271*, 746-747.

Bradshaw, G. J., & Hicks, R. E. Word recognition, lexical decision and visual field. *Bulletin of the Psychonomic Society*, 1977, *10*, 266.

Bradshaw, G. J., Hicks, R. E., & Rose, B. Lexical discrimination and letter-string identification in the two visual fields. *Brain and Language*, 1979, *8*, 10-18.

Bradshaw, J. L. Peripherally-presented and unreported words may bias the perceived meaning of a centrally-fixated homograph. *Journal of Experimental Psychology*, 1974, *103*, 1200-1202.

Bradshaw, J. L. Right-hemisphere language: Familial and non-familial sinistrals, cognitive deficits and writing hand position in sinistrals, and concrete-abstract, imageable-nonimageable dimensions in word recognition. A review of interrelated issues. *Brain and Language*, 1980, *10*, 172-188. (a)

Bradshaw, J. L. Sex and side: A double dichotomy interacts. *Behavioral and Brain Sciences*, 1980, *3*, 229-230. (b)

Bradshaw, J. L., Bradley, D., Gates, E. A., & Patterson, K. Serial, parallel or holistic identification of single words in the two visual fields? *Perception and Psychophysics*, 1977, *21*, 431-438.

Bradshaw, J. L., Bradley, D., & Patterson, K. The perception and identification of mirror-reversed patterns. *Quarterly Journal of Experimental Psychology*, 1976, *28*, 667-681.

Bradshaw, J. L., Farrelly, J., & Taylor, M. J. Synonym and antonym pairs in the detection of dichotically and monaurally presented targets: Competing monaural stimulation can generate a REA. *Acta Psychologica*, 1981, *47*, 189-205.

Bradshaw, J. L., & Gates, E. A. Visual field differences in verbal tasks: Effects of task familiarity and sex of subject. *Brain and Language*, 1978, *5*, 166-187.

Bradshaw, J. L., Gates, E. A., & Nettleton, N. C. Bihemispheric involvement in lexical decisions: Handedness and a possible sex difference. *Neuropsychologia*, 1977, *15*, 277-286.

Bradshaw, J. L., Gates, E. A., & Patterson, K. Hemispheric differences in processing visual patterns. *Quarterly Journal of Experimental Psychology*, 1976, *28*, 667-681.

Bradshaw, J. L., & Mapp, A. Laterally presented words: Orthographic analysis and serial, parallel or holistic modes of processing. *Australian Journal of Psychology*, 1982, *34*, 71-90.

Bradshaw, J. L., & Nettleton, N. C. The nature of hemispheric specialization in man. *Behavioral and Brain Sciences*, 1981, *4*, 51-63.

Bradshaw, J. L., Nettleton, N. C., & Geffen, G. Ear differences and delayed auditory feedback: Effects on a speech and a music task. *Journal of Experimental Psychology*, 1971, *91*, 85-92.

Bradshaw, J. L., Nettleton, N. C., & Geffen, G. Ear asymmetry and delayed auditory feedback. Effects of task requirements and competitive stimulation. *Journal of Experimental Psychology*, 1972, *94*, 269-275.

Bradshaw, J. L., Nettleton, N. C., & Taylor, M. J. Right hemisphere language and cognitive deficit in sinistrals? *Neuropsychologia,* 1981, *19,* 113–132. (a)

Bradshaw, J. L., Nettleton, N. C., & Taylor, M. J. The use of laterally presented words in research into cerebral asymmetry: Is directional scanning likely to be a source of artifact? *Brain and Language,* 1981, *14,* 1–14. (b)

Bradshaw, J. L., & Perriment, A. D. Laterality effects and choice reaction time in a unimanual two-finger task. *Perception and Psychophysics,* 1970, *7,* 185–188.

Bradshaw, J. L., & Sherlock, D. Bugs and faces in the two visual fields: Task order, difficulty, practice and the analytic/holistic dichotomy. *Cortex,* 1982, in press.

Bradshaw, J. L., & Taylor, M. A word naming deficit in nonfamilial sinistrals? Laterality effects of vocal responses to tachistoscopically-presented letter strings. *Neuropsychologia,* 1979, *17,* 21–32.

Bradshaw, J. L., Taylor, M. J., Patterson, K., & Nettleton, N. C. Upright and inverted faces, and housefronts, in the two visual fields: A right and a left hemisphere contribution. *Journal of Clinical Neuropsychology,* 1980, *2,* 245–257.

Briggs, G. G., & Nebes, R. D. Patterns of hand preference in a student population. *Cortex,* 1975, *11,* 230–238.

Briggs, G. G., & Nebes, R. D. The effects of handedness, family history and sex on the performance of a dichotic listening task. *Neuropsychologia,* 1976, *14,* 129–134.

Brinkman, J., & Kuypers, H. G. J. M. Cerebral control of contralateral and ipsilateral arm, hand and finger movements in the split-brain rhesus monkey. *Brain,* 1973, *96,* 653–674.

Brizzolara, D., Umiltà, C., Marzi, C. A., Berlucchi, G., & Rizzolatti, G. A verbal response in a discriminative reaction time task with lateralised visual stimuli is compatible with a right-hemispheric superiority. *Brain Research,* 1975, *85,* 185.

Broadbent, D. E., & Gregory, M. Accuracy of recognition for speech presented to the right and left ears. *Quarterly Journal of Experimental Psychology,* 1964, *16,* 359–360.

Brown, J. W. Brain structure and language production: A dynamic view. In D. Caplan (Ed.), *Biological studies of mental processes.* Cambridge, Mass.: MIT Press, 1980.

Brugge, J. F., & Merzenich, M. M. Responses of neurones in auditory cortex of the macaque monkey to monaural and binaural stimulation. *Journal of Neurophysiology,* 1973, *36,* 1138–1158.

Brust, J. C. M. Music and language: Musical alexia and agraphia. *Brain,* 1980, *103,* 367–392.

Bryden, M. P. Ear preference in auditory perception. *Journal of Experimental Psychology,* 1963, *65,* 103–105.

Bryden, M. P. Tachistoscopic recognition, handedness, and cerebral dominance. *Neuropsychologia,* 1965, *3,* 1–8.

Bryden, M. P. Accuracy and order of report in tachistoscopic recognition. *Canadian Journal of Psychology,* 1966, *20,* 262–272.

Bryden, M. P. Binaural competition and division of attention as determinants of the laterality effect in dichotic listening. *Canadian Journal of Psychology,* 1969, *23,* 101–113.

Bryden, M. P. Laterality effects in dichotic listening: Relations with handedness and reading ability in children. *Neuropsychologia,* 1970, *8,* 443–450.

Bryden, M. P. Perceptual asymmetry in vision: Relation to handedness, eyedness, and speech lateralization. *Cortex,* 1973, *9,* 419–435.

Bryden, M. P. Speech lateralization in families: A preliminary study using dichotic listening. *Brain and Language,* 1975, *2,* 201–211.

Bryden, M. P. Response bias and hemispheric differences in dot localization. *Perception and Psychophysics,* 1976, *19,* 23–28.

Bryden, M. P. Strategy effects in the assessment of hemispheric asymmetry. In G. Underwood (Ed.), *Strategies of information processing.* London: Academic Press, 1978.

Bryden, M. P. Evidence for sex-related differences in cerebral organization. In M. A. Wittig & A. C. Petersen (Eds.), *Sex-related differences in cognitive functioning.* New York: Academic Press, 1979.

Bryden, M. P. Sex differences in brain organization: Different brains or different strategies? *Behavioral and Brain Sciences,* 1980, *3,* 230–231.

Bryden, M. P., & Allard, F. Visual hemifield differences depend upon typeface. *Brain and Language,* 1976, *3,* 191–200.

Bryden, M. P., & Allard, F. Dichotic listening and the development of linguistic processes. In

M. Kinsbourne (Ed.), *Asymmetrical function of the brain*. Cambridge: Cambridge University Press, 1978.

Bryden, M. P., & Rainey, C. A. Left-right differences in tachistoscopic recognition. *Journal of Experimental Psychology*, 1963, *66*, 568-571.

Buffery, A. W. H., & Gray, J. A. Sex differences in the development of spatial and linguistic skills. In C. Ounsted & D. C. Taylor (Eds.), *Gender differences: Their ontogeny and significance*. Edinburgh: Churchill-Livingstone, 1972.

Bunt, A. H., Minckler, D. S., & Johanson, G. W. Demonstration of bilateral projection of the central retina of the monkey with horseradish peroxidase neuronography. *Journal of Comparative Neurology*, 1977, *171*, 619-630.

Burklund, C. W., & Smith, A. Language and the cerebral hemispheres. *Neurology*, 1977, *27*, 627-633.

Burstein, B., Bank, L., & Jarvik, L. F. Sex differences in cognitive functioning: Evidence, determinants, implications. *Human Development*, 1980, *23*, 289-313.

Burt, C. L. *The backward child*. London: University of London Press, 1937.

Butler, S. R., & Glass, A. Asymmetries in the CNV over left and right hemispheres while subjects await numeric information. *Biological Psychology*, 1974, *2*, 1-16. (a)

Butler, S. R., & Glass, A. Asymmetries in the electroencephalogram associated with cerebral dominance. *Electroencephalography and Clinical Neurophysiology*, 1974, *36*, 481-491. (b)

Butler, S. R., & Glass, A. EEG correlates of cerebral dominance. In A. H. Riesen & R. F. Thompson (Eds.), *Advances in psychobiology* (Vol. 3). New York: John Wiley, 1976.

Byrne, B., & Sinclair, J. Memory for tonal sequence and timbre: A correlation with familial handedness. *Neuropsychologia*, 1979, *17*, 539-542.

Cacioppo, J. T., Petty, R. E., & Snyder, C. W. Cognitive and affective response as a function of relative hemispheric involvement. *International Journal of Neuroscience*, 1979, *9*, 81-89.

Cain, D. P., & Wada, J. A. An anatomical asymmetry in the baboon brain. *Brain, Behavior and Evolution*, 1979, *16*, 222-226.

Campain, R., & Minckler, J. A note on the gross configurations of the human auditory cortex. *Brain and Language*, 1976, *3*, 318-323.

Campbell, R. Asymmetries in interpreting and expressing a posed facial expression. *Cortex*, 1978, *14*, 327-342.

Caplan, P., & Kinsbourne, M. Baby drops the rattle: Asymmetry of duration of grasp by infants. *Child Development*, 1976, *47*, 532-534.

Caramazza, A., & Broner, I. Lexical access in bilinguals. *Bulletin of the Psychonomic Society*, 1979, *13*, 212-214.

Carey, S. A case study: Face recognition. In E. Walker (Ed.), *Explorations in the biology of language*. Sussex: Harvester Press, 1978.

Carey, S., & Diamond, R. From piecemeal to configurational representation of faces. *Science*, 1977, *195*, 312-314.

Carey, S., & Diamond, R. Maturational determination of the developmental course of face encoding. In D. Caplan (Ed.), *Biological studies of mental processes*. Cambridge, Mass.: MIT Press, 1980.

Carmon, A. Spatial and temporal factors in visual perception of patients with unilateral cerebral lesions. In M. Kinsbourne (Ed.), *Asymmetrical function of the brain*. Cambridge: Cambridge University Press, 1978.

Carmon, A., & Bechtoldt, H. P. Dominance of the right cerebral hemisphere for stereopsis. *Neuropsychologia*, 1969, *7*, 29-39.

Carmon, A., & Gombos, G. M. A physiological vascular correlate of hand preference: Possible implications with respect to hemispheric cerebral dominance. *Neuropsychologia*, 1970, *8*, 119-128.

Carmon, A., Gordon, H. W., Bental, E., & Harness, B. Z. Retraining in literal alexia: Substitution of a right hemisphere perceptual strategy for impaired left hemisphere processing. *Bulletin of the Los Angeles Neurological Societies*, 1977, *42*, 41-50.

Carmon, A., Harishanu, Y., Lowinger, E., & Lavy, S. Asymmetries in hemispheric blood volume and cerebral dominance. *Behavioral Biology*, 1972, *7*, 853-859.

Carmon, A., Kleiner, M., & Nachshon, I. Visual hemifield effects in dichoptic presentations of digits. *Neuropsychologia*, 1975, *13*, 289-295.

Carmon, A., & Nachshon, I. Ear asymmetry in perception of emotional non-verbal stimuli. *Acta Psychologica*, 1973, *37*, 351-357.

Carmon, A., Nachshon, I., Isseroff, A., & Kleiner, M. Visual field differences in reaction time to Hebrew letters. *Psychonomic Science*, 1972, *28*, 222–224.

Carmon, A., Nachshon, I., & Starinsky, R. Developmental aspects of visual hemifield differences in perception of verbal material. *Brain and Language*, 1976, *3*, 463–469.

Carroll, L. *The annotated Alice, with an introduction and notes by Martin Gardner*. New York: Bramhall House, 1960.

Carter, G. L., & Kinsbourne, M. The ontogeny of right cerebral lateralization of spatial mental set. *Developmental Psychology*, 1979, *15*, 241–245.

Carter-Saltzman, L. Patterns of cognitive abilities and lateralization in adoptive and biological families. Paper presented at Sixth Annual Meeting of the Behavior Genetics Association, Boulder, Colorado, 1976.

Carter-Saltzman, L. Patterns of cognitive functioning in relation to handedness and sex-related differences. In M. A. Wittig & A. C. Petersen (Eds.), *Sex-related differences in cognitive functioning*. New York: Academic Press, 1979.

Carter-Saltzman, L. Biological and sociocultural effects on handedness: Comparison between biological and adoptive families. *Science*, 1980, *209*, 1263–1265.

Castro-Caldas, A., & Botelho, M. A. S. Dichotic listening in the recovery of aphasia after stroke. *Brain and Language*, 1980, *10*, 145–151.

Catlin, J., & Neville, H. The laterality effect in reaction time to speech stimuli. *Neuropsychologia*, 1976, *14*, 141–143.

Catlin, J., Vanderveer, N. J., & Teicher, R. D. Monaural right-ear advantage in a target-identification task. *Brain and Language*, 1976, *3*, 470–481.

Chakrabarti, J., & Barker, D. G. Lateral dominance and reading ability. *Perceptual and Motor Skills*, 1966, *22*, 881–882.

Chamberlain, H. D. The inheritance of left-handedness. *Journal of Heredity*, 1928, *19*, 557–559.

Chaney, R. B., & Webster, J. C. Information in certain multidimensional sounds. *The Journal of the Acoustical Society of America*, 1966, *40*, 447–455.

Chapple, W. D. Role of asymmetry in the functioning of invertebrate nervous systems. In S. Harnad, R. W. Doty, L. Goldstein, J. Jaynes, & G. Krauthamer (Eds.), *Lateralization in the nervous system*. New York: Academic Press, 1977.

Chen, L. C. Y. Manual communication by combined alphabet and gestures. *Archives of Physical Medicine and Rehabilitation*, 1971, *52*, 381–384.

Chi, Je. G., Dooling, E. C., & Gilles, F. H. Left-right asymmetries of the temporal speech areas of the human fetus. *Archives of Neurology*, 1977, *34*, 346–348.

Chiarello, C. A house divided? Cognitive functioning with callosal agenesis. *Brain and Language*, 1980, *11*, 128–158.

Chui, H. Chang, & Damasio, A. R. Human cerebral asymmetries evaluated by computed tomography. *Journal of Neurology, Neurosurgery, and Psychiatry*, 1980, *43*, 873–878.

Churchill, J. A., Igna, E., & Senf, R. The association of position at birth and handedness. *Paediatrics*, 1962, *29*, 307–309.

Clifton-Everest, I. M. The immediate recognition of tachistoscopically presented visual patterns by backward readers. *Genetic Psychology Monographs*, 1974, *89*, 221–239.

Cohen, G. Hemispheric differences in a letter classification task. *Perception and Psychophysics*, 1972, *11*, 139–142.

Cohen, G. Hemispheric differences in serial versus parallel processing. *Journal of Experimental Psychology*, 1973, *97*, 349–356.

Cohen, G. Hemispheric differences in the effects of cuing in visual recognition tasks. *Journal of Experimental Psychology: Human Perception and Performance*, 1975, *1*, 366–373. (a)

Cohen, G. Hemispheric differences in the utilization of advance information. In P. M. A. Rabbitt & S. Dornic (Eds.), *Attention and performance V*. New York: Academic Press, 1975. (b)

Cohen, G. Components of the laterality effect in letter recognition: Asymmetries in iconic storage. *Quarterly Journal of Experimental Psychology*, 1976, *28*, 105–114.

Cohen, G. Comment on "Information processing in the cerebral hemispheres: Selective activation and capacity limitations" by Hellige, Cox, and Litvac. *Journal of Experimental Psychology: General*, 1979, *108*, 309–315.

Cohen, G., & Freeman, R. Individual differences in reading strategies in relation to cerebral asymmetry. In J. Requin (Ed.), *Attention and performance VII*. Hillsdale, N.J.: Lawrence Erlbaum, 1978.

Cohen, G., & Martin, M. Hemisphere differences in an auditory Stroop test. *Perception and Psychophysics,* 1975, *17,* 79–83.

Cohen, H. J., Birch, H. G., & Taft, L. T. Some considerations for evaluating the Doman-Delacato "Patterning" method. *Pediatrics,* 1970, *45,* 302–314.

Coles, P. R. Profile orientation and social distance in portrait painting. *Perception,* 1974, *3,* 303–308.

Collins, R. L. Toward an admissible genetic model for the inheritance of the degree and direction of asymmetry. In S. Harnad, R. W. Doty, L. Goldstein, J. Jaynes, & G. Krauthamer (Eds.), *Lateralization in the nervous system.* New York: Academic Press, 1977. (a)

Collins, R. L. Origins of the sense of asymmetry: Mendelian and non-Mendelian models of inheritance. *Annals of the New York Academy of Sciences,* 1977, *299,* 283–305. (b)

Coltheart, M. Mysteries of reading in brain defects. *New Scientist,* 1979, *8,* 368–370.

Coltheart, M. Deep dyslexia: A right-hemisphere hypothesis. In M. Coltheart, K. Patterson, & J. C. Marshall (Eds.), *Deep dyslexia.* London: Routledge & Kegan Paul, 1980. (a)

Coltheart, M. Reading, phonological recoding, and deep dyslexia. In M. Coltheart, K. Patterson, & J. C. Marshall (Eds.), *Deep dyslexia.* London: Routledge & Kegan Paul, 1980. (b)

Coltheart, M., Patterson, K., & Marshall, J. C. *Deep dyslexia.* London: Routledge & Kegan Paul, 1980.

Cooper, W. E. The analytic/holistic distinction applied to the speech of patients with hemispheric brain damage. *Behavioral and Brain Sciences,* 1981, *4,* 68–69.

Corballis, M. C. Laterality and myth. *American Psychologist,* 1980, *35,* 284–295. (a)

Corballis, M. C. Is left-handedness genetically determined? In J. Herron (Ed.), *Neuropsychology of left-handedness.* New York: Academic Press, 1980. (b)

Corballis, M. C. Toward an evolutionary perspective on hemispheric specialization. *Behavioral and Brain Sciences,* 1981, *4,* 69–70.

Corballis, M. C., Anuza, T., & Blake, L. Tachistoscopic perception under head tilt. *Perception and Psychophysics,* 1978, *24,* 274–284.

Corballis, M. C., & Beale, I. L. Bilateral symmetry and behavior. *Psychological Review,* 1970, *77,* 451–464. (a)

Corballis, M. C., & Beale, I. L. Monocular discrimination of mirror image obliques by pigeons: Evidence for lateralized stimulus control. *Animal Behavior,* 1970, *18,* 563–566. (b)

Corballis, M. C., & Beale, I. L. On telling left from right. *Scientific American,* 1971, *224,* 96–104.

Corballis, M. C., & Beale, I. L. *The psychology of left and right.* Hillsdale, N.J.: Lawrence Erlbaum, 1976.

Corballis, M. C., & Morgan, M. J. On the biological basis of human laterality: I. Evidence for a maturational left-right gradient. *Behavioral and Brain Sciences,* 1978, *2,* 261–336.

Coren, S., & Porac, C. Fifty centuries of right handedness: The historical record. *Science,* 1977, *198,* 631–632.

Coren, S., & Porac, C. Normative data on hand position during writing. *Cortex,* 1979, *15,* 679–682.

Coren, S., & Porac, C. Birth factors and laterality: The effect of birth order, parental age and birth stress on four indices of lateral preference. *Behavior Genetics,* 1980, *10,* 123–138. (a)

Coren, S., & Porac, C. Family patterns in four dimensions of lateral preference. *Behavior Genetics,* 1980, *10,* 333–348. (b)

Corkin, S. Serial ordering deficits in inferior readers. *Neuropsychologia,* 1974, *12,* 347–354.

Coryell, J. F., & Michel, G. F. How supine postural preferences of infants can contribute toward the development of handedness. *Infant Behaviour and Development,* 1978, *1,* 245–257.

Cotton, B., Tzeng, O. J. L., & Wang, C. Role of cerebral hemispheric processing in the visual half field: Stimulus-response compatibility effect. *Journal of Experimental Psychology: Human Perception and Performance,* 1980, *6,* 13–23.

Coughlan, A. K., & Warrington, E. K. Word-comprehension and word-retrieval in patients with localized cerebral lesions. *Brain,* 1978, *101,* 163–185.

Craig, J. D. A dichotic rhythm task: Advantage for the left-handed. *Cortex,* 1980, *16,* 613–621.

Crighton-Browne, J. On the weight of the brain and its component parts in the insane. *Brain,* 1880, *2,* 42–67.

Critchley, M. Speech and speech-loss in relation to the duality of the brain. In V. B. Mountcastle (Ed.), *Interhemispheric relations and cerebral dominance.* Baltimore: Johns Hopkins University Press, 1962.

Critchley, M. *The dyslexic child.* London: William Heinemann, 1970.

Critchley, M., & Critchley, E. A. *Dyslexia defined.* London: William Heinemann Medical Books, 1978.

Crovitz, H. F., & Zener, K. A group-test for assessing hand- and eye-dominance. *American Journal of Psychology,* 1962, *75,* 271–276.

Crowell, D. H., Jones, R. H., Kapuniai, L. E., & Nakagawa, J. K. Unilateral cortical activity in newborn humans: An early index of cerebral dominance? *Science,* 1973, *180,* 205–207.

Cunningham, D. F. *Contribution to the surface anatomy of the cerebral hemispheres.* Dublin: Royal Irish Academy, 1892.

Curry, F. K. W. A comparison of left-handed and right-handed subjects on verbal and non-verbal dichotic listening tasks. *Cortex,* 1967, *3,* 343–352.

Curry, F. K. W. A comparison of performances of a right hemispherectomized subject and 25 normals on four dichotic listening tasks. *Cortex,* 1968, *4,* 144–153.

Cutting, J. A parallel between degree of encodedness and the ear advantage: Evidence from an ear-monitoring task. *The Journal of the Acoustical Society of America,* 1973, *53,* 368 (A).

Cutting, J. E. Two left-hemisphere mechanisms in speech perception. *Perception and Psychophysics,* 1974, *16,* 601–612.

Cutting, J. E. There may be nothing peculiar to perceiving in a speech mode. In J. Requin (Ed.), *Attention and performance, VII.* New York: John Wiley, 1979.

Cutting, J. E. Sign language and spoken language. *Nature,* 1980, *284,* 661–662.

Czopf, J. Uber die Rolle der nicht dominanten Hemisphäre in der Restitution der Sprache der Aphasischen. *Archiv fur Psychiatrie und Nervenkrankheiten* (Berlin), 1972, *216,* 162–171.

Dabbs, L., & Choo, R. Carotid blood flow predicts specialized mental ability. *Neuropsychologia,* 1980, *18,* 711–713.

Damasio, A. R., & Damasio, H. Musical faculty and cerebral dominance. In M. Critchley & R. A. Henson (Eds.), *Music and the brain.* London: Heinemann, 1977.

Dart, R. A. The predatory implemental technique of Australopithecus. *American Journal of Physical Anthropology,* 1949, *7,* 1–38.

Darwin, C. J. Auditory perception and cerebral dominance. Doctoral dissertation, University of Cambridge, 1969.

Darwin, C. J. Ear differences in the recall of fricatives and vowels. *Quarterly Journal of Experimental Psychology,* 1971, *23,* 46–62.

Darwin, C. J., & Baddeley, A. D. Acoustic memory and the perception of speech. *Cognitive Psychology,* 1974, *6,* 41–60.

Davidoff, J. B. Hemispheric differences in the perception of lightness. *Neuropsychologia,* 1975, *13,* 121–124.

Davidoff, J. B. Hemispheric sensitivity differences in the perception of colour. *Quarterly Journal of Experimental Psychology,* 1976, *28,* 387–394.

Davidoff, J. B. Hemispheric differences in dot detection. *Cortex,* 1977, *13,* 434–444.

Davidson, R. J., & Schwartz, G. E. The influence of musical training on patterns of EEG asymmetry during musical and nonmusical self-generation tasks. *Psychophysiology,* 1977, *14,* 58–63.

Davis, A. E., & Wada, J. A. Hemisphere asymmetries of visual and auditory information processing. *Neuropsychologia,* 1977, *15,* 799–806. (a)

Davis, A. E., & Wada, J. A. Hemispheric asymmetries in human infants: Spectral analysis of flash and click evoked potentials. *Brain and Language,* 1977, *4,* 23–31. (b)

Davis, R., & Schmit, V. Timing the transfer of information between hemispheres in man. *Acta Psychologica,* 1971, *35,* 335–346.

Davis, R., & Schmit, V. Visual and verbal coding in the interhemispheric transfer of information. *Acta Psychologica,* 1973, *37,* 229–240.

Dawson, J. L. M. B. An anthropological perspective on the evolution and lateralization of the brain. *Annals of the New York Academy of Sciences,* 1977, *299,* 424–447.

Day, J. Right hemisphere language processing in normal right handers. *Journal of Experimental Psychology: Human Perception and Performance,* 1977, *3,* 518–528.

Day, J. Visual half field recognition as a function of syntactic class and imageability. *Neuropsychologia,* 1979, *17,* 515–519.

Dean, R. S. Cerebral laterality and reading comprehension. *Neuropsychologia,* 1978, *16,* 633–636.

Dee, H. L. Auditory asymmetry and strength of manual preference. *Cortex,* 1971, *7,* 236–245.

Dee, H. L., & Fontenot, D. J. Cerebral dominance and lateral differences in perception and memory. *Neuropsychologia*, 1973, *11*, 167–173.

DeFries, J. C., Johnson, R. C., Kuse, A. R., McClearn, G. E., Polovina, J., Vandenberg, S. G., & Wilson, J. R. Familial resemblance for specific cognitive abilities. *Behavior Genetics*, 1979, *9*, 23–43.

Delacato, C. H. *The treatment and prevention of reading problems (The neuropsychological approach)*. Springfield, Ill.: Charles C Thomas, 1959.

Delacato, C. H. *The diagnosis and treatment of speech and reading problems*. Springfield, Ill.: Charles C Thomas, 1963.

Delacato, C. H. *Neurological organization and reading*. Springfield, Ill.: Charles C Thomas, 1966.

Delacato, C. H. *A new start for the child with reading problems: A manual for parents*. New York: D. McKay, 1970.

Demarest, J., & Demarest, L. Auditory asymmetry and strength of manual preference reexamined. *International Journal of Neuroscience*, 1980, *11*, 121–124.

Denckla, M. B. Development of speed in repetitive and successive finger movements in normal children. *Developmental Medicine and Child Neurology*, 1973, *15*, 635–645.

Denckla, M. B. Development of motor coordination in normal children. *Developmental Medicine and Child Neurology*, 1974, *16*, 729–741.

Denckla, M. B., Rudel, R. G., & Broman, M. The development of a spatial orientation skill in normal, learning-disabled, and neurologically impaired children. In D. Caplan (Ed.), *Biological studies of mental processes*. Cambridge, Mass.: MIT Press, 1980.

Denenberg, V. H. Hemispheric laterality in animals and the effects of early experience. *Behavioral and Brain Sciences*, 1981, *4*, 1–49.

Denenberg, V. H., Garbanati, J., Sherman, G., Yutzey, D. A., & Kaplan, R. Infantile stimulation induces brain lateralization in rats. *Science*, 1978, *201*, 1150–1152.

Dennis, M. Impaired sensory and motor differentiation with corpus callosum agenesis: A lack of callosal inhibition during ontogeny? *Neuropsychologia*, 1976, *14*, 455–469.

Dennis, M. Capacity and strategy for syntactic comprehension after left or right hemidecortication. *Brain and Language*, 1980, *10*, 287–317. (a)

Dennis, M. Language acquisition in a single hemisphere: Semantic organization. In D. Caplan (Ed.), *Biological studies of mental processes*. Cambridge, Mass.: MIT Press, 1980. (b)

Dennis, M., & Kohn, B. Comprehension of syntax in infantile hemiplegics after cerebral hemidecortication: Left-hemisphere superiority. *Brain and Language*, 1975, *2*, 472–482.

Dennis, M., Lovett, M., & Wiegel-Crump, C. A. Written language acquisition after left or right hemidecortication in infancy. *Brain and Language*, 1981, *12*, 54–91.

Dennis, M., & Whitaker, H. A. Language acquisition following hemidecortication: Linguistic superiority of the left over the right hemisphere. *Brain and Language*, 1976, *3*, 404–433.

Dennis, M., & Whitaker, H. A. Hemispheric equipotentiality and language acquisition. In S. J. Segalowitz & F. A. Gruber (Eds.), *Language development and neurological theory*. New York: Academic Press, 1977.

De Renzi, E. Hemispheric asymmetry as evidenced by spatial disorders. In M. Kinsbourne (Ed.), *Asymmetrical function of the brain*. Cambridge: Cambridge University Press, 1978.

Deutsch, D. An auditory illusion. *Nature*, 1974, *251*, 307–309.

Deutsch, D. Pitch memory: An advantage for the left handed. *Science*, 1978, *199*, 559–560.

Deutsch, D. Handedness and memory for tonal pitch. In J. Herron (Ed.), *Neuropsychology of left-handedness*. New York: Academic Press, 1980.

Deutsch, D., & Roll, P. L. Separate "what" and "where" decision mechanisms in processing a dichotic tonal sequence. *Journal of Experimental Psychology: Human Perception and Performance*, 1976, *2*, 23–29.

Dewson, J. H. Preliminary evidence of hemispheric asymmetry of auditory function in monkeys. In S. Harnad, R. W. Doty, L. Goldstein, J. Jaynes, & G. Krauthamer (Eds.), *Lateralization in the nervous system*. New York: Academic Press, 1977.

Diamond, M. C., Dowling, G. A., & Johnson, R. E. Morphological cerebral asymmetry in male and female rats. Unpublished manuscript, 1980.

Diekhoff, G. M., Garland, J., Dansereau, D. F., & Walker, C. A. Muscle tension, skin conductance, and finger pulse volume. *Acta Psychologica*, 1978, *42*, 83–93.

Dimond, S. J. Hemisphere function and immediate memory. *Psychonomic Science*, 1969, *16*, 111–112.

Dimond, S. J. Hemisphere refractoriness and control of reaction time. *Quarterly Journal of Experimental Psychology*, 1970, *22*, 610–617.

Dimond, S. J. Evolution and lateralization of the brain: Concluding remarks. *Annals of the New York Academy of Sciences*, 1977, *299*, 477–501.

Dimond, S. J. Tactual and auditory vigilance on splitbrain man. *Journal of Neurology, Neurosurgery and Psychiatry*, 1979, *42*, 70–74. (a)

Dimond, S. J. Performance by splitbrain humans on lateralized vigilance tasks. *Cortex*, 1979, *15*, 43–50. (b)

Dimond, S. J. *Neuropsychology: A textbook of systems and psychological functions of the human brain*. London: Butterworths, 1980.

Dimond, S. J., & Beaumont, J. G. Use of two cerebral hemispheres to increase brain capacity. *Nature*, 1971, *232*, 270–271.

Dimond, S. J., & Beaumont, J. G. Hemisphere function and color naming. *Journal of Experimental Psychology*, 1972, *96*, 87–91. (a)

Dimond, S. J., & Beaumont, J. G. Processing in perceptual integration between and within the cerebral hemispheres. *British Journal of Psychology*, 1972, *63*, 509–514. (b)

Dimond, S. J., & Beaumont, J. G. A right hemisphere basis for calculation in the human brain. *Psychonomic Science*, 1972, *26*, 137–138. (c)

Dimond, S. J., & Beaumont, J. G. Differences in the vigilance performance of the right and left hemispheres. *Cortex*, 1973, *9*, 259–266.

Dimond, S. J., & Beaumont, J. G. Experimental studies of hemisphere function in the human brain. In S. J. Dimond & J. G. Beaumont (Eds.), *Hemisphere function in the human brain*. London: Elek Science, 1974.

Dimond, S. J., & Farrington, J. Emotional response to films shown to the right or left hemisphere of the brain measured by heart rate. *Acta Psychologica*, 1977, *41*, 255–260.

Dingwall, W. O. The evolution of human communication systems. In H. Whitaker & H. A. Whitaker (Eds.), *Studies in neurolinguistics* (Vol. 4). New York: Academic Press, 1979.

Diringer, D. *The alphabet: A key to the history of mankind* (3rd ed.). London: Hutchinson, 1968.

Dirks, D. Perception of dichotic and monaural verbal material and cerebral dominance for speech. *Acta Oto-Laryngologica*, 1964, *58*, 73–80.

Di Stefano, M., Morelli, M., Marzi, C. A., & Berlucchi, G. Hemispheric control of unilateral and bilateral movements of proximal and distal parts of the arm as inferred from simple reaction time to lateralized light stimuli in man. *Experimental Brain Research*, 1980, *38*, 197–204.

Divenyi, P. L., & Efron, R. Spectral versus temporal features in dichotic listening. *Brain and Language*, 1979, *7*, 375–386.

Dodds, A. G. Hemispheric differences in tactuo-spatial processing. *Neuropsychologia*, 1978, *16*, 247–254.

Doehring, D. G., & Hoshko, I. M. Classification of reading problems by the Q-technique of factor analysis. *Cortex*, 1977, *13*, 281–294.

Doehring, D. C., & Ling, D. Matching to sample of three-tone simultaneous and successive sounds, by musical and nonmusical subjects. *Psychonomic Science*, 1971, *25*, 103–105.

Doman, G. *What to do about your brain-injured child*. London: Cape, 1974.

Donchin, E., Kutas, M., & McCarthy, G. Electrocortical indices of hemispheric utilization. In S. Harnad, R. W. Doty, L. Goldstein, J. Jaynes, & G. Krauthamer (Eds.), *Lateralization in the nervous system*. New York: Academic Press, 1977.

Donchin, E., McCarthy, G., & Kutas, M. Electroencephalographic investigations of hemispheric specialization. In J. E. Desmedt (Ed.), *Language and hemispheric specialization in man: Cerebral event related potentials*. Basel: Karger, 1977.

Duda, P. D., & Kirby, H. W. Effects of eye-movement controls and frequency levels on accuracy of word recognition. *Perceptual and Motor Skills*, 1980, *50*, 979–985.

Dumas, R., & Morgan, A. EEG asymmetry as a function of occupation, task, and task difficulty. *Neuropsychologia*, 1975, *13*, 219–228.

Dunlop, D. B., Dunlop, P., & Fenelon, B. Vision-laterality analysis in children with reading disability: The results of new techniques of examination. *Cortex*, 1973, *9*, 227–236.

Eagleson, H. M., Vaughn, G. R., & Knudson, A. B. C. Hand signals for dysphasia. *Archives of Physical Medicine and Rehabilitation,* 1970, *51,* 111–113.

Eccles, J. C. Brain, speech and consciousness. *Naturwissenschaften,* 1973, *60,* 167–176.

Efron, R. The effect of handedness on the perception of simultaneity and temporal order. *Brain,* 1963, *86,* 261–284. (a)

Efron, R. Temporal perception, aphasia and déjà vu. *Brain,* 1963, *86,* 403–424. (b)

Egeth, H. E. Parallel versus serial processes in multidimensional stimulus discrimination. *Perception and Psychophysics,* 1966, *1,* 245–252.

Ehrlichman, H., & Weinberger, A. Lateral eye movements and hemispheric asymmetry: A critical review. *Psychological Bulletin,* 1978, *85,* 1080–1101.

Eisenson, J. Language and intellectual modifications associated with right cerebral damage. *Language and Speech,* 1962, *5,* 49–53.

Elithorn, A., & Barnett, T. J. Apparent individual differences in channel capacity. *Acta Psychologica,* 1967, *27,* 75–83.

Ellenberg, L., & Sperry, R. W. Capacity for holding sustained attention following commissurotomy. *Cortex,* 1979, *15,* 421–438.

Ellenberg, L., & Sperry, R. W. Lateralized division of attention in the commissurotomized and intact brain. *Neuropsychologia,* 1980, *18,* 411–418.

Ellis, A. W. Developmental and acquired dyslexia: Some observations on Jorm (1979). *Cognition,* 1979, *7,* 413–420.

Ellis, H. D., & Shepherd, J. W. Recognition of abstract and concrete words presented in left and right visual fields. *Journal of Experimental Psychology,* 1974, *103,* 1035–1036.

Ellis, H. D., & Shepherd, J. W. Recognition of upright and inverted faces presented in the left and right visual fields. *Cortex,* 1975, *11,* 3–7.

Ellis, H. D., & Young, A. W. Age of acquisition and recognition of nouns presented in left and right visual fields: A failed hypothesis. *Neuropsychologia,* 1977, *15,* 825–828.

Entus, A. K. Hemispheric asymmetry in processing of dichotically presented speech and non-speech stimuli by infants. In S. J. Segalowitz & F. A. Gruber (Eds.), *Language development and neurological theory.* New York: Academic Press, 1977.

Ettlinger, G., Jackson, C. V., & Zangwill, O. L. Cerebral dominance in sinistrals. *Brain,* 1956, *79,* 569–588.

Fairweather, H. Sex differences in cognition. *Cognition,* 1976, *4,* 231–280.

Falk, D. Language, handedness and primitive brains. Did the australopithecines sign? *American Anthropologist,* 1980, *82,* 72–78.

Fechner, G. T. *Elemente der Psychophysik* (Vol. 2). Leipzig: Breitkopf and Härtel, 1860.

Fedio, P., & Weinberg, L. K. Dysnomia and impairment of verbal memory following intracarotid injection of sodium amytal. *Brain Research,* 1971, *31,* 159–168.

Fennell, E. B., Bowers, D., & Satz, P. Within-modal and cross-modal reliabilities of two laterality tests. *Brain and Language,* 1977, *4,* 63–69.

Fennell, E., Satz, P., Van Den Abell, T., Bowers, D., & Thomas, R. Visuospatial competency, handedness, and cerebral dominance. *Brain and Language,* 1978, *5,* 206–214.

Ferris, G. S., & Dorsen, M. M. Agenesis of the corpus callosum. 1. Neuropsychological studies. *Cortex,* 1975, *11,* 95–122.

Field, M., Ashton, R., & White, K. Agenesis of the corpus callosum: Report of two pre-school children and review of the literature. *Developmental Medicine and Child Neurology,* 1978, *20,* 47–61.

Finger, S., Walbran, B., & Stein, D. G. Brain damage and behavioral recovery: Serial lesion phenomena. *Brain Research,* 1973, *63,* 1–18.

Finlayson, M. A. J. A behavioral manifestation of the development of interhemispheric transfer of learning in children. *Cortex,* 1976, *12,* 290–295.

Finucci, J. M., Guthrie, J. T., Childs, A. L., Abbey, H., & Childs, B. The genetics of specific reading disability. *Annals of Human Genetics,* 1976, *40,* 1–23.

Fischer, F. W., Liberman, I. Y., & Shankweiler, D. Reading reversals and developmental dyslexia: A further study. *Cortex,* 1978, *14,* 496–510.

Flanery, R. C., & Balling, J. D. Developmental changes in hemispheric specialization for tactile spatial ability. *Developmental Psychology,* 1979, *15,* 364–372.

Fleminger, J. J., Dalton, R., & Standage, K. F. Age as a factor in handedness of adults. *Neuropsychologia,* 1977, *15,* 471–473.

Flor-Henry, P. Psychosis and temporal lobe epilepsy: A controlled investigation. *Epilepsia,* 1969, *10,* 363–395.

Fontenot, D. J. Visual field differences in the recognition of verbal and nonverbal stimuli in man. *Journal of Comparative and Physiological Psychology,* 1973, *85,* 564–569.

Franco, L., & Sperry, R. W. Hemisphere lateralization for cognitive processing of geometry. *Neuropsychologia,* 1977, *15,* 107–114.

Frankfurter, A., & Honeck, R. P. Ear differences in the recall of monaurally presented sentences. *Quarterly Journal of Experimental Psychology,* 1973, *25,* 138–146.

Freimuth, M., & Wapner, S. The influence of lateral organization on the evaluation of paintings. *British Journal of Psychology,* 1979, *70,* 211–218.

Fried, I., Tanguay, P. E., Boder, E., Doubleday, L., & Greensite, M. Developmental dyslexia: Electrophysiological evidence of clinical subgroups. *Brain and Language,* 1981, *12,* 14–22.

Fromkin, V., Krashen, S., Curtiss, S., Rigler, D., & Rigler, M. The development of language in Genie: A case of language acquisition beyond the "critical period." *Brain and Language,* 1974, *1,* 81–107.

Fry, D. B. Right ear advantage for speech presented monaurally. *Language and Speech,* 1974, *17,* 142–151.

Gaddes, W. H. *Learning disabilities and brain function: A neuropsychological approach.* New York: Springer-Verlag, 1980.

Gaede, S. E., Parsons, O. A., & Bertera, J. H. Hemispheric differences in musical perception: Aptitude vs experience. *Neuropsychologia,* 1978, *16,* 369–373.

Gainotti, G. Affectivity and brain dominance: A survey. In J. Obiols, C. Ballús, E. González Monclús, & J. Pujol (Eds.), *Biological psychiatry today.* Amsterdam: Elsevier/North-Holland Biomedical Press, 1979.

Galaburda, A. M. Paper presented at 13th Annual Winter Conference on Brain Research. Keystone, Colo., Jan. 19–26, 1980.

Galaburda, A. M., LeMay, M., Kemper, T. L., & Geschwind, N. Right-left asymmetries in the brain. *Science,* 1978, *199,* 852–856.

Galaburda, A. M., Sanides, F., & Geschwind, N. Human brain: Cytoarchitectonic left-right asymmetries in the temporal speech region. *Archives of Neurology,* 1978, *35,* 812–817.

Galin, D. Implications for psychiatry of left and right cerebral specialization: A neuro-physiological context for unconscious processes. *Archives of General Psychiatry,* 1974, *31,* 572–583.

Galin, D. Lateral specialization and psychiatric issues: Speculations on development and the evolution of consciousness. *Annals of the New York Academy of Sciences,* 1977, *299,* 397–411.

Galin, D., Diamond, R., & Herron, J. Development of crossed and uncrossed tactile localization on the fingers. *Brain and Language,* 1977, *4,* 588–590.

Galin, D., & Ellis, R. R. Indices of lateralized cognitive processes. Relationship of evoked potential asymmetries to EEG alpha asymmetry. In J. E. Desmedt (Ed.), *Language and hemispheric specialization in man: Cerebral event-related potentials.* Basel: Karger, 1977.

Galin, D., Johnstone, J., Nakell, L., & Herron, J. Development of the capacity for tactile information transfer between hemispheres in normal children. *Science,* 1979, *204,* 1330–1332.

Gardner, E. B., & Branski, D. M. Unilateral cerebral activation and perception of gaps: A signal detection analysis. *Neuropsychologia,* 1976, *14,* 43–54.

Gardner, E. B., English, A. G., Flannery, B. M., Hartnett, M. B., McCormick, J. K., & Wilhelmy, B. B. Shape-recognition accuracy and response latency in a bilateral tactile task. *Neuropsychologia,* 1977, *15,* 607–616.

Gardner, H., Zurif, E. B., Berry, T., & Baker, E. Visual communication in aphasia. *Neuropsychologia,* 1976, *14,* 275–292.

Gardner, R. A., & Gardner, B. T. Teaching sign-language to a chimpanzee. *Science,* 1969, *165,* 664–672.

Garner, W. R. Aspects of a stimulus: Features, dimensions, and configurations. In E. Rosch & B. B. Lloyd (Eds.), *Cognition and categorization.* Hillsdale, N.J.: Lawrence Erlbaum, 1978.

Gates, A., & Bradshaw, J. L. The role of the cerebral hemispheres in music. *Brain and Language,* 1977, *4,* 403–431. (a)

Gates, A., & Bradshaw, J. L. Music perception and cerebral asymmetries. *Cortex,* 1977, *13,* 390–401. (b)

Gazzaniga, M. S. *The bisected brain.* New York: Appleton-Century-Crofts, 1970.

Gazzaniga, M. S., Bogen, J. E., & Sperry, R. W. Some functional effects of sectioning the cerebral commissures in man. *Proceedings of the National Academy of Sciences*, 1962, *48*, 1765–1769.

Gazzaniga, M. S., & Hillyard, S. A. Language and speech capacity of the right hemisphere. *Neuropsychologia*, 1971, *9*, 273–280.

Gazzaniga, M. S., & LeDoux, J. E. *The integrated mind.* New York: Plenum Press, 1978.

Gazzaniga, M. S., & Sperry, R. W. Simultaneous double discrimination response following brain bisection. *Psychonomic Science*, 1966, *4*, 261–262.

Gazzaniga, M. S., & Sperry, R. W. Language after section of the cerebral commissures. *Brain*, 1967, *90*, 131–148.

Geffen, G. Development of hemispheric specialization for speech perception. *Cortex*, 1976, *12*, 337–346.

Geffen, G. The development of the right ear advantage in dichotic listening with focused attention. *Cortex*, 1978, *14*, 169–177.

Geffen, G., Bradshaw, J. L., & Nettleton, N. C. Hemispheric asymmetry: Verbal and spatial encoding of visual stimuli. *Journal of Experimental Psychology*, 1972, *95*, 25–31.

Geffen, G., Bradshaw, J. L., & Nettleton, N. C. Attention and hemispheric differences in reaction time during simultaneous audiovisual tasks. *Quarterly Journal of Experimental Psychology*, 1973, *25*, 404–412.

Geffen, G., Bradshaw, J. L., & Wallace, G. Interhemispheric effects on reaction time to verbal and nonverbal visual stimuli. *Journal of Experimental Psychology*, 1971, *87*, 415–422.

Geffen, G., & Sexton, M. A. The development of auditory strategies of attention. *Developmental Psychology*, 1978, *14*, 11–17.

Geffen, G., & Traub, E. Preferred hand and familial sinistrality in dichotic monitoring. *Neuropsychologia*, 1979, *17*, 527–531.

Geffen, G., & Traub, E. The effects of duration of stimulation, preferred hand and familial sinistrality in dichotic monitoring. *Cortex*, 1980, *16*, 83–96.

Geffen, G., Traub, E., & Stierman, I. Language laterality assessed by unilateral ECT and dichotic monitoring. *Journal of Neurology, Neurosurgery, and Psychiatry*, 1978, *41*, 354–360.

Geffen, G., & Wale, J. The development of selective listening and hemispheric asymmetry. *Developmental Psychology*, 1979, *15*, 138–146.

Geschwind, N. Disconnexion syndromes in animals and man. *Brain*, 1965, *88*, 237–294.

Geschwind, N. The organization of language and the brain. *Science*, 1970, *170*, 940–944.

Geschwind, N. Language and the brain. *Scientific American*, 1972, *226*, 76–83.

Geschwind, N., & Levitsky, W. Human brain: Left-right asymmetries in temporal speech region. *Science*, 1968, *461*, 186–187.

Gesell, A., & Ames, L. B. The development of handedness. *Journal of Genetic Psychology*, 1947, *70*, 155–175.

Gevins, A. S., Zeitlin, G. M., Doyle, J. C., Yingling, C. D., Schaffer, R. E., Callaway, E., & Yeager, C. L. EEG correlates of higher cortical functions. *Science*, 1979, *203*, 665–668.

Giannitrapani, D. Developing concepts of lateralization of cerebral functions. *Cortex*, 1967, *3*, 353–370.

Gilbert, C. Nonverbal perceptual abilities in relation to left-handedness and cerebral lateralization. *Neuropsychologia*, 1977, *15*, 779–791.

Gilbert, C., & Bakan, P. Visual asymmetry in perception of faces. *Neuropsychologia*, 1973, *11*, 355–362.

Gimbutas, M. *The gods and goddesses of Old Europe: 7,000–3,500 B.C.* London: Thames & Hudson, 1974.

Ginsburg, G. P., & Hartwick, A. Directional confusion as a sign of dyslexia. *Perceptual and Motor Skills*, 1971, *32*, 535–543.

Glanville, B. B., Best, C. T., & Levenson, R. A cardiac measure of cerebral asymmetries in infant auditory perception. *Developmental Psychology*, 1977, *13*, 54–59.

Glass, A. V., Gazzaniga, M. S., & Premack, D. Artificial language training in global aphasics. *Neuropsychologia*, 1973, *11*, 95–103.

Glick, S. D., Jerussi, T. P., & Zimmerberg, B. Behavioral and neuropharmacological correlates of nigrostriatal asymmetry in rats. In S. Harnad, R. W. Doty, L. Goldstein, J. Jaynes, & G. Krauthamer (Eds.), *Lateralization in the nervous system.* New York: Academic Press, 1977.

Glick, S. D., Meibach, R. C., Cox, R. D., & Maayani, S. Multiple and interrelated functional asymmetries in rat brain. *Life Sciences*, 1979, *25*, 395–400.

Glick, S. D., Schonfield, A. R., & Strumpf, A. J. Sex differences in brain asymmetry of the rodent. *Behavioral and Brain Sciences*, 1980, *3*, 236.

Godfrey, J. J. Perceptual difficulty and the right ear advantage for vowels. *Brain and Language*, 1974, *1*, 323–335.

Goldberg, E., & Costa, L. Hemisphere differences in the acquisition of descriptive systems. *Brain and Language*, 1981, *14*, 144–173.

Goldman, P. S. Development determinants of cortical plasticity. *Acta Neurobiologiae Experimentalis*, 1972, *32*, 495–511.

Goldstein, K. *Language and language disturbances.* New York: Grune & Stratton, 1948.

Goodglass, H., & Calderon, M. Parallel processing of verbal and musical stimuli in right and left hemispheres. *Neuropsychologia*, 1977, *15*, 397–407.

Goodman, D. M., Beatty, J., & Mulholland, T. B. Detection of cerebral lateralization of function using EEG alpha contingent visual stimulation. *Electroencephalography and Clinical Neurophysiology*, 1980, *48*, 418–431.

Gordon, H. W. Hemispheric asymmetries in the perception of musical chords. *Cortex*, 1970, *6*, 387–398.

Gordon, H. Verbal and nonverbal cerebral processing in man for audition. Unpublished doctoral dissertation, California Institute of Technology, 1973.

Gordon, H. W. Auditory specialization of the right and left hemispheres. In M. Kinsbourne & W. L. Smith (Eds.), *Hemispheric disconnection and cerebral function.* Springfield, Ill.: Charles C Thomas, 1974.

Gordon, H. W. Hemispheric asymmetry and musical performance. *Science*, 1975, *189*, 68–69.

Gordon, H. W. Hemispheric asymmetry for dichotically presented chords in musicians and nonmusicians. *Acta Psychologica*, 1978, *42*, 383–395. (a)

Gordon, H. W. Left hemisphere dominance for rhythmic elements in dichotically presented melodies. *Cortex*, 1978, *14*, 58–76. (b)

Gordon, H. W. Right hemisphere comprehension of verbs in patients with complete forebrain commissurotomy: Use of the dichotic method and manual performance. *Brain and Language*, 1980, *11*, 76–86. (a)

Gordon, H. W. Cognitive asymmetry in dyslexic families. *Neuropsychologia*, 1980, *18*, 645–656. (b)

Gordon, H. W. Cerebral organization in bilinguals. I. Lateralization. *Brain and Language*, 1980, *9*, 255–268. (c)

Gordon, H. W., & Bogen, J. E. Hemispheric lateralization of singing after intracarotid sodium amylobarbitone. *Journal of Neurology, Neurosurgery, and Psychiatry*, 1974, *37*, 727–738.

Gordon, H. W., & Carmon, A. Transfer of dominance in speed of verbal response to visually presented stimuli from right to left hemisphere. *Perceptual and Motor Skills*, 1976, *42*, 1091–1100.

Gott, P. S. Language after dominant hemispherectomy. *Journal of Neurology, Neurosurgery and Psychiatry*, 1973, *36*, 1082–1088.

Goyen, J. D., & Lyle, J. G. Short-term memory and visual discrimination in retarded readers. *Perceptual and Motor Skills*, 1973, *36*, 403–408.

Grant, D. W. Visual asymmetry on a color-naming task: A developmental perspective. *Perceptual and Motor Skills*, 1980, *50*, 475–480.

Gross, M. M. Hemispheric specialization for processing visually presented verbal and spatial stimuli. *Perception and Psychophysics*, 1972, *12*, 357–363.

Gross, Y., Franko, R., & Lewin, I. Effects of voluntary eye movements on hemispheric activity and choice of cognitive mode. *Neuropsychologia*, 1978, *16*, 653–657.

Gruzelier, J. H., & Flor-Henry, P., (Eds.). *Hemisphere asymmetries of function in psychopathology.* Amsterdam: Elsevier/North-Holland Biomedical Press, 1979.

Gruzelier, J. H., & Hammond, N. V. Gains, losses and lateral differences in the hearing of schizophrenic patients. *British Journal of Psychology*, 1979, *70*, 319–330.

Guiard, Y. Cerebral hemispheres and selective attention. *Acta Psychologica*, 1980, *46*, 41–61.

Gur, R. E. Cognitive concomitants of hemispheric dysfunction in schizophrenia. *Archives of General Psychiatry*, 1979, *36*, 269–274.

Gur, R. C., & Gur, R. E. Correlates of conjugate lateral eye movements in man. In S. Harnad, R. W. Doty, L. Goldstein, J. Jaynes, & G. Krauthamer (Eds.), *Lateralization in the nervous system.* New York: Academic Press, 1977. (a)

Gur, R. E., & Gur, R. C. Sex differences in the relations among handedness, sighting-dominance and eye-acuity. *Neuropsychologia,* 1977, *15,* 585–590. (b)

Gur, R. C., & Gur, R. E. Handedness and individual differences in hemispheric activation. In J. Herron (Ed.), *Neuropsychology of left-handedness.* New York: Academic Press, 1980.

Gur, R. C., Packer, I. K., Hungerbuhler, J. P., Reivich, M., Obrist, W. D., Amarnek, W. S., & Sackeim, H. A. Differences in the distribution of gray and white matter in human cerebral hemispheres. *Science,* 1980, *207,* 1226–1228.

Gur, R. C., & Reivich, M. Cognitive task effects on hemispheric blood flow in humans: Evidence for individual differences in hemispheric activation. *Brain and Language,* 1980, *9,* 78–92.

Haggard, M. P. Encoding and the REA for speech signals. *Quarterly Journal of Experimental Psychology,* 1971, *23,* 34–45.

Haggard, M. P., & Parkinson, A. M. Stimulus and task factors as determinants of ear advantage. *Quarterly Journal of Experimental Psychology,* 1971, *23,* 168–177.

Hall, J. L., & Goldstein, M. H. Representation of binaural stimuli by single units in primary auditory cortex of unanaesthetized cats. *Journal of the Acoustical Society of America,* 1968, *43,* 456–461.

Hallgren, B. Specific dyslexia: A clinical and genetic study. *Acta Psychiatrica et Neurologica,* 1950, Suppl., *65,* 1–287.

Halperin, Y., Nachshon, I., & Carmon, A. Shift of ear superiority in dichotic listening to temporally patterned nonverbal stimuli. *Journal of the Acoustical Society of America,* 1973, *53,* 46–50.

Hamilton, C. R. An assessment of hemispheric specialization in monkeys. *Annals of the New York Academy of Sciences,* 1977, *299,* 222–232.

Hamsher, K. de S., & Benton, A. L. The reliability of reaction time determinations. *Cortex,* 1977, *13,* 306–310.

Hannay, H. J. Asymmetry in reception and retention of colors. *Brain and Language,* 1979, *8,* 191–201.

Hannay, H. J., & Malone, D. R. Visual field effects and short-term memory for verbal material. *Neuropsychologia,* 1976, *14,* 203–209.

Hannay, H. J., Rogers, J. P., & Durant, R. F. Complexity as a determinant of visual field effects for random forms. *Acta Psychologica,* 1976, *40,* 29–34.

Hannay, H. J., & Smith, A. C. Dichaptic perception of forms by normal adults. *Perceptual and Motor Skills,* 1979, *49,* 991–1000.

Hansch, E. C., & Pirozzolo, F. J. Task relevant effects on the assessment of cerebral specialization for facial emotion. *Brain and Language,* 1980, *10,* 51–59.

Harburg, E., Feldstein, A., & Papsdorf, J. Handedness and smoking. *Perceptual and Motor Skills,* 1978, *47,* 1171–1174.

Hardyck, C. A model of individual differences in hemispheric functioning. In H. Whitaker & H. A. Whitaker (Eds.), *Studies in neurolinguistics* (Vol. 3). New York: Academic Press, 1977. (a)

Hardyck, C. Laterality and intellectual ability: A just not noticeable difference? *British Journal of Educational Psychology,* 1977, *47,* 305–311. (b)

Hardyck, C., & Petrinovich, L. F. Left-handedness. *Psychological Bulletin,* 1977, *84,* 385–404.

Hardyck, C., Tzeng, O. J. L., & Wang, W. S. Y. Cerebral lateralization of function and bilingual decision processes: Is thinking lateralized? *Brain and Language,* 1978, *5,* 56–71.

Harlap, S. Gender of infants conceived on different days of the menstrual cycle. *New England Journal of Medicine,* 1979, *300,* 1445–1448.

Harriman, J., & Buxton, H. The influence of prosody on the recall of monaurally presented sentences. *Brain and Language,* 1979, *8,* 62–68.

Harris, L. J. Sex differences in the growth and use of language. In E. Donelson & J. Gullahorn (Eds.), *Woman: A psychological perspective.* New York: John Wiley, 1977.

Harris, L. J. Sex differences in spatial ability: Possible environmental, genetic, and neurological factors. In M. Kinsbourne (Ed.), *Asymmetrical function of the brain*. Cambridge: Cambridge University Press, 1978.

Harris, L. J. Left-handedness: Early theories, facts, and fancies. In J. Herron (Ed.), *Neuropsychology of left-handedness*. New York: Academic Press, 1980. (a)

Harris, L. J. Which hand is the "eye" of the blind?–A new look at an old question. In J. Herron (Ed.), *Neuropsychology of left-handedness*. New York: Academic Press, 1980. (b)

Harris, L. J., & Carr, T. H. Implications of differences between perceptual systems for the analysis of hemispheric specialization. *Behavioral and Brain Sciences*, 1981, *4*, 71-72.

Hartlage, L. C., & Green, J. B. EEG differences in children's reading, spelling and arithmetic abilities. *Perceptual and Motor Skills*, 1971, *32*, 133-134.

Harvey, L. O. Single representation of the visual midline in humans. *Neuropsychologia*, 1978, *16*, 601-610.

Hatta, T. Hemisphere asymmetries in the perception and memory of random forms. *Psychologia*, 1976, *19*, 157-162.

Hatta, T. Functional hemisphere asymmetries in an inferential thought task. *Psychologia*, 1977, *20*, 145-150. (a)

Hatta, T. Recognition of Japanese kanji in the left and right visual fields. *Neuropsychologia*, 1977, *15*, 685-688. (b)

Hatta, T. Recognition of Japanese Kanji and Hirakana in the left and right visual fields. *Japanese Psychological Research*, 1978, *20*, 51-59. (a)

Hatta, T. The functional asymmetry of tactile pattern learning in normal subjects. *Psychologia*, 1978, *21*, 83-89. (b)

Haun, F. Functional dissociation of the hemispheres using foveal visual input. *Neuropsychologia*, 1978, *16*, 725-733.

Hawn, P. R., & Harris, L. J. Hand asymmetries in grasp duration and reaching in two- and five-month-old infants. Paper presented at the biennial meeting of the Society for Research in Child Development, San Francisco, 1979.

Hayashi, T., & Bryden, M. P. Ocular dominance and perceptual asymmetry. *Perceptual and Motor Skills*, 1967, *25*, 605-612.

Hécaen, H. Acquired aphasia in children and the ontogenesis of hemispheric functional specialization. *Brain and Language*, 1976, *3*, 114-134.

Hécaen, H. Right hemisphere contribution to language functions. In P. A. Buser & A. Rougeul-Buser (Eds.), *Cerebral correlates of conscious experience*. Inserm Symposium No. 6. Amsterdam: Elsevier/North-Holland Biomedical Press, 1978.

Hécaen, H., Ajuriaguerra, J. de, & David M. Les deficits fonctionnels après lobectomie occipitale. *Monatsschrift für Psychiatrie und Neurologie*, 1952, *123*, 239-290.

Hécaen, H., & Albert, M. L. *Human neuropsychology*. New York: John Wiley, 1978.

Hécaen, H., & Marcie, P. Disorders of written language following right hemisphere lesions: Spatial dysgraphia. In S. J. Dimond & J. G. Beaumont (Eds.), *Hemisphere function in the human brain*. London: Elek Science, 1974.

Hécaen, H., & Sauguet, J. Cerebral dominance in left-handed subjects. *Cortex*, 1971, *7*, 19-48.

Heilman, K. M. Apraxia. In K. M. Heilman & E. Valenstein (Eds.), *Clinical neuropsychology*. Oxford: Oxford University Press, 1979. (a)

Heilman, K. M. Neglect and related disorders. In K. M. Heilman & E. Valenstein (Eds.), *Clinical neuropsychology*. Oxford: Oxford University Press, 1979. (b)

Heilman, K. M., & Van Den Abell, T. Right hemispheric dominance for mediating cerebral activation. *Neuropsychologia*, 1979, *17*, 315-321.

Hellige, J. B. Changes in same-different laterality patterns as a function of practice and stimulus quality. *Perception and Psychophysics*, 1976, *20*, 267-273.

Hellige, J. B. Visual laterality and cerebral hemisphere specialization: Methodological and theoretical considerations. In J. B. Sidowski (Ed.), *Conditioning, cognition, and methodology: Contemporary issues in experimental psychology*. Hillsdale, N.J.: Lawrence Erlbaum, 1980. (a)

Hellige, J. B. Effects of perceptual quality and visual field of probe stimulus presentation on memory search for letters. *Journal of Experimental Psychology: Human Perception and Performance*, 1980, *6*, 639-651. (b)

Hellige, J. B., & Cox, P. J. Effects of concurrent verbal memory on recognition of stimuli from left and right visual fields. *Journal of Experimental Psychology: Human Perception and Performance,* 1976, *2,* 210–221.

Hellige, J. B., Cox, P. J., & Litvac, L. Information processing in the cerebral hemispheres: Selective hemispheric activation and capacity limitations. *Journal of Experimental Psychology: General,* 1979, *108,* 251–279.

Hellige, J. B., & Webster, R. Right hemisphere superiority for initial stages of letter processing. *Neuropsychologia,* 1979, *17,* 653–660.

Henderson, L., & Chard, J. The reader's implicit knowledge of orthographic structure. In U. Frith (Ed.), *Cognitive processes in spelling.* New York: Academic Press, 1980.

Hermann, K. *Reading disability.* Springfield, Ill.: Charles C Thomas, 1959.

Hermelin, B., & O'Connor, N. Right and left-handed reading of Braille. *Nature,* 1971, *231,* 470. (a)

Hermelin, B., & O'Connor, N. Functional asymmetry in the reading of Braille. *Neuropsychologia,* 1971, *9,* 431–435. (b)

Heron, W. Perception as a function of retinal locus and attention. *American Journal of Psychology,* 1957, *70,* 38–48.

Herrman, D. J., & Van Dyke, K. Handedness and the mental rotation of perceived patterns. *Cortex,* 1978, *14,* 521–529.

Hertz, R. La préeminence de la main droite: Etude sur la polarité religieuse. *Revue Philosophique,* 1909, *68,* 553–580.

Hewes, G. W. Primate communication and the gestural origin of language. *Current Anthropology,* 1973, *14,* 5–24.

Hewitt, W. The development of the human corpus callosum. *Journal of Anatomy,* 1962, *96,* 355–358.

Hicks, R. A., Elliott, D., Garbesi, L., & Martin, S. Multiple birth risk factors and the distribution of handedness. *Cortex,* 1979, *15,* 135–137.

Hicks, R. A., Pellegrini, R. J., & Evans, E. A. Handedness and birth risk. *Neuropsychologia,* 1978, *16,* 243–245.

Hicks, R. A., Pellegrini, R. J., Evans, E. A., & Moore, J. D. Birth risk and left-handedness reconsidered. *Archives of Neurology,* 1979, *36,* 119–120.

Hicks, R. E. Intrahemispheric response competition between vocal and unimanual performance in normal adult human males. *Journal of Comparative and Physiological Psychology,* 1975, *89,* 50–60.

Hicks, R. E., & Kinsbourne, M. On the genesis of human handedness: A review. *Journal of Motor Behavior,* 1976, *8,* 257–266. (a)

Hicks, R. E., & Kinsbourne, M. Human handedness: A partial cross-fostering study. *Science,* 1976, *192,* 908–910. (b)

Hicks, R. E., & Kinsbourne, M. Human handedness. In M. Kinsbourne (Ed.), *Asymmetrical function of the brain.* Cambridge: Cambridge University Press, 1978.

Hicks, R. E., Provenzano, F. J., & Rybstein, E. D. Generalized and lateralized effects of concurrent verbal rehearsal upon performance of sequential movements of the fingers by the left and right hands. *Acta Psychologica,* 1975, *39,* 119–130.

Hier, D. B., & Kaplan, J. Are sex differences in cerebral organization clinically significant? *Behavioral and Brain Sciences,* 1980, *3,* 238–239.

Hier, D. B., LeMay, M., Rosenberger, P. B., & Perlo, V. P. Developmental dyslexia. *Archives of Neurology,* 1978, *35,* 90–92.

Hilliard, R. D. Hemispheric laterality effects on a facial recognition task in normal subjects. *Cortex,* 1973, *9,* 246–258.

Hines, D. Bilateral tachistoscope recognitions of verbal and nonverbal stimuli. *Cortex,* 1972, *8,* 315–322. (a)

Hines, D. A brief reply to McKeever, Suberi and Van Deventer's comment on "Bilateral tachistoscopic recognitions of verbal and nonverbal stimuli." *Cortex,* 1972, *8,* 480–482. (b)

Hines, D. Recognition of verbs, abstract nouns and concrete nouns from the left and right visual half fields. *Neuropsychologia,* 1976, *14,* 211–216.

Hines, D. Differences in tachistoscopic recognition between abstract and concrete words as a function of visual half field and frequency. *Cortex,* 1977, *13,* 66–73.

Hines, D. Visual information processing in the left and right hemispheres. *Neuropsychologia,* 1978, *16,* 593–600.

Hines, D., Fennell, E. B., Bowers, D., & Satz, P. Left-handers show greater test-retest variability in auditory and visual asymmetry. *Brain and Language*, 1980, *10*, 208–211.

Hines, D., & Satz, P. Superiority of right visual half-fields in right handers for recall of digits presented at varying rates. *Neuropsychologia*, 1971, *9*, 21–25.

Hines, D., & Satz, P. Cross modal asymmetries in perception related to asymmetry in cerebral function. *Neuropsychologia*, 1974, *12*, 239–247.

Hines, D., Satz, P., & Clementino, T. Perceptual and memory components of the superior recall of letters from the right visual half-fields. *Neuropsychologia*, 1973, *11*, 175–180.

Hines, D., Satz, P., Schell, B., & Schmidlin, S. Differential recall of digits in the left and right visual half-fields under free and fixed order of recall. *Neuropsychologia*, 1969, *7*, 13–22.

Hirata, K., & Bryden, M. P. Right visual field superiority for letter recognition with partial report. *Canadian Journal of Psychology*, 1976, *30*, 134–139.

Hirsch, S. M., & Anderson, R. P. The effects of perceptual motor training on reading achievement. In R. P. Anderson & C. G. Halcomb (Eds.), *Learning disability/minimal brain dysfunction syndrome*. Springfield, Ill.: Charles C Thomas, 1976.

Hirshkowitz, M., Earle, J., & Paley, B. EEG alpha asymmetry in musicians and nonmusicians: A study of hemispheric specialization. *Neuropsychologia*, 1978, *16*, 125–128.

Hiscock, M. Eye-movement asymmetry and hemispheric function: An examination of individual differences. *Journal of Psychology*, 1977, *97*, 49–52.

Hiscock, M., & Kinsbourne, M. Ontogeny of cerebral dominance: Evidence from time-sharing asymmetry in children. *Developmental Psychology*, 1978, *14*, 321–329.

Hiscock, M., & Kinsbourne, M. Asymmetry of verbal-manual time sharing in children: A follow up study. *Neuropsychologia*, 1980, *18*, 151–162.

Hochberg, F. H., & LeMay, M. Arteriographic correlates of handedness. *Neurology*, 1975, *25*, 218–222.

Holmes, D. R., & McKeever, W. F. Material specific serial memory deficit in adolescent dyslexics. *Cortex*, 1979, *15*, 51–62.

Honda, H. Shift of visual laterality differences by loading of auditory discrimination tasks. *Japanese Journal of Psychology*, 1978, *49*, 8–14.

Hubbard, J. I. Handedness not a function of birth order. *Nature*, 1971, *232*, 276–277.

Hublet, C., Morais, J., & Bertelson, P. Spatial effects in speech perception in the absence of spatial competition. *Perception*, 1977, *6*, 461–466.

Hudson, P. T. W. The genetics of handedness: A reply to Levy and Nagylaki. *Neuropsychologia*, 1975, *13*, 331–339.

Humphrey, N., & McManus, C. Status and the left cheek. *New Scientist*, 1973, *59*, 437–439.

Hutt, C. *Sex differences*. St. Albans, England: Crosby Lockwood Staples, 1975.

Hynd, G. W., Obrzut, J. E., Weed, W., & Hynd, C. R. Development of cerebral dominance: Dichotic listening asymmetry in normal and learning-disabled children. *Journal of Experimental Child Psychology*, 1979, *28*, 445–454.

Ingle, D. Animal models for lateralized sex differences. *Behavioral and Brain Sciences*, 1980, *3*, 240.

Inglis, J. Dichotic stimulation, temporal-lobe damage, and the perception and storage of auditory stimuli—A note on Kimura's findings. *Canadian Journal of Psychology*, 1962, *16*, 11–17.

Inglis, J., & Sykes, D. H. Some sources of variation in dichotic listening performance in children. *Journal of Experimental Child Psychology*, 1967, *5*, 480–488.

Ingram, D. Motor asymmetries in young children. *Neuropsychologia*, 1975, *13*, 95–102.

Isaac, G. The emergence of man. *Nature*, 1980, *285*, 72.

Isseroff, A., Carmon, A., & Nachshon, I. Dissociation of hemifield reaction time differences from verbal stimulus directionality. *Journal of Experimental Psychology*, 1974, *103*, 145–149.

Jarvella, R. J., & Herman, S. J. Speed and accuracy of sentence recall: Effects of ear presentation, semantics, and grammar. *Journal of Experimental Psychology*, 1973, *97*, 108–110.

Jeeves, M. A. A comparison of interhemispheric transmission times in acallosals and normals. *Psychonomic Science*, 1969, *16*, 245–246.

Jeeves, M. A. Hemisphere differences in response rates to visual stimuli in children. *Psychonomic Science*, 1972, *27*, 201–203.

Jeeves, M. A. Some limits to interhemispheric integration in cases of callosal agenesis and partial commissurotomy. In I. Steele Russel, M. W. Hof, & G. Berlucchi (Eds.), *Structure and function of cerebral commissures*. London: Macmillan, 1979.

Jeeves, M. A., & Dixon, N. F. Hemisphere differences in response rates to visual stimuli. *Psychonomic Science*, 1970, *20*, 249–251.

Jensen, H. *Sign, symbol and script: An account of man's efforts to write.* London: Allen & Unwin, 1970.

Johnson, D. J., & Myklebust, H. R. *Learning disabilities: Educational principles and practices.* New York: Grune & Stratton, 1967.

Johnson, O., & Harley, C. Handedness and sex differences in cognitive tests of brain laterality. *Cortex*, 1980, *16*, 73–82.

Johnson, O., & Kozma, A. Effects of concurrent verbal and musical tasks on a unimanual skill. *Cortex*, 1977, *13*, 11–16.

Johnson, P. Dichotically stimulated ear differences in musicians and nonmusicians. *Cortex*, 1977, *13*, 385–389.

Johnson, R. C., Bowers, J. K., Gamble, M., Lyons, F. M., Presbrey, T. W., & Vetter, R. R. Ability to transcribe music and ear superiority for tone sequences. *Cortex*, 1977, *13*, 295–299.

Johnstone, J., Galin, D., & Herron, J. Choice of handedness measures in studies of hemispheric specialization. *International Journal of Neuroscience*, 1979, *9*, 71–80.

Jones, B. Sex and visual field effects on accuracy and decision making when subjects classify male and female faces. *Cortex*, 1979, *15*, 551–560.

Jones, B., & Santi, A. Lateral asymmetries in visual perception with and without eye movements. *Cortex*, 1978, *14*, 164–168.

Jones, R. K. Observations on stammering after localized cerebral injury. *Journal of Neurology, Neurosurgery and Psychiatry*, 1966, *29*, 192–195.

Jones-Gotman, M., & Milner, B. Design fluency: The invention of nonsense drawings after focal cortical lesions. *Neuropsychologia*, 1977, *15*, 653–674.

Jonides, J. Left and right visual field superiority for letter classification. *Quarterly Journal of Experimental Psychology*, 1979, *31*, 423–439.

Jorm, A. F. The cognitive and neurological basis of developmental dyslexia: A theoretical framework and review. *Cognition*, 1979, *7*, 19–33.

Joynt, R. J., & Goldstein, M. N. The minor cerebral hemisphere. In W. J. Friedlander (Ed.), *Advances in Neurology, Vol. 7, Current reviews of higher nervous system dysfunction.* New York: Raven Press, 1975.

Kagan, J., & Kogen, N. Individual variation in cognitive processes. In P. H. Mussen (Ed.), *Carmichael's manual of child psychology* (Vol. 1, 3rd ed.). New York: John Wiley, 1970.

Kallman, H. J. Ear asymmetries with monaurally-presented sounds. *Neuropsychologia*, 1977, *15*, 833–835.

Kallman, H. J. Can expectancy explain reaction time ear asymmetries? *Neuropsychologia*, 1978, *16*, 225–228.

Kallman, H. J., & Corballis, M. C. Ear asymmetry in reaction time to musical sounds. *Perception and Psychophysics*, 1975, *17*, 368–370.

Katz, A. N. Cognitive arithmetic: Evidence for right hemispheric mediation in an elementary component stage. *Quarterly Journal of Experimental Psychology*, 1980, *32*, 69–84.

Keefe, B., & Swinney, D. On the relationship of hemispheric specialization and developmental dyslexia. *Cortex*, 1979, *15*, 471–481.

Keele, S. W. *Attention and human performance.* Pacific Palisades, Calif.: Goodyear Publishing Co., 1973.

Kellar, L. A., & Bever, T. G. Hemispheric asymmetries in the perception of musical intervals as a function of musical experience and family handedness background. *Brain and Language*, 1980, *10*, 24–38.

Kershner, J. R. Cerebral dominance in disabled readers, good readers and gifted children: Search for a valid model. *Child Development*, 1977, *48*, 61–67.

Kershner, J. R. Rotation of mental images and asymmetries in word recognition in disabled readers. *Canadian Journal of Psychology*, 1979, *33*, 39–50.

Kershner, J. R., & Jeng, A. G. R. Dual functional hemispheric asymmetry in visual perception: Effects of ocular dominance and post exposural processes. *Neuropsychologia*, 1972, *10*, 437–445.

Kershner, J., Thomae, R., & Callaway, R. Nonverbal fixation control in young children induces a left-field advantage in digit recall. *Neuropsychologia*, 1977, *15*, 569–576.

Kertesz, A. Recovery and treatment. In K. M. Heilman & E. Valenstein (Eds.), *Clinical neuropsychology*. New York: Oxford University Press, 1979.

Kertesz, A., & Geschwind, N. Patterns of pyramidal decussation and their relationship to hand-edness. *Archives of Neurology,* 1971, *24,* 326–332.

Kertesz, A., & McCabe, P. Recovery patterns and prognosis in aphasia. *Brain,* 1977, *100,* 1–18.

Ketterer, M. W., & Smith, B. D. Bilateral electrodermal activity, lateralized cerebral processing and sex. *Psychophysiology,* 1977, *14,* 513–516.

Keuss, P. J. G. Processing of geometrical dimensions in a binary classification task: Evidence for a dual process model. *Perception and Psychophysics,* 1977, *21,* 371–376.

Kim, Y., Royer, F., Boustelle, C., & Boller, F. Temporal sequencing of verbal and nonverbal materials: Effect of laterality of lesion. *Cortex,* 1980, *16,* 135–143.

Kimura, D. Some effects of temporal-lobe damage on auditory perception. *Canadian Journal of Psychology,* 1961, *15,* 156–165. (a)

Kimura, D. Cerebral dominance and the perception of verbal stimuli. *Canadian Journal of Psychology,* 1961, *15,* 166–171. (b)

Kimura, D. Speech lateralization in young children as determined by an auditory task. *Journal of Comparative and Physiological Psychology,* 1963, *56,* 899–902.

Kimura, D. Left-right differences in the perception of melodies. *Quarterly Journal of Experimental Psychology,* 1964, *16,* 355–358.

Kimura, D. Dual functional asymmetry of the brain in visual perception. *Neuropsychologia,* 1966, *4,* 275–285.

Kimura, D. Functional asymmetry of the brain in dichotic listening. *Cortex,* 1967, *3,* 163–178.

Kimura, D. Spatial localization in left and right visual fields. *Canadian Journal of Psychology,* 1969, *23,* 445–458.

Kimura, D. The asymmetry of the human brain. *Scientific American,* 1973, *228,* 70–78. (a)

Kimura, D. Manual activity during speaking. I. Right handers. *Neuropsychologia,* 1973, *11,* 45–50. (b)

Kimura, D. The neural basis of language qua gesture. In H. Whitaker & H. A. Whitaker (Eds.), *Studies in neurolinguistics* (Vol. 1). New York: Academic Press, 1976.

Kimura, D. Acquisition of a motor skill after left hemisphere damage. *Brain,* 1977, *100,* 527–542.

Kimura, D., & Archibald, Y. Motor functions of the left hemisphere. *Brain,* 1974, *97,* 337–350.

Kimura, D., & Durnford, M. Normal studies on the function of the right hemisphere in vision. In S. J. Dimond & J. G. Beaumont (Eds.), *Hemisphere function in the human brain.* London: Elek Science, 1974.

Kimura, D., & Folb, S. Neural processing of backwards speech sounds. *Science,* 1968, *161,* 395–396.

King, F. L., & Kimura, D. Left-ear superiority in dichotic perception of vocal nonverbal sounds. *Canadian Journal of Psychology,* 1972, *26,* 111–116.

Kinsbourne, M. The cerebral basis of lateral asymmetries in attention. *Acta Psychologica,* 1970, *33,* 193–201.

Kinsbourne, M. The minor cerebral hemisphere as a source of aphasic speech. *Archives of Neurology,* 1971, *25,* 302–306.

Kinsbourne, M. Eye and head turning indicates cerebral lateralization. *Science,* 1972, *176,* 539–541.

Kinsbourne, M. The control of attention by interaction between the cerebral hemispheres. In S. Kornblum (Ed.), *Attention and performance II.* New York: Academic Press, 1973.

Kinsbourne, M. The mechanism of hemispheric control of the lateral gradient of attention. In P. M. A. Rabbit & S. Dornic (Eds.), *Attention and performance V.* New York: Academic Press, 1975.

Kinsbourne, M. Evolution of language in relation to lateral action. In M. Kinsbourne (Ed.), *Asymmetrical function of the brain.* Cambridge: Cambridge University Press, 1978.

Kinsbourne, M., & Cook, J. Generalized and lateralized effects of concurrent verbalization on a unimanual skill. *Quarterly Journal of Experimental Psychology,* 1971, *23,* 341–345.

Kinsbourne, M., & Hicks, R. E. Functional cerebral space: A model for overflow transfer and interference effects in human performance: A tutorial overview. In J. Requin (Ed.), *Attention and performance VII.* Hillsdale, N.J.: Lawrence Erlbaum, 1978. (a)

Kinsbourne, M., & Hicks, R. E. Mapping cerebral functional space: Competiton and collaboration in human performance. In M. Kinsbourne (Ed.), *Asymmetrical function of the brain.* Cambridge: Cambridge University Press, 1978. (b)

Kinsbourne, M., & Hiscock, M. Does cerebral dominance develop? In S. Segalowitz & F. A.

Gruber (Eds.), *Language development and neurological theory.* New York: Academic Press, 1977.

Kinsbourne, M., & McMurray, J. The effect of cerebral dominance on time sharing between speaking and tapping by preschool children. *Child Development,* 1975, *46,* 240–242.

Kinsbourne, M., & Warrington, E. K. Developmental factors in reading and writing backwardness. *British Journal of Psychology,* 1963, *54,* 145–156.

Kirsner, K. H. Hemisphere specific processes in letter matching. *Journal of Experimental Psychology: Human Perception and Performance,* 1980, *6,* 167–179.

Klatzky, R. L., & Atkinson, R. C. Specialization of the cerebral hemispheres in scanning for information in short-term memory. *Perception and Psychophysics,* 1971, *10,* 335–338.

Klein, D., Moscovitch, M., & Vigna, C. Attentional mechanisms and perceptual asymmetries in tachistoscopic recognition of words and faces. *Neuropsychologia,* 1976, *14,* 55–66.

Klisz, D. K. Visual field differences between a fricative and a stop consonant. *Cortex,* 1980, *16,* 169–173.

Knights, R. M., & Moule, A. D. Normative and reliability data on finger and foot tapping in children. *Perceptual and Motor Skills,* 1967, *25,* 717–720.

Knopman, D. S., Rubens, A. B., Klassen, A. C., Meyer, M. W., & Niccum, N. Regional cerebral blood flow patterns during verbal and nonverbal auditory activation. *Brain and Language,* 1980, *9,* 93–112.

Knox, A. W., & Boone, D. R. Auditory laterality and tested handedness. *Cortex,* 1970, *7,* 164–173.

Knox, C., & Kimura, D. Cerebral processing of nonverbal sounds in boys and girls. *Neuropsychologia,* 1970, *8,* 227–237.

Kocel, K. Cognitive abilities: Handedness, familial sinistrality and sex. *Annals of the New York Academy of Sciences,* 1977, *299,* 233–242.

Koerner, F., & Teuber, H. L. Visual field defects after missile injuries to the geniculo-striate pathway in man. *Experimental Brain Research,* 1973, *18,* 88–113.

Kolakowski, D., & Malina, R. M. Spatial ability, throwing accuracy and man's hunting heritage. *Nature,* 1974, *251,* 410–412.

Kopp, N., Michel, F., Carrier, H., Biron, A., & Duvillard, P. Etude de certaines asymmétries hémisphériques du cerveau humain. *Journal of the Neurological Sciences,* 1977, *34,* 340–363.

Krashen, S. D. Mental abilities underlying linguistic and nonlinguistic functions. *Linguistics,* 1973, *115,* 39–53. (a)

Krashen, S. D. Lateralization, language learning, and the critical period: Some new evidence. *Language Learning,* 1973, *23,* 63–74. (b)

Krashen, S. D. Cerebral asymmetry. In H. Whitaker & H. A. Whitaker (Eds.), *Studies in neurolinguistics* (Vol. 1). New York: Academic Press, 1976.

Krashen, S. D. The left hemisphere. In M. C. Wittrock (Ed.), *The human brain.* Englewood Cliffs, N.J.: Prentice-Hall, 1977.

Kreuter, C., Kinsbourne, M., & Trevarthen, C. Are deconnected cerebral hemispheres independent channels? A preliminary study of the effect of unilateral loading on bilateral finger tapping. *Neuropsychologia,* 1972, *10,* 453–461.

Kriss, A., Blumhardt, L. D., Halliday, A. M., & Pratt, R. T. C. Neurological asymmetries immediately after unilateral ECT. *Journal of Neurology, Neurosurgery and Psychiatry,* 1978, *41,* 1135–1144.

Krueger, L. E. Effect of bracketing lines on speed of 'same'–'different' judgment of two adjacent letters. *Journal of Experimental Psychology,* 1970, *84,* 324–330.

Krueger, L. E. A theory of perceptual matching. *Psychological Review,* 1978, *85,* 278–304.

Krynicki, V. E., & Nahas, A. D. Differing lateralized perceptual-motor patterns in schizophrenic and non-psychotic children. *Perceptual and Motor Skills,* 1979, *49,* 603–610.

Kuhn, G. M. The Phi coefficient as an index of ear differences in dichotic listening. *Cortex,* 1973, *9,* 447–457.

Kutas, M., & Donchin, E. Studies of squeezing: Handedness, responding hand, response force, and asymmetry of readiness potential. *Science,* 1974, *186,* 545–548.

Kutas, M., & Hillyard, S. A. Reading between the lines: Event-related brain potentials during natural sentence processing. *Brain and Language,* 1980, *11,* 354–373.

Lacroix, J. M., & Comper, P. Lateralization in the electrodermal system as a function of cognitive/hemispheric manipulations. *Psychophysiology,* 1979, *16,* 116–129.

Lake, D. A., & Bryden, M. P. Handedness and sex differences in hemispheric asymmetry. *Brain and Language*, 1976, *3*, 266-282.

Lansdell, H. Verbal and nonverbal factors in right-hemisphere speech: Relation to early neurological history. *Journal of Comparative and Physiological Psychology*, 1969, *69*, 734-738.

Lashley, K. S. In search of the engram. In F. A. Beach, D. O. Hebb, C. T. Morgan, & H. W. Nissen (Eds.), *The neuropsychology of Lashley*. New York: McGraw-Hill, 1960.

Lassen, N. A., Ingvar, D. H., & Skinhøj, F. Brain function and blood flow. *Scientific American*, 1978, *239*, 50-59.

Lecours, A. R. Myelogenetic correlates of the development of speech and language. In E. H. Lenneberg & C. Lenneberg (Eds.), *Foundations of language development: A multidisciplinary approach* (Vol. 1). New York: Academic Press, 1975.

Ledlow, A., Swanson, J. M., & Kinsbourne, M. Reaction times and evoked potentials as indicators of hemispheric differences for laterally presented name and physical matches. *Journal of Experimental Psychology: Human Perception and Performance*, 1978, *4*, 440-454.

LeDoux, J. E., Wilson, D. H., & Gazzaniga, M. S. Manipulo-spatial aspects of cerebral lateralization: Clues to the origin of lateralization. *Neuropsychologia*, 1977, *15*, 743-750.

Leehey, S., Carey, S., Diamond, R., & Cahn, A. Upright and inverted faces: The right hemisphere knows the difference. *Cortex*, 1978, *14*, 411-419.

Leehey, S. C., & Cahn, A. Lateral asymmetries in the recognition of words, familiar faces and unfamiliar faces. *Neuropsychologia*, 1979, *17*, 619-635.

Lehman, R. A. W. The handedness of rhesus monkeys III. Consistency within and across activities. *Cortex*, 1980, *16*, 197-204.

Leiber, L. Lexical decisions in the right and left cerebral hemispheres. *Brain and Language*, 1976, *3*, 443-450.

Leisman, G., & Ashkenazi, M. Aetiological factors in dyslexia: IV. Cerebral hemispheres are functionally equivalent. *International Journal of Neuroscience*, 1980, *11*, 157-164.

LeMay, M. Morphological cerebral asymmetries of modern man, fossil man, and nonhuman primate. *Annals of the New York Academy of Sciences*, 1976, *280*, 349-366.

LeMay, M. Asymmetries of the skull and handedness: Phrenology revisited. *Journal of the Neurological Sciences*, 1977, *32*, 243-253.

LeMay, M., & Culebras, A. Human brain morphologic differences in the hemispheres demonstrable by carotid angiography. *New England Journal of Medicine*, 1972, *287*, 168-170.

LeMay, M., & Geschwind, N. Hemispheric differences in the brains of Great Apes. *Brain, Behavior and Evolution*, 1975, *11*, 48-52.

LeMay, M., & Geschwind, N. Asymmetries of the human cerebral hemispheres. In A. Caramazza & E. B. Zurif (Eds.), *Language acquisition and language breakdown*. Baltimore, Md.: Johns Hopkins University Press, 1978.

Lenneberg, E. H. *Biological foundations of language.* New York: John Wiley, 1967.

Levin, H. S. The acalculias. In K. M. Heilman & E. Valenstein (Eds.), *Clinical neuropsychology*. Oxford: Oxford University Press, 1979.

Levy, J. Possible basis for the evolution of lateral specialization of the human brain. *Nature*, 1969, *224*, 614-615.

Levy, J. Information processing and higher psychological functions in the disconnected hemispheres of commissurotomy patients. Unpublished doctoral dissertation, California Institute of Technology, 1970.

Levy, J. Cerebral lateralization and spatial ability. *Behavior Genetics*, 1976, *6*, 171-188.

Levy, J. The correlation of the $\emptyset$ function of the difference score with performance and its relevance to laterality experiments. *Cortex*, 1977, *13*, 458-464. (a)

Levy, J. The mammalian brain and the adaptive advantage of cerebral asymmetry. *Annals of the New York Academy of Sciences*, 1977, *229*, 266-272. (b)

Levy, J., & Levy, J. M. Human lateralization from head to foot: Sex-related factors. *Science*, 1978, *200*, 1291-1292.

Levy, J., & Nagylaki, T. A model for the genetics of handedness. *Genetics*, 1972, *72*, 117-128.

Levy, J., & Reid, M. Variations in writing posture and cerebral organization. *Science*, 1976, *194*, 337-339.

Levy, J., & Reid, M. Variations in cerebral organization as a function of handedness, hand posture in writing, and sex. *Journal of Experimental Psychology: General*, 1978, *107*, 119-144.

Levy, J., & Trevarthen, C. Metacontrol of hemispheric function in human split-brain patients.

Journal of Experimental Psychology: Human Perception and Performance, 1976, *2*, 299-312.

Levy, J., & Trevarthen, C. B. Perceptual, semantic and phonetic aspects of elementary language processes in split-brain patients. *Brain*, 1977, *100*, 105-118.

Levy, J., Trevarthen, C. B., & Sperry, R. W. Perception of bilateral chimeric figures following hemispheric deconnexion. *Brain*, 1972, *95*, 61-78.

Levy, R. S. The question of electrophysiological asymmetries preceding speech. In H. Whitaker & H. A. Whitaker (Eds.), *Studies in neurolinguistics* (Vol. 3). New York: Academic Press, 1977.

Levy-Agresti, J., & Sperry, R. W. Differential perceptual capacities in major and minor hemispheres. *Proceedings of the National Academy of Science U.S.A.*, 1968, *61*, 1151.

Ley, R. G., & Bryden, M. P. Hemispheric differences in processing emotional stimuli? *Bulletin of the Psychonomic Society*, 1977, *10*, (239) 261.

Ley, R. G., & Bryden, M. P. The right hemisphere and emotion. In G. Underwood & R. Stevens (Eds.), *Aspects of consciousness* (Vol. 2). New York: Academic Press, 1981.

Lieberman, P. Hominid evolution, supralaryngeal vocal tract physiology and the fossil evidence for reconstructions. *Brain and Language*, 1979, *7*, 101-126.

Liederman, J., & Kinsbourne, M. Rightward motor bias in newborns depends upon parental right-handedness. *Neuropsychologia*, 1980, *18*, 579-584. (a)

Liederman, J., & Kinsbourne, M. Rightward turning biases in neonates reflect a single neural asymmetry in motor programming: A reply to Turkewitz. *Infant Behavior and Development*, 1980, *3*, 245-251. (b)

Lishman, W. A., & McMeekan, E. R. L. Handedness in relation to direction and degree of cerebral dominance for language. *Cortex*, 1977, *13*, 30-43.

Lloyd, B., & Archer, J. *Exploring sex differences*. New York: Academic Press, 1976.

Lloyd, G. E. R. *Polarity and analogy: Two types of argumentation in early Greek thought*. Cambridge: Cambridge University Press, 1966.

Locke, S., & Kellar, L. Categorical perception in a nonlinguistic mode. *Cortex*, 1973, *9*, 353-367.

Loehlin, J. C., Sharan, S., & Jacobs, R. In pursuit of the "spatial gene": A family study. *Behavioral Genetics*, 1978, *8*, 27-41.

Lomas, J. Competition within the left hemisphere between speaking and unimanual tasks performed without visual guidance. *Neuropsychologia*, 1980, *18*, 141-149.

Lomas, J., & Kimura, D. Intrahemispheric interaction between speaking and sequential manual activity. *Neuropsychologia*, 1976, *14*, 23-33.

Lombroso, C. Left-handedness and left-sidedness. *North American Review*, 1903, *177*, 440-444.

Longden, K., Ellis, C., & Iversen, S. D. Hemispheric differences in the discrimination of curvature. *Neuropsychologia*, 1976, *14*, 195-202.

Loo, R., & Schneider, R. An evaluation of the Briggs-Nebes modified version of Annett's handedness inventory. *Cortex*, 1979, *15*, 683-686.

Lovegrove, W. J., Bowling, A., Badcock, C., & Blackwood, M. Specific reading disability: Differences in contrast sensitivity as a function of spatial frequency. *Science*, 1980, *210*, 439-440.

Lovegrove, W. J., Heddle, M., & Slaghuis, W. Reading disability: Spatial frequency specific deficits in visual information store. *Neuropsychologia*, 1980, *18*, 111-115.

Luria, A. R. *Traumatic aphasia*. The Hague: Mouton, 1970.

Lyle, J. G., & Goyen, J. D. Visual recognition, developmental lag, and strephosymbolia in reading retardation. *Journal of Abnormal Psychology*, 1968, *73*, 25-29.

McBride, W. G., Black, B. P., Brown, C. J., Dolby, R. M., Murray, A. D., & Thomas, D. B. Method of delivery and developmental outcome at 5 years of age. *Medical Journal of Australia*, 1979, *1*, 301-304.

Maccoby, E. E., & Jacklin, C. N. *The psychology of sex differences*. Stanford, Calif.: Stanford University Press, 1974.

McDonough, S. H. The psychology of musical processes as a function of the two cerebral hemispheres and handedness. M.Sc. thesis, University of Edinburgh, 1973.

McDougall, W. *Body and mind*. London: Methuen, 1911.

McFarland, K., & Ashton, R. The influence of concurrent task difficulty on manual performance. *Neuropsychologia*, 1978, *16*, 735-741. (a)

McFarland, K., & Ashton, R. The lateralized effects of concurrent cognitive and motor performance. *Perception and Psychophysics*, 1978, *23*, 344-349. (b)

McGee, M. G. Human spatial abilities: Psychometric studies and environmental, genetic, hormonal, and neurological influences. *Psychological Bulletin,* 1979, *86,* 889-918.

McGee, M. G. The effect of brain asymmetry on cognitive functions depends upon what ability, for which sex, at what point in development. *Behavioral and Brain Sciences,* 1980, *3,* 243-244.

McGlone, J. Sex differences in human brain asymmetry: A critical survey. *Behavioral and Brain Sciences,* 1980, *3,* 215-263.

McIlwain, J. T. Central vision: Visual cortex and superior colliculus. *Annual Review of Physiology,* 1972, *34,* 291-314.

MacKavey, W., Curcio, F., & Rosen, J. Tachistoscopic word recognition performance under conditions of simultaneous bilateral presentation. *Neuropsychologia,* 1975, *13,* 27-33.

McKeever, W. F. Lateral word recognition: Effects of unilateral and bilateral presentation, asynchrony of bilateral presentation, and forced order of report. *Quarterly Journal of Experimental Psychology,* 1971, *23,* 410-416.

McKeever, W. F., & Gill, K. M. Visual half-field differences in the recognition of bilaterally presented single letters and vertically spelled words. *Perceptual and Motor Skills,* 1972, *34,* 815-818. (a)

McKeever, W. F., & Gill, K. M. Visual half-field differences in masking effects for sequential letter stimuli in the right and left handed. *Neuropsychologia,* 1972, *10,* 111-117. (b)

McKeever, W. F., Gill, K. M., & Van Deventer, A. D. Letter versus dot stimuli as tools for splitting the normal brain with reaction time. *Quarterly Journal of Experimental Psychology,* 1975, *27,* 363-373.

McKeever, W. F., Hoemann, H. W., Florian, V. A., & Van Deventer, A. D. Evidence of minimal cerebral asymmetries for the processing of English words and American sign language in the congenitally deaf. *Neuropsychologia,* 1976, *14,* 413-423.

McKeever, W. F., & Huling, M. D. Lateral dominance in tachistoscopic word recognition performances obtained with simultaneous bilateral input. *Neuropsychologia,* 1971, *9,* 15-20. (a)

McKeever, W. F., & Huling, M. D. Bilateral tachistoscopic word recognition as a function of hemisphere stimulation and interhemispheric transfer time. *Neuropsychologia,* 1971, *9,* 281-288. (b)

McKeever, W. F., & Jackson, T. L. Cerebral dominance assessed by object and color naming latencies: Sex and familial sinistrality effects. *Brain and Language,* 1979, *7,* 175-190.

McKeever, W. F., & Suberi, M. Parallel but temporally displaced visual half-field metacontrast functions. *Quarterly Journal of Experimental Psychology,* 1974, *26,* 258-265.

McKeever, W. F., Suberi, M., & Van Deventer, A. D. Fixation control in tachistoscopic studies of laterality effects: Comment and data relevant to Hines' Experiment. *Cortex,* 1972, *8,* 473-479.

McKeever, W. F., & Van Deventer, A. D. Dyslexic adolescents: Evidence of impaired visual and auditory language processing associated with normal lateralization and visual responsivity. *Cortex,* 1975, *11,* 361-378.

McKeever, W. F., & Van Deventer, A. D. Visual and auditory language processing asymmetries: Influence of handedness, familial sinistrality and sex. *Cortex,* 1977, *13,* 225-241. (a)

McKeever, W. F., & Van Deventer, A. D. Familial sinistrality and degree of left handedness. *British Journal of Psychology,* 1977, *68,* 469-471. (b)

McKeever, W. F., Van Deventer, A. D., & Suberi, M. Avowed assessed and familial handedness and differential hemispheric processing of brief sequential and non-sequential visual stimuli. *Neuropsychologia,* 1973, *11,* 235-238.

McManus, I. C. Scrotal asymmetry in man and ancient sculpture. *Nature,* 1976, *259,* 426.

McManus, I. C. Human laterality. Unpublished doctoral dissertation, Cambridge University, 1979.

McManus, I. C. Handedness in twins: A critical review. *Neuropsychologia,* 1980, *18,* 347-355.

McManus, I. C., & Humphrey, N. K. Turning the left cheek. *Nature,* 1973, *243,* 271-272.

MacNeilage, P. F., Sussman, H. M., & Stolz, W. Incidence of laterality effects in mandibular and manual performance in dichoptic visual pursuit tracking. *Cortex,* 1975, *11,* 251-258.

Maddess, R. J. Reaction time to hemiretinal stimulation. *Neuropsychologia,* 1975, *13,* 213-218.

Magoun, H. W. Discussion of brain mechanisms in speech. In E. C. Carterette (Ed.), *Brain Function: Speech language and communication* (Vol. 3). Berkeley: University of California Press, 1966.

Majkowski, J., Bochenek, Z., Bochenek, W., Knapik-Fijalkowska, D., & Kopec, J. Latency of averaged evoked potentials to contralateral and ipsilateral auditory stimulation in normal subjects. *Brain Research*, 1971, *25*, 416–419.

Mancuso, R. P., Lawrence, A. F., Hintze, R. W., & White, C. T. Effect of altered central and peripheral visual field stimulation on correct recognition and visual evoked response. *International Journal of Neuroscience*, 1979, *9*, 113–122.

Manning, A. A., Goble, W., Markman, R., & LaBreche, T. Lateral cerebral differences in the deaf in response to linguistic and nonlinguistic stimuli. *Brain and Language*, 1977, *4*, 309–321.

Marcel, T., Katz, L., & Smith, M. Laterality and reading proficiency. *Neuropsychologia*, 1974, *12*, 131–139.

Marcel, T., & Patterson, K. Word recognition and production: Reciprocity in clinical and normal studies. In J. Requin (Ed.), *Attention and performance VII*. Hillsdale, N.J.: Lawrence Erlbaum, 1978.

Marcel, T., & Rajan, P. Lateral specialization for recognition of words and faces in good and poor readers. *Neuropsychologia*, 1975, *13*, 489–497.

Marcie, P., & Hécaen, H. Agraphia: Writing disorders associated with unilateral cortical lesions. In K. M. Heilman & E. Valenstein (Eds.), *Clinical neuropsychology*. New York: Oxford University Press, 1979.

Marcie, P., Hécaen, H., Dubois, J., & Angelergues, R. Les troubles de la réalisation de la parole au cours des lésions de l'hémisphère droit. *Neuropsychologia*, 1965, *3*, 217–247.

Marin, O. S. M., Schwartz, M. F., & Saffran, E. M. Origins and distribution of language. In M. S. Gazzaniga (Ed.), *Handbook of behavioral neurobiology, Vol. 2. Neuropsychology*. New York: Plenum, 1979.

Markowitz, H., & Weitzman, D. O. Monocular recognition of letters and Landolt Cs in left and right visual hemifields. *Journal of Experimental Psychology*, 1969, *72*, 187–189.

Marsh, G. R. Asymmetry of electrophysiological phenomena and its relation to behavior in humans. In M. Kinsbourne (Ed.), *Asymmetrical function of the brain*. Cambridge: Cambridge University Press, 1978.

Marshall, J. C. On the biology of language acquisition. In D. Caplan (Ed.), *Biological studies of mental processes*. Cambridge, Mass.: MIT Press, 1980.

Marshall, J. C., Caplan, D., & Holmes, J. M. The measure of laterality. *Neuropsychologia*, 1975, *13*, 315–321.

Martin, M. Hemispheric asymmetries for physical and semantic selection of visually presented words. *Neuropsychologia*, 1978, *16*, 717–724.

Marzi, C. A., Brizzolara, D., Rizzolatti, G., Umiltà, C., & Berlucchi, G. Left hemisphere superiority for the recognition of well known faces. *Brain Research*, 1974, *66*, 358.

Marzi, I. A., & Berlucchi, G. Right visual field superiority for accuracy of recognition of famous faces in normals. *Neuropsychologia*, 1977, *15*, 751–756.

Massaro, D. Primary and secondary recognition in reading. In D. Massaro (Ed.), *Understanding language: An information processing analysis of speech perception, reading, and psycholinguistics*. New York: Academic Press, 1975.

Mateer, C. Impairments of nonverbal oral movements after left hemisphere damage: A follow-up of analysis of errors. *Brain and Language*, 1978, *6*, 334–341.

Mazziotta, J. C., Phelps, M. E., Miller, J., & Kuhl, D. E. Tomographic mapping of human cerebral metabolism: Normal unstimulated state. *Neurology*, 1981, *31*, 503–516.

Mebert, C. J., & Michel, G. F. Handedness in artists. In J. Herron (Ed.), *Neuropsychology of left-handedness*. New York: Academic Press, 1980.

Meij, H. S., & Meij, J. C. P. Functional asymmetry in the motor system of the horse. *South African Journal of Science*, 1980, *76*, 552–556.

Meikle, T. H., & Sechzer, J. A. Interocular transfer of brightness discrimination in "split-brain" cats. *Science*, 1960, *132*, 734–735.

Merrell, D. J. Dominance of hand and eye. *Human Biology*, 1957, *29*, 314–328.

Metzger, R. L., & Antes, J. R. Sex and coding strategy effects on reaction time to hemispheric probes. *Memory and Cognition*, 1976, *4*, 167–171.

Meyer, D. E., & Schvaneveldt, R. W. Facilitation in recognizing pairs of words: Evidence of a dependence between retrieval operations. *Journal of Experimental Psychology*, 1971, *90*, 227–234.

Meyer, G. E. Right hemisphere sensitivity for the McCollough effect. *Nature*, 1976, *264*, 751–753.

Meyer, L. B. *Emotion and meaning in music*. Chicago: University of Chicago Press, 1956.

Miller, L. K., & Butler, D. The effect of set size on hemifield asymmetries in letter recognition. *Brain and Language,* 1980, *9,* 307–314.

Mills, L., & Rollman, G. B. Left hemisphere selectivity for processing duration in normal subjects. *Brain and Language,* 1979, *7,* 320–335.

Mills, L., & Rollman, G. B. Hemispheric asymmetry for auditory perception of temporal order. *Neuropsychologia,* 1980, *18,* 41–47.

Milner, A. D., & Dunne, J. J. Lateralized perception of bilateral chimaeric faces by normal subjects. *Nature,* 1977, *268,* 175–176.

Milner, A. D., & Jeeves, M. A. A review of behavioural studies of agenesis of the corpus callosum. In I. Steele Russell, M. W. Hof, & G. Berlucchi (Eds.), *Structure and function of cerebral commissures.* London: Macmillan, 1979.

Milner, B. Laterality effects in audition. In V. B. Mountcastle (Ed.), *Interhemispheric relations and cerebral dominance.* Baltimore: Johns Hopkins University Press, 1962.

Milner, B. Visual recognition and recall after right temporal-lobe excision in man. *Neuropsychologia,* 1968, *6,* 191–209.

Milner, B. Clues to the cerebral organization of memory. In P. A. Buser & A. Rougeul-Buser (Eds.), *Cerebral correlates of conscious experience.* Inserm Symposium No. 6. Amsterdam: Elsevier/North-Holland Biomedical Press, 1977.

Milner, B., Taylor, L., & Sperry, R. W. Lateralized suppression of dichotically presented digits after commissural section in man. *Science,* 1968, *161,* 184–186.

Mittwoch, U. To be right is to be born male. *New Scientist,* 1977, *73,* 74–77.

Mohr, J. P. Rapid amelioration of motor aphasia. *Archives of Neurology,* 1973, *28,* 77–82.

Molfese, D. L. Hemispheric specialization for temporal information. Implications for the perception of voicing cues during speech perception. *Brain and Language,* 1980, *11,* 285–299.

Molfese, D. L., & Molfese, V. J. Hemisphere and stimulus differences as reflected in the cortical responses of newborn infants to speech stimuli. *Developmental Psychology,* 1979, *15,* 505–511. (a)

Molfese, D. L., & Molfese, V. J. VOT distinctions in infants: Learned or innate? In H. Whitaker & H. A. Whitaker (Eds.), *Studies in neurolinguistics, IV.* New York: Academic Press, 1979. (b)

Moore, W. H., & Weidner, W. E. Bilateral tachistoscopic word perception in aphasic and normal subjects. *Perceptual and Motor Skills,* 1974, *39,* 1003–1011.

Morais, J. Monaural ear differences for reaction times to speech with a many-to-one mapping paradigm. *Perception and Psychophysics,* 1976, *19,* 144–148.

Morais, J. Spatial constraints on attention to speech. In J. Requin (Ed.), *Attention and performance VII.* Hillsdale, N.J.: Lawrence Erlbaum, 1978.

Morais, J., & Bertelson, P. Laterality effects in diotic listening. *Perception,* 1973, *2,* 107–111.

Morais, J., & Bertelson, P. Spatial position versus ear of entry as determinant of the auditory laterality effects: A stereophonic test. *Journal of Experimental Psychology: Human Perception and Performance,* 1975, *104,* 253–262.

Morais, J., & Landercy, M. Listening to speech while retaining music: What happens to the right-ear advantage? *Brain and Language,* 1977, *4,* 295–308.

Morgan, M. Embryology and inheritance of asymmetry. In S. Harnad, R. W. Doty, L. Goldstein, J. Jaynes, & G. Krauthamer (Eds.), *Lateralization in the nervous system.* New York: Academic Press, 1977.

Morgan, M. J. Influences of sex on variation in human brain asymmetry. *Behavioral and Brain Sciences,* 1980, *3,* 244–245.

Morgan, W. P. A case of congenital word blindness. *British Medical Journal,* 1896, *2,* 1378.

Mortillet, G. de. Formations des variétés. Albinisme et gauchissement. *Bulletins de la Société d'Anthropologie de Paris,* 1890, *1,* 4 serie, 570–580.

Moscovitch, M. Choice reaction-time study assessing the verbal behavior of the minor hemisphere in normal adult humans. *Journal of Comparative and Physiological Psychology,* 1972, *80,* 66–74.

Moscovitch, M. On the representation of language in the right hemisphere of right-handed people. *Brain and Language,* 1976, *3,* 47–71.

Moscovitch, M. The development of lateralization of language functions and its relation to cognitive and linguistic development: A review and some theoretical speculations. In S. J. Segalowitz & F. A. Gruber (Eds.), *Language development and neurological theory.* New York: Academic Press, 1977.

Moscovitch, M. Information processing and the cerebral hemispheres. In M. S. Gazzaniga (Ed.),

Handbook of behavioral neurobiology, Vol. 2: Neuropsychology. New York: Plenum, 1979.

Moscovitch, M., & Catlin, J. Interhemispheric transmission of information: Measurement in normal man. *Psychonomic Science,* 1970, *18,* 211–213.

Moscovitch, M., & Klein, D. Material specific perceptual interference for visual words and faces: Implications for models of capacity limitations, attention and laterality. *Journal of Experimental Psychology: Human Perception and Performance,* 1980, *6,* 590–604.

Moscovitch, M., Scullion, D., & Christie, D. Early versus late stages of processing and their relation to functional hemisphere asymmetries in face recognition. *Journal of Experimental Psychology: Human Perception and Performance,* 1976, *2,* 401–416.

Murray, M. R., & Richards, S. J. A right-ear advantage in monotic shadowing. *Acta Psychologica,* 1978, *42,* 495–504.

Myers, R. E. Interocular transfer of pattern discrimination in cats following section of crossed optic fibres. *Journal of Comparative and Physiological Psychology,* 1955, *48,* 470–473.

Myers, R. E. Function of corpus callosum in interocular transfer. *Brain,* 1956, *79,* 358–363.

Myslobodsky, M. S., & Rattok, J. Asymmetry of electrodermal activity in man. *Bulletin of the Psychonomic Society,* 1975, *6,* 501–502.

Myslobodsky, M. S., & Rattok, J. Bilateral electrodermal activity in waking man. *Acta Psychologica,* 1977, *41,* 273–282.

Nachshon, I., & Carmon, A. Hand preference in sequential and spatial discrimination tasks. *Cortex,* 1975, *11,* 123–131.

Naeser, M. A., Levine, H. L., Benson, D. F., Stuss, D. T., & Weir, W. S. Frontal leukotomy size and hemispheric asymmetries on computerized tomographic scans of schizophrenics with variable recovery. *Archives of Neurology,* 1981, *38,* 30–37.

Naidoo, S. *Specific dyslexia.* London: Pitman, 1972.

Nash, J. *Developmental psychology: A psychobiological approach* (2nd ed.). Englewood Cliffs, N.J.: Prentice-Hall, 1978.

Natale, M. Perception of nonlinguistic auditory rhythms by the speech hemisphere. *Brain and Language,* 1977, *4,* 32–44.

National Health and Medical Research Council. *Report on methods used by I.A.H.P.* Woden, Canberra: Author, 1976.

Nava, P. L., Butler, S. R., & Glass, A. Asymmetries of the alpha rhythm associated with functions of the right hemisphere. *Electroencephalography and Clinical Neurophysiology,* 1975, *39,* 221.

Naylor, H. Reading disability and lateral asymmetry: An information-processing analysis. *Psychological Bulletin,* 1980, *87,* 531–545.

Nebes, R. D. Superiority of the minor hemisphere in commissurotomized man for the perception of part-whole relations. *Cortex,* 1971, *7,* 333–349. (a)

Nebes, R. D. Handedness and the perception of part-whole relationships. *Cortex,* 1971, *7,* 350–356. (b)

Nebes, R. D. Dominance of the minor hemisphere in commissurotomized man on a test of figural unification. *Brain,* 1972, *95,* 633–638.

Nebes, R. D. Perception of dot patterns by the disconnected right and left hemisphere in man. *Neuropsychologia,* 1973, *11,* 285–290.

Nebes, R. D. Hemispheric specialization in commissurotomized man. *Psychological Bulletin,* 1974, *81,* 1–14.

Nebes, R. D. Direct examination of cognitive function in the right and left hemispheres. In M. Kinsbourne (Ed.), *Asymmetrical function of the brain.* Cambridge: Cambridge University Press, 1978.

Nebes, R. D., & Sperry, R. W. Hemispheric deconnection syndrome with cerebral birth injury in the dominant arm area. *Neuropsychologia,* 1971, *9,* 247–259.

Neill, D. O., Sampson, H., & Gribben, J. A. Hemiretinal effects in tachistoscopic letter recognition. *Journal of Experimental Psychology,* 1971, *91,* 129–135.

Neisser, U. *Cognitive psychology.* Englewood Cliffs, N.J.: Prentice-Hall, 1967.

Neman, R., Roos, P., Menolascino, F. J., McCann, B. M., & Heal, L. W. Experimental evaluation of sensorimotor patterning used with mentally retarded children. *American Journal of Mental Deficiency,* 1975, *79,* 372–384.

Neville, A. C. *Animal asymmetry: Studies in biology.* London: Edward Arnold, 1976.

Newcombe, F., & Ratcliff, G. G. Handedness, speech lateralization and ability. *Neuropsychologia*, 1973, *11*, 399–407.

Newcombe, F. G., Ratcliff, G. G., Carrivick, P. J., Hiorns, R. W., Harrison, G. A., & Gibson, J. B. Hand preference and I.Q. in a group of Oxfordshire villages. *Annals of Human Biology*, 1975, *2*, 235–242.

Newell, A. You can't play 20 questions with nature and win: Projective comments on the papers in the symposium. In W. G. Chase (Ed.), *Visual information processing*. New York: Academic Press, 1973.

Newland, J. Children's knowledge of left and right. Unpublished master's thesis, University of Auckland, 1972.

Nicholson, J. *A question of sex*. London: Fontana, 1979.

Nickerson, R. S. On the time it takes to tell things apart. In J. Requin (Ed.), *Attention and performance VII*. Hillsdale, N.J.: Lawrence Erlbaum, 1978.

Neilsen, J. M. *Agnosia, apraxia, aphasia: Their value in cerebral localization*. New York: Hafner, 1946.

Nilsson, J., Glencross, D., & Geffen, G. The effects of familial sinistrality and preferred hand on dichaptic and dichotic tasks. *Brain and Language*, 1980, *10*, 390–404.

Nottebohm, F. Origins and mechanisms in the establishment of cerebral dominance. In M. S. Gazzaniga (Ed.), *Handbook of behavioral neurobiology, Vol. 2, Neuropsychology*. New York: Plenum, 1979.

Obrzut, J. E., Hynd, G. W., Obrzut, A., & Leitgeb, J. L. Time sharing and dichotic listening in normal and learning disabled children. *Brain and Language*, 1980, *11*, 181–194.

Obrzut, J. E., Hynd, G. W., Obrzut, A., & Pirozzolo, F. J. Effect of directed attention on cerebral asymmetries in normal and learning disabled children. *Developmental Psychology*, 1981, *17*, 118–125.

O'Connor, J. *Structural visualization*. Boston: Human Engineering Laboratory, 1943.

O'Connor, K. P., & Shaw, J. C. Field dependence, laterality and EEG. *Biological Psychology*, 1978, *6*, 93–109.

Ohgishi, M. Hemispheric differences in the mode of information processing. *Japanese Journal of Psychology*, 1978, *49*, 257–264.

Ojemann, G. A. Subcortical language mechanisms. In H. Whitaker & H. A. Whitaker (Eds.), *Studies in neurolinguistics* (Vol. 1). New York: Academic Press, 1976.

Ojemann, G. A. Asymmetric function of the thalamus in man. *Annals of the New York Academy of Sciences*, 1977, *299*, 380–396.

Ojemann, G., & Mateer, C. Human language cortex: Localization of memory, syntax, and sequential motor-phoneme identification systems. *Science*, 1979, *205*, 1401–1403.

Ojemann, G. A., & Whitaker, H. A. Language localization and variability. *Brain and Language*, 1978, *6*, 239–260. (a)

Ojemann, G. A., & Whitaker, H. A. The bilingual brain. *Archives of Neurology*, 1978, *35*, 409–412. (b)

Oke, A., Keller, R., Mefford, I., & Adams, R. N. Lateralization of norepinephrine in human thalamus. *Science*, 1978, *200*, 1411–1413.

Oldfield, R. C. The assessment and analysis of handedness: The Edinburgh inventory. *Neuropsychologia*, 1971, *9*, 97–113.

Olson, M. E. Laterality differences in tachistoscopic word recognition in normal and delayed readers in elementary school. *Neuropsychologia*, 1973, *11*, 343–350.

Orbach, J. Differential recognition of Hebrew and English words in right and left visual fields as a function of cerebral dominance and reading habits. *Neuropsychologia*, 1967, *5*, 127–134.

Orenstein, H. B., & Meighan, W. B. Recognition of bilaterally presented words varying in concreteness and frequency: Lateral dominance or sequential processing? *Bulletin of the Psychonomic Society*, 1976, *7*, 179–180.

Orgass, B., Poeck, K., Kerschensteiner, M., & Hartje, W. Visuo-cognitive performances in patients with unilateral hemispheric lesions: An investigation with three factorial reference tests. *Zeitschrift für Neurologie*, 1972, *202*, 177–195.

Ornstein, R. E. *The psychology of consciousness*. San Francisco: W. H. Freeman & Co., Publishers, 1972.

Ornstein, R. E. *The psychology of consciousness*. New York: Harcourt Brace Jovanovich, 1977.

Orton, J. L. "Word-blindness" in school children and other papers on strephosymbolia (Specific language disability–dyslexia). *Orton Society Monograph* (No. 2). Towson, Md.: Orton Society, 1966.

Orton, S. T. "Word-blindness" in school children. *Archives of Neurology and Psychiatry*, 1925, *14*, 581–615.

Orton, S. T. Specific reading disability–strephosymbolia. *Journal of the American Medical Association*, 1928, *90*, 1095–1099.

Orton, S. T. *Reading, writing and speech problems in children.* New York: W. W. Norton & Co., 1937.

Osaka, N. Naso-temporal differences in human reaction time in the peripheral visual field. *Neuropsychologia*, 1978, *16*, 299–303.

Oscar-Berman, M., Goodglass, H., & Cherlow, D. G. Perceptual laterality and iconic recognition of visual materials by Korsakoff patients and normal adults. *Journal of Comparative and Physiological Psychology*, 1973, *82*, 316–321.

Oscar-Berman, M., Rehbein, L., Porfert, A., & Goodglass, H. Dichaptic hand-order effects with verbal and nonverbal tactile stimuli. *Brain and Language*, 1978, *6*, 323–333.

Oscar-Berman, M., Zurif, E. B., & Blumstein, S. Effects of unilateral brain damage on the processing of speech sounds. *Brain and Language*, 1975, *2*, 345–355.

Overton, W., & Weiner, M. Visual field position and word-recognition threshold. *Journal of Experimental Psychology*, 1966, *71*, 249–253.

Paivio, A. *Imagery and verbal processes.* New York: Holt, Rinehart & Winston, 1971.

Palmer, R. D. Dimensions of differentiation in handedness. *Journal of Clinical Psychology*, 1974, *30*, 545–552.

Papçun, G., Krashen, S., Terbeek, D., Remington, R., & Harshman, R. Is the left hemisphere specialized for speech, language and/or something else? *Journal of the Acoustical Society of America*, 1974, *55*, 319–327.

Paredes, J. A., & Hepburn, M. J. The split brain and the culture-and-cognition paradox. *Current Anthropology*, 1976, *17*, 121–127.

Parker, S. T., & Gibson, K. R. A developmental model for the evolution of language and intelligence in early hominids. *Behavioral and Brain Sciences*, 1979, *2*, 367–381.

Paterson, A., & Zangwill, O. L. Disorders of visual space perception associated with lesions of the right cerebral hemisphere. *Brain*, 1944, *67*, 331–358.

Patterson, K., & Bradshaw, J. L. Differential hemispheric mediation of nonverbal visual stimuli. *Journal of Experimental Psychology: Human Perception and Performance*, 1975, *1*, 246–252.

Patterson, K. E. What is right with "deep" dyslexic patients? *Brain and Language*, 1979, *8*, 111–129.

Pavlidis, G. T. Do eye movements hold the key to dyslexia? *Neuropsychologia*, 1981, *19*, 57–64.

Pearson, R., & Pearson, L. *The vertebrate brain.* London: Academic Press, 1976.

Penfield, W. *The excitable cortex in conscious man.* Springfield, Ill.: Charles C Thomas, 1958.

Pennal, B. E. Human cerebral asymmetry in color discrimination. *Neuropsychologia*, 1977, *15*, 563–568.

Perecman, E., & Kellar, L. The effect of voice and place among aphasic, nonaphasic, right damaged and normal subjects on a metalinguistic task. *Brain and Language*, 1981, *12*, 213–223.

Perelló, J. Digressions on the biological foundations of language. *Journal of Communication Disorders*, 1970, *3*, 140–149.

Perl, N., & Haggard, M. Practice and strategy in a measure of cerebral dominance. *Neuropsychologia*, 1975, *13*, 347–352.

Peters, M. Why the preferred hand taps more quickly than the non-preferred hand: Three experiments on handedness. *Canadian Journal of Psychology*, 1980, *34*, 62–67.

Peters, M., & Durding, B. M. Footedness of left- and right-handers. *American Journal of Psychology*, 1979, *92*, 133–142.

Peters, M., & Petrie, B. F. Functional asymmetries in the stepping reflex of human neonates. *Canadian Journal of Psychology*, 1979, *33*, 198–200.

Petersen, M. R., Beecher, M. D., Zoloth, S. R., Moody, D. B., & Stebbins, W. C. Neural lateralization of species-specific vocalizations by Japanese macaques (Macaca fuscata). *Science*, 1978, *202*, 324–327.

Peterson, J. M. Left-handedness: Differences between student artists and scientists. *Perceptual and Motor Skills*, 1979, *48*, 961–962.

Peterson, J. M., & Lansky, L. M. Left-handedness among architects: Some facts and some speculations. *Perceptual and Motor Skills,* 1974, *38,* 547–550.

Pettit, J. M., & Noll, J. D. Cerebral dominance in aphasia recovery. *Brain and Language,* 1979, *7,* 191–200.

Phelps, M. E., Mazziotta, J. C., Kuhl, D. E., Nuwer, M., Packwood, J., Metter, J., & Engel, J. (Jr.). Tomographic mapping of human cerebral metabolism, visual stimulation and deprivation. *Neurology,* 1981, *31,* 517–529.

Phillips, R. J. Some explanatory experiments on memory for photographs of faces. *Acta Psychologica,* 1979, *43,* 39–56.

Phillips, R. J., & Rawles, R. E. Recognition of upright and inverted faces: A correlational study. *Perception,* 1979, *8,* 577–583.

Piazza, D. M. Cerebral lateralization in young children as measured by dichotic listening and finger tapping tasks. *Neuropsychologia,* 1977, *15,* 417–425.

Pinsky, S. D., & McAdam, D. W. Electroencephalographic and dichotic indices of cerebral laterality in stutterers. *Brain and Language,* 1980, *11,* 374–397.

Pirozzolo, F. J. Lateral asymmetries in visual perception: A review of tachistoscopic half field studies. *Perceptual and Motor Skills,* 1977, *45,* 695–701.

Pirozzolo, F. J. *The neuropsychology of developmental reading disorders.* New York: Holt, Rinehart & Winston, 1979.

Pirozzolo, F. J., & Rayner, K. Hemispheric specialization in reading and word recognition. *Brain and Language,* 1977, *4,* 248–261.

Poffenberger, A. T. Reaction time to retinal stimulation with special reference to the time lost in conduction through nervous centers. *Archives of Psychology,* 1912, *23,* 1–173.

Pohl, P. Dichotic listening in a child recovering from acquired aphasia. *Brain and Language,* 1979, *8,* 372–379.

Poizner, H., Battison, R., & Lane, H. Cerebral asymmetry for American Sign Language: The effects of moving stimuli. *Brain and Language,* 1979, *7,* 351–362.

Poizner, H., & Lane, H. Cerebral asymmetry in the perception of American Sign Language. *Brain and Language,* 1979, *7,* 210–226.

Polich, J. M. Hemispheric differences in stimulus identification. *Perception and Psychophysics,* 1978, *24,* 49–57.

Polich, J. M. Left hemisphere superiority for visual search. *Cortex,* 1980, *16,* 39–50.

Pomerantz, A. P., & Harris, L. J. Are there sex-related asymmetries in foot size? *Perceptual and Motor Skills,* 1980, *51,* 675–678.

Porac, C., & Coren, S. The dominant eye. *Psychological Bulletin,* 1976, *83,* 880–897.

Porac, C., & Coren, S. Individual and familial patterns in four dimensions of lateral preference. *Neuropsychologia,* 1979, *17,* 543–548. (a)

Porac, C., & Coren, S. A test of the validity of offsprings' report of parental handedness. *Perceptual and Motor Skills,* 1979, *49,* 227–231. (b)

Porac, C., Coren, S., & Duncan, P. Life-span age trends in laterality. *Journal of Gerontology,* 1980, *35,* 715–721.

Porac, C., Coren, S., Steiger, J. H., & Duncan, P. Human laterality: A multidimensional approach. *Canadian Journal of Psychology,* 1980, *34,* 91–96.

Porter, R. J., & Berlin, C. I. On interpreting developmental changes in the dichotic right-ear advantage. *Brain and Language,* 1975, *2,* 186–200.

Porteus, S. D. *Porteus Maze Test: Fifty years' application.* Palo Alto, Calif.: Pacific Books, 1965.

Pratt, R. T. C., Warrington, E. K., & Halliday, A. M. Unilateral ECT as a test for cerebral dominance, with a strategy for treating left-handers. *British Journal of Psychiatry,* 1971, *119,* 79–83.

Preilowski, B. F. B. Possible contribution of the anterior forebrain commissures to bilateral motor coordination. *Neuropsychologia,* 1972, *10,* 267–277.

Preilowski, B. Consciousness after complete surgical section of the fore-brain commissures in man. In I. Steele Russell, M. W. Hof., & G. Berlucchi (Eds.), *Structure and function of cerebral commissures.* London: Macmillan, 1979.

Premack, D. Language in the chimpanzee? *Science,* 1971, *172,* 808–822.

Prince, J. H. *Unusual habits of Australian animals.* Sydney: Reed, 1980.

Provine, R. R., & Westerman, J. A. Crossing the midline: Limits of early eye-hand behavior. *Child Development,* 1979, *50,* 437–441.

Provins, K. A. Motor skills, handedness, and behaviour. *Australian Journal of Psychology*, 1967, *19*, 137–150.

Provins, K. A., & Cunliffe, P. The reliability of some motor performance tests of handedness. *Neuropsychologia*, 1972, *10*, 199–206.

Provins, K. A., & Jeeves, M. A. Hemisphere differences in response time to simple auditory stimuli. *Neuropsychologia*, 1975, *13*, 207–211.

Puccetti, R. The case for mental duality: Evidence from split-brain data and other considerations. *Behavioral and Brain Sciences*, 1981, *4*, 93–123.

Qureshi, R., & Dimond, S. J. Calculation and the right hemisphere. *Lancet*, 1979, *1*, 322–323.

Ramsay, D. S. Beginnings of bimanual handedness and speech in infants. *Infant Behavior and Development*, 1980, *3*, 67–77.

Ramsay, D. S., Campos, J. J., & Fenson, L. Onset of bimanual handedness in infants. *Infant Behavior and Development*, 1979, *2*, 69–76.

Rapaczynki, W., & Ehrlichman, H. Opposite visual hemifield superiorities in face recognition as a function of cognitive style. *Neuropsychologia*, 1979, *17*, 645–652.

Rasmussen, T., & Milner, B. The role of early left-brain injury in determining lateralization of cerebral speech functions. *Annals of the New York Academy of Sciences*, 1977, *299*, 355–369.

Ratcliff, G., Dila, C., Taylor, L., & Milner, B. The morphological asymmetry of the hemispheres and cerebral dominance for speech: A possible relation. *Brain and Language*, 1980, *11*, 87–98.

Rayner, K. Eye movements and cognitive psychology: On-line computer approaches to studying visual information processing. *Behavior Research Methods and Instrumentation*, 1979, *11*, 164–171.

Rayner, K., Well, A. D., & Pollatsek, A. Asymmetry of the effective visual field in reading. *Perception and Psychophysics*, 1980, *27*, 537–544.

Rebert, C. S. Neuroelectric measures of lateral specialization in relation to performance. *Contemporary Clinical Neurophysiology*, 1978 (EEG Supplement No. 34), 231–238.

Repp, B. H. Measuring laterality effects in dichotic listening. *Journal of the Acoustical Society of America*, 1977, *62*, 720–737.

Reynolds, D. McQ., & Jeeves, M. A. A developmental study of hemisphere specialization for recognition of faces in normal subjects. *Cortex*, 1978, *14*, 511–520.

Richardson, J. T. E. Further evidence on the effect of word imageability in dyslexia. *Quarterly Journal of Experimental Psychology*, 1975, *27*, 445–449.

Richardson, J. T. E. The effects of stimulus attributes upon latency of word recognition. *British Journal of Psychology*, 1976, *67*, 315–325.

Richardson, J. T. E., & Firlej, M. D. E. Laterality and reading attainment. *Cortex*, 1979, *15*, 581–595.

Reige, W. H., Mettler, E. D., & Williams, M. V. Age and hemispheric asymmetry in nonverbal tactual memory. *Neuropsychologia*, 1980, *18*, 707–710.

Rife, D. C. Handedness, with special reference to twins. *Genetics*, 1940, *25*, 178–186.

Riklan, M., & Levita, E. Psychological studies of thalamic lesions in humans. *Journal of Nervous and Mental Disease*, 1970, *150*, 251–265.

Risberg, J., Halsey, J. H., Wills, E. L., & Wilson, E. M. Hemispheric specialization in normal man studied by bilateral measurements of the regional cerebral blood flow. *Brain*, 1975, *98*, 511–524.

Risse, G. L., & Gazzaniga, M. S. Verbal retrieval of right hemisphere memories established in the absence of language. *Neurology*, 1976, *26*, 354.

Rivers, D. L., & Love, R. J. Language performance on visual processing tasks in right hemisphere lesion cases. *Brain and Language*, 1980, *10*, 348–366.

Rizzolatti, G. Interfield differences in reaction times to lateralised visual stimuli in normal subjects. In I. Steele Russell, M. W. Hof., & G. Berlucchi (Eds.), *Structure and function of cerebral commissures*. London: Macmillan, 1979.

Rizzolatti, G., Bertoloni, G., & Buchtel, H. A. Interference of concomitant motor and verbal tasks on simple reaction time: A hemispheric difference. *Neuropsychologia*, 1979, *17*, 323–330.

Rizzolatti, G., & Buchtel, H. A. Hemispheric superiority in reaction time to faces: A sex difference. *Cortex*, 1977, *13*, 300–305.

Rizzolatti, G., Umiltà, C., & Berlucchi, G. Opposite superiorities of the right and left cerebral hemispheres in discriminative reaction time to physiognomical and alphabetical material. *Brain,* 1971, *94,* 431–442.

Robbins, M. P. A study of the validity of Delacato's theory of neurological organization. *Exceptional Children,* 1966, *32,* 517–523.

Robbins, M. P., & Glass, G. V. The Doman-Delacato rationale: A critical analysis. In J. Hellmuth (Ed.), *Educational therapy* (Vol. 2). Seattle, Wash.: Special Child Publications, 1969.

Roberts, L. D., & Gregory, A. H. Ear differences and delayed auditory feedback: Effect on a simple verbal repetition task and a non-verbal tapping task. *Journal of Experimental Psychology,* 1973, *101,* 269–272.

Robin, D. E., & Shortridge, R. T. J. Lateralization of tumors of the nasal cavity and paranasal sinuses and its relation to aetiology. *Lancet,* 1979, *8118*(1), 695–696.

Robinson, G. M., & Solomon, D. J. Rhythm is processed by the speech hemisphere. *Journal of Experimental Psychology,* 1974, *102,* 508–511.

Robinson, R. G. Differential behavioural and biochemical effects of right and left hemispheric cerebral infarction in the rat. *Science,* 1979, *205,* 707–710.

Rogers, L. J. Lateralisation in the avian brain. *Bird Behaviour,* 1980, *2,* 1–12.

Rosen, J. J., Curcio, F., MacKavey, W., & Herbert, J. Superior recall of letters in the right visual field with bilateral presentation and partial report. *Cortex,* 1975, *11,* 144–154.

Rosenberg, B. A. Mental-task instructions and optokinetic nystagmus to the left and right. *Journal of Experimental Psychology: Human Perception and Performance,* 1980, *6,* 459–472.

Rosenzweig, M. R. Representations of the two ears at the auditory cortex. *American Journal of Physiology,* 1951, *167,* 147–158.

Rosenzweig, M. R. Cortical correlates of auditory localization and of related perceptual phenomena. *Journal of Comparative and Physiological Psychology,* 1954, *47,* 269–276.

Ross, P., Pergament, L., & Anisfield, M. Cerebral lateralization of deaf and hearing individuals for linguistic comparison judgments. *Brain and Language,* 1979, *8,* 69–80.

Rossing, H. Zur sprachlichen leistung der rechten (nicht-dominanten) hemisphäre. *Zeitschrift für Dialectologie and Linguistik,* 1975, *13,* 172–197.

Rourke, B. P. Reading retardation in children: Developmental lag or deficit? In R. M. Knights & D. J. Bakker (Eds.), *The neuropsychology of learning disorders.* Baltimore: University Park Press, 1976.

Rourke, B. P. Neuropsychological research in reading retardation: A review. In A. L. Benton & D. Pearl (Eds.), *Dyslexia: An appraisal of current knowledge.* Oxford: Oxford University Press, 1978.

Rozin, P., Poritsky, S., & Sotsky, R. American children with reading problems can easily learn to read English represented by Chinese characters. *Science,* 1971, *171,* 1264–1267.

Rubens, A. B. Anatomical asymmetries of human cerebral cortex. In S. Harnad, R. W. Doty, L. Goldstein, J. Jaynes, & G. Krauthamer (Eds.), *Lateralization in the nervous system.* New York: Academic Press, 1977.

Rubin, D. A., & Rubin, R. T. Differences in asymmetry of facial expression between left- and right-handed children. *Neuropsychologia,* 1980, *18,* 373–377.

Russell, I. S., & Ochs, S. Localization of a memory trace in one cortical hemisphere and transfer to the other hemisphere. *Brain,* 1963, *86,* 37–54.

Rutter, M. Prevalence and types of dyslexia. In A. L. Benton & D. Pearl (Eds.), *Dyslexia: An appraisal of current knowledge.* Oxford: Oxford University Press, 1978.

Sabatino, D. A., & Ysseldyke, J. E. Effect of extraneous "background" on visual-perceptual performance of readers and non-readers. *Perceptual and Motor Skills,* 1972, *35,* 323–328.

Sackeim, H. A., Gur, R. C., & Saucy, M. C. Emotions are expressed more intensely on the left side of the face. *Science,* 1978, *202,* 434–436.

Saffran, E. M., Bogyo, L. C., Schwartz, M. F., & Marin, O. S. M. Does deep dyslexia reflect right-hemisphere reading? In M. Coltheart, K. Patterson, & J. C. Marshall (Eds.), *Deep dyslexia.* London: Routledge & Kegan Paul, 1980.

Salmaso, D. Hemispheric differences on a novel task requiring attention. *Perceptual and Motor Skills,* 1980, *51,* 383–391.

Sarnat, H. B., & Netsky, M. G. *Evolution of the nervous system.* Oxford: Oxford University Press, 1974.

Sarno, J. E., Swisher, L. P., & Sarno, M. T. Aphasia in a congenitally deaf man. *Cortex,* 1969, *5,* 398–414.

Sasanuma, S. Kana and Kanji processing in Japanese aphasics. *Brain and Language,* 1975, *2,* 369–383.

Sasanuma, S. Acquired dyslexia in Japanese: Clinical features and underlying mechanisms. In M. Coltheart, K. Patterson, & J. C. Marshall (Eds.), *Deep dyslexia.* London: Routledge & Kegan Paul, 1980.

Sasanuma, S., & Fujimura, O. Selective impairment of phonetic and non-phonetic transcription of words in Japanese aphasic patients: Kana vs. Kanji in visual recognition and writing. *Cortex,* 1971, *7,* 1–18.

Sasanuma, S., Itoh, M., Mori, K., & Kobayashi, Yo. Tachistoscopic recognition of Kana and Kanji words. *Neuropsychologia,* 1977, *15,* 547–553.

Sasse, M. A.N.S.U.A. A new start for the under achiever. *Australian Journal of Mental Retardation,* 1977, *4,* 7–11.

Satz, P. Left-handedness and early brain insult: An explanation. *Neuropsychologia,* 1973, *11,* 115–117.

Satz, P. A test of some models of hemispheric speech organization in the left- and right-handed. *Science,* 1979, *203,* 1131–1133.

Satz, P. Incidence of aphasia in left-handers: A test of some hypothetical models of cerebral speech organization. In J. Herron (Ed.), *Neuropsychology of left-handedness.* New York: Academic Press, 1980.

Satz, P., Achenbach, K., & Fennell, E. Correlations between assessed manual laterality and predicted speech laterality in a normal population. *Neuropsychologia,* 1967, *5,* 295–310.

Satz, P., Bakker, D. J., Teunissen, J., Goebel, R., & Van der Vlugt, H. Developmental parameters of the ear asymmetry: A multivariate approach. *Brain and Language,* 1975, *2,* 171–185.

Satz, P., Baymur, L., & Van der Vlugt, H. Pathological left-handedness: Cross-cultural tests of a model. *Neuropsychologia,* 1979, *17,* 77–81.

Satz, P., & Morris, R. The search for subtype classification in learning disabled children. In R. E. Tarter (Ed.), *The child at risk.* Oxford: Oxford University Press, 1980.

Satz, P., Taylor, H. G., Friel, J., & Fletcher, J. M. Some developmental and predictive precursors of reading disabilities: A six year follow-up. In A. L. Benton & D. Pearl (Eds.), *Dyslexia: An appraisal of current knowledge.* Oxford: Oxford University Press, 1978.

Savage-Rumbaugh, E., Rumbaugh, D. M., & Boysen, S. Do apes use language? *American Scientist,* 1980, *68,* 49–61.

Schaller, G. B. *The mountain gorilla: Ecology and behavior.* Chicago: University of Chicago Press, 1963.

Schmit, V., & Davis, R. The role of hemispheric specialization in the analysis of Stroop stimuli. *Acta Psychologica,* 1974, *38,* 149–158.

Schmuller, J. Hemispheric asymmetry for alphabetic identification: Scaling analyses. *Brain and Language,* 1979, *8,* 263–274.

Schmuller, J., & Goodman, R. Bilateral tachistoscopic perception, handedness, and laterality. *Brain and Language,* 1979, *8,* 81–91.

Schmuller, J., & Goodman, R. Bilateral tachistoscopic perception, handedness, and laterality II, Nonverbal stimuli. *Brain and Language,* 1980, *11,* 12–18.

Schneider, G. E. Two visual systems. *Science,* 1969, *163,* 895–902.

Scholes, R. J., & Fischler, I. Hemispheric function and linguistic skill in the deaf. *Brain and Language,* 1979, *7,* 336–350.

Scholfield, W. N. Do children find movements which cross the body midline difficult? *Quarterly Journal of Experimental Psychology,* 1976, *28,* 571–582.

Schouten, M. E. H. The case against a speech mode of perception. *Acta Psychologica,* 1980, *44,* 71–98.

Schuell, H., Jenkins, J. J., & Jiménez-Pabōn, E. *Aphasia in adults.* New York: Harper & Row, 1964.

Schulhoff, C., & Goodglass, H. Dichotic listening, side of brain injury and cerebral dominance. *Neuropsychologia,* 1969, *7,* 149–160.

Schwartz, J., & Tallal, P. Rate of acoustic change may underlie hemispheric specialization for speech perception. *Science,* 1980, *207,* 1380–1381.

Schwartz, M. Left-handedness and high-risk pregnancy. *Neuropsychologia,* 1977, *15,* 341–344.

Schwartz, M., & Smith, M. L. Visual asymmetries with chimeric faces. *Neuropsychologia,* 1980, *18,* 103–106.

Scott, S., Hynd, G. W., Hunt, L., & Weed, W. Cerebral speech lateralization in the American Navajo. *Neuropsychologia*, 1979, *17*, 89–92.

Seamon, J. G., & Gazzaniga, M. S. Coding strategies and cerebral laterality effects. *Cognitive Psychology*, 1973, *5*, 249–256.

Searleman, A. A review of right hemisphere linguistic capabilities. *Psychological Bulletin*, 1977, *84*, 503–528.

Searleman, A. Subject variables and cerebral organization for language. *Cortex*, 1980, *16*, 239–254.

Searleman, A., Tweedy, J., & Springer, S. P. Interrelationships among subject variables believed to predict cerebral organization. *Brain and Language*, 1979, *7*, 267–276.

Seitz, M. R., Weber, B. A., Jacobson, J. T., & Morehouse, R. The use of averaged electroencephalographic response techniques in the study of auditory processing related to speech and language. *Brain and Language*, 1980, *11*, 261–284.

Seliger, H. W. Implications of a multiple critical periods hypothesis for second language learning. In W. C. Ritchie (Ed.), *Second language acquisition: Issues and implications*. New York: Academic Press, 1978.

Selnes, O. A. The corpus callosum: Some anatomical and functional considerations with special reference to language. *Brain and Language*, 1974, *1*, 111–139.

Semmes, J. Hemispheric specialization: A possible clue to mechanism. *Neuropsychologia*, 1968, *6*, 11–26.

Sexton, M. A., & Geffen, G. The development of three strategies of attention in dichotic monitoring. *Developmental Psychology*, 1979, *15*, 299–310.

Shakhnovich, A. R., Serbinenko, F. A., Razumovsky, A. Ye., Rodionov, I. M., & Oskolok, L. N. The dependence of cerebral blood flow on mental activity and on emotional state in man. *Neuropsychologia*, 1980, *18*, 465–476.

Shankweiler, D. Defects in recognition and reproduction of familiar tunes after unilateral temporal lobectomy. Paper presented at the 37th annual meeting of the Eastern Psychological Association, New York, April, 1966.

Shankweiler, D., & Studdert-Kennedy, M. Identification of consonants and vowels presented to left and right ears. *Quarterly Journal of Experimental Psychology*, 1967, *19*, 59–63.

Shankweiler, D., & Studdert-Kennedy, M. A continuum of lateralization for speech perception? *Brain and Language*, 1975, *2*, 212–225.

Shanon, B. Lateralization effects in musical decision tasks. *Neuropsychologia*, 1980, *18*, 21–31.

Shefsky, M. W., Stenson, H. H., & Miller, L. K. Hemispheric asymmetry: A signal detection analysis. *Perceptual and Motor Skills*, 1980, *51*, 599–604.

Sherman, G. F., Garbanati, J. A., Rosen, G. D., Yutzey, D. A., & Denenberg, V. H. Brain and behavioral asymmetries for spatial preference in rats. *Brain Research*, 1980, *192*, 61–67.

Sherman, J. A. Field articulation, sex, spatial visualization, dependency, practice, laterality of the brain and birth order. *Perceptual and Motor Skills*, 1974, *38*, 1223–1235.

Sherman, J. A. *Sex-related cognitive differences: An essay on theory and evidence*. Springfield, Ill.: Charles C Thomas, 1978.

Sherman, J. L., Kulhavy, R. W., & Burns, K. Cerebral laterality and verbal processes. *Journal of Experimental Psychology: Human Learning and Memory*, 1976, *2*, 720–727.

Shevrin, H., Smokler, I. A., & Wolf, E. Field independence, lateralization and defensive style. *Perceptual and Motor Skills*, 1979, *49*, 195–202.

Sidtis, J. J. On the nature of the cortical function underlying right hemisphere auditory perception. *Neuropsychologia*, 1980, *18*, 321–330.

Sidtis, J. J. The complex tone test: Implications for the assessment of auditory laterality effects. *Neuropsychologia*, 1981, *19*, 103–112.

Sidtis, J. J., & Bryden, M. P. Asymmetrical perception of language and music: Evidence for independent processing strategies. *Neuropsychologia*, 1978, *16*, 627–632.

Silverberg, R., Bentin, S., Gaziel, T., Obler, L. K., & Albert, M. L. Shift of visual field preference for English words in native Hebrew speakers. *Brain and Language*, 1979, *8*, 184–190.

Silverberg, R., Gordon, H. W., Pollack, S., & Bentin, S. Shift of visual field preference for Hebrew words in native speakers learning to read. *Brain and Language*, 1980, *11*, 99–105.

Silverman, A., Adevai, G., & McGough, W. Some relationships between handedness and perception. *Journal of Psychosomatic Research*, 1966, *10*, 151–158.

Simernitskaya, E. G. On two forms of writing defect following local brain lesions. In S. J.

Dimond & J. G. Beaumont (Eds.), *Hemispheric function in the human brain.* London: Paul Elek, 1974.

Simion, F., Bagnara, S., Bisiacchi, P., Roncato, S., & Umiltà, C. Laterality effects, levels of processing, and stimulus properties. *Journal of Experimental Psychology: Human Perception and Performance,* 1980, *6,* 184–195.

Smith, A. Speech and other functions after left (dominant) hemispherectomy. *Journal of Neurology, Neurosurgery and Psychiatry,* 1966, *29,* 467–471.

Smith, A. Nondominant hemispherectomy. *Neurology,* 1969, *19,* 442–445.

Smith, A., & Burklund, C. W. Dominant hemispherectomy: Preliminary report on neuropsychological sequelae. *Science,* 1966, *153,* 1280–1282.

Smith, A., & Sugar, O. Development of above normal language and intelligence. 21 years after left hemispherectomy. *Neurology,* 1975, *25,* 813–818.

Smith, M. O., Chu, J., & Edmonston, W. E. Cerebral lateralization of haptic perception: Interaction of responses to braille and music reveals a functional basis. *Science,* 1977, *197,* 689–690.

Southgate, V., & Roberts, G. R. *Reading–Which approach?* London: University of London Press, 1970.

Sparks, R., & Geschwind, N. Dichotic listening in man after section of the neocortical commissures. *Cortex,* 1968, *4,* 3–16.

Sparks, R., Helm, N., & Albert, M. Aphasia rehabilitation resulting from melodic intonation therapy. *Cortex,* 1974, *10,* 303–316.

Sparrow, S. S., & Satz, P. Dyslexia, laterality and neuropsychological development. In D. J. Bakker & P. Satz (Eds.), *Specific reading disability: Advances in theory and method.* Rotterdam, the Netherlands: University of Rotterdam Press, 1970.

Spellacy, F. Lateral preferences in the identification of patterned stimuli. *Journal of the Acoustical Society of America,* 1970, *47,* 574–578.

Spellacy, F., & Blumstein, S. The influence of language set on ear preference in phoneme recognition. *Cortex,* 1970, *6,* 430–439.

Sperry, R. W. The great cerebral commissure. *Scientific American,* 1964, *210,* 42–52.

Sperry, R. W. Mental unity following surgical disconnection of the cerebral hemispheres. *The Harvey Lectures: Series 62.* New York: Academic Press, 1968.

Sperry, R. W. Consciousness, freewill and personal identity. In D. A. Oakley & H. C. Plotkin (Eds.), *Brain, behaviour and evolution.* London: Methuen, 1979.

Sperry, R. W., & Gazzaniga, M. S. Language following surgical disconnection of the commissures. In C. H. Millikan & F. L. Darley (Eds.), *Brain mechanisms underlying speech and language.* New York: Grune & Stratton, 1967.

Sperry, R. W., Gazzaniga, M. S., & Bogen, J. E. Interhemispheric relationships: The neocortical commissures, syndromes of hemispheric disconnection. In P. J. Vinken & G. W. Bruyn (Eds.), *Handbook of clinical neurology, Vol. 4. Disorders of speech, perception and symbolic behavior.* Amsterdam: Elsevier/North-Holland Biomedical Press, 1969.

Sperry, R. W., Zaidel, E., & Zaidel, D. Self recognition and social awareness in the deconnected minor hemisphere. *Neuropsychologia,* 1979, *17,* 153–166.

Spreen, O., Spellacy, F. J., & Reid, J. R. The effect of interstimulus interval and intensity on ear asymmetry for nonverbal stimuli in dichotic listening. *Neuropsychologia,* 1970, *8,* 245–250.

Springer, S. P. Hemispheric specialization for speech opposed by contralateral noise. *Perception and Psychophysics,* 1973, *13,* 391–393.

Springer, S. P. Tachistoscopic and dichotic-listening investigations of laterality in normal human subjects. In S. Harnad, R. W. Doty, L. Goldstein, J. Jaynes, & G. Krauthamer (Eds.), *Lateralization in the nervous system.* New York: Academic Press, 1977.

Springer, S. P. Speech perception and the biology of language. In M. S. Gazzaniga (Ed.), *Handbook of behavioral neurobiology, Vol. 2: Neuropsychology.* New York: Plenum, 1979.

Springer, S. P., & Gazzaniga, M. S. Dichotic testing of partial and complete split brain subjects. *Neuropsychologia,* 1975, *13,* 341–346.

Springer, S. P., & Searleman, A. The ontogeny of hemispheric specialization: Evidence from dichotic listening in twins. *Neuropsychologia,* 1978, *16,* 269–281.

Springer, S. P., & Searleman, A. Left-handedness in twins: Implications for the mechanisms underlying cerebral asymmetry of function. In J. Herron (Ed.), *Neuropsychology of left-handedness.* New York: Academic Press, 1980.

Starr, B. Mirror image transfer in optic chiasm sectioned monkeys. In I. Steele Russell, M. W. Van Hof, & G. Berlucchi (Eds.), *Structure and function of cerebral commissures.* London: Macmillan, 1979.

Stein, J., & Fowler, S. Visual dyslexia. *Trends in the Neurosciences,* 1981, *4,* 77–80.

Sternberg, S. Memory scanning: New findings and current controversies. In D. Deutsch & J. A. Deutsch (Eds.), *Short term memory.* New York: Academic Press, 1975.

Stone, J., Leicester, J., & Sherman, S. M. The naso-temporal division of the monkey's retina. *Journal of Comparative Neurology,* 1973, *150,* 333–348.

Stone, M. A. Measures of laterality and spurious correlation. *Neuropsychologia,* 1980, *18,* 339–345.

Studdert-Kennedy, M. A right-ear advantage in choice reaction time to monaurally presented vowels: A pilot study. *Status report on speech research (Haskins Laboratories),* July–December 1972, 75–81.

Studdert-Kennedy, M. The beginnings of speech. In G. B. Barlow, K. Immelmann, M. Main, & L. Petrinovich (Eds.), *Behavioral development: The Bielefeld Interdisciplinary Project.* Cambridge: Cambridge University Press, 1980. (a)

Studdert-Kennedy, M. Speech perception. *Language and Speech,* 1980, *23,* 45–65. (b)

Studdert-Kennedy, M., & Shankweiler, D. Hemispheric specialization for speech perception. *Journal of the Acoustical Society of America,* 1970, *48,* 579–594.

Studdert-Kennedy, M., Shankweiler, D., & Schulman, S. Opposed effects of a delayed channel on perception of dichotically and monotonically presented CV syllables. *Journal of the Acoustical Society of America,* 1970, *48,* 599–602.

Suberi, M., & McKeever, W. F. Differential right hemisphere memory storage of emotional and nonemotional faces. *Neuropsychologia,* 1977, *15,* 757–768.

Subirana, A. The prognosis in aphasia in relation to cerebral dominance and handedness. *Brain,* 1958, *81,* 415–425.

Subirana, A. The relationship between handedness and language function. *International Journal of Neurology,* 1964, *4,* 215–234.

Subirana, A. Handedness and cerebral dominance. In P. J. Vinken & G. W. Bruyn (Eds.), *Handbook of clinical neurology* (Vol. 4). Amsterdam: Elsevier/North-Holland Biomedical Press, 1969.

Summers, J. J., & Sharp. C. A. Bilateral effects of concurrent verbal and spatial rehearsal on complex motor sequencing. *Neuropsychologia,* 1979, *17,* 331–343.

Sussman, H. M. Respiratory tracking of dichotically presented tonal amplitudes. *Journal of Speech and Hearing Research,* 1977, *20,* 555–564.

Sussman, H. M., & Westbury, J. R. A laterality effect in isometric and isotonic labial tracking. *Journal of Speech and Hearing Research,* 1978, *21,* 563–579.

Swadlow, H. A., Geschwind, N., & Waxman, S. G. Commissural transmission in humans. *Science,* 1979, *204,* 530–531.

Swanson, J., Ledlow, A., & Kinsbourne, M. Lateral asymmetries revealed by simple reaction time. In M. Kinsbourne (Ed.), *Asymmetrical function of the brain.* Cambridge: Cambridge University Press, 1978.

Swanson, J. M., Kinsbourne, M., & Horn, J. M. Cognitive deficit and left-handedness: A cautionary note. In J. Herron (Ed.), *Neuropsychology of left-handedness.* New York: Academic Press, 1980.

Symmes, J. S., & Rapoport, J. L. Unexpected reading failure. *American Journal of Orthopsychiatry,* 1972, *42,* 82–91.

Takeda, M., & Yoshimura, H. Lateral eye movement while eyes are closed. *Perceptual and Motor Skills,* 1979, *48,* 1227–1231.

Tallal, P. Auditory perceptual factors in language and learning disabilities. In R. M. Knights & D. J. Bakker (Eds.), *The neuropsychology of learning disorders: Theoretical approaches.* Baltimore: University Park Press, 1976.

Tallal, P., & Piercy, M. Defects of auditory perception in children with developmental dysphasia. In M. A. Wyke (Ed.), *Developmental dysphasia.* New York: Academic Press, 1978.

Tallal, P., Stark, R. E., Kallman, C., & Mellits, D. Developmental dysphasia: Relation between acoustic deficits and verbal processing. *Neuropsychologia,* 1980, *18,* 273–284.

Tan, L. E., & Nettleton, N. C. Left handedness, birth order and birth stress. *Cortex,* 1980, *16,* 363–374.

Taylor, D. C. Differential rates of cerebral maturation between sexes and between hemispheres. Evidence from epilepsy. *Lancet,* 1969, *2,* 140–142.

Teng, E. L. Dichotic pairing of digits with tones: High performance level and lack of ear effect. *Quarterly Journal of Experimental Psychology,* 1980, *32,* 287–293.

Teng, E. L., Lee, P. H., Yang, K., & Chang, P. C. Handedness in a Chinese population: Biological, social, and pathological factors. *Science,* 1976, *193,* 1148–1150.

Teng, E. L., Lee, P. H., Yang, K. S., & Chang, P. C. Lateral preferences for hand, foot and eye, and their lack of association with scholastic achievement, in 4143 Chinese. *Neuropsychologia,* 1979, *17,* 41–48.

Teng, E. L., & Sperry, R. W. Interhemispheric interaction during simultaneous bilateral presentation of letters or digits in commissurotomized patients. *Neuropsychologia,* 1973, *11,* 131–140.

Terrace, H. S. *Nim: A chimpanzee who learned sign language.* New York: Knopf, 1980.

Terrace, H. S., Petitto, L. A., Sanders, R. J., & Bever, T. G. Can an ape create a sentence? *Science,* 1979, *206,* 891–902.

Teszner, D. Etude anatomique de l'asymétrie droite-gauche du planum temporale sur 100 cerveaux d'adultes. Doctoral thesis, University of Paris, 1972.

Teszner, D., Tzavaras, A., Gruner, J., & Hécaen, H. L'asymétrie droit-gauche du planum temporale, à propos de l'étude anatomique de 100 cerveaux. *Revue Neurologique,* 1972, *126,* 444–449.

Teuber, H. L. Why two brains? In F. O. Schmitt & F. G. Worden (Eds.), *The neurosciences: Third study program.* Cambridge, Mass.: MIT Press, 1974.

Thomas, D. G., & Campos, J. J. The relationship of handedness to a "lateralized" task. *Neuropsychologia,* 1978, *16,* 511–515.

Thompson, A. L., & Marsh, J. F. Probability sampling of manual asymmetry. *Neuropsychologia,* 1976, *14,* 217–223.

Thompson, L. J. Language disabilities in men of eminence. *Bulletin of the Orton Society,* 1969, *19,* 113–120.

Thompson, L. J. Language disabilities in men of excellence. *Journal of Learning Disabilities,* 1971, *4,* 34–45.

Thomson, M. E. A comparison of laterality effects in dyslexics and controls using verbal dichotic listening tasks. *Neuropsychologia,* 1976, *14,* 243–246.

Thomson, W. J., & Clausnitzer, S. Effects of a concurrent musical task on a unimanual skill. *Bulletin of the Psychonomic Society,* 1980, *16,* 469–470.

Thorson, J., Lange, G. D., & Biederman-Thorson, M. Objective measure of the dynamics of a visual movement illusion. *Science,* 1969, *164,* 1087–1088.

Tomer, R., Mintz, M., Levi, A., & Myslobodsky, M. S. Reactive gaze laterality in schizophrenic patients. *Biological Psychology,* 1979, *9,* 115–127.

Tomlinson-Keasey, C., & Kelly, R. R. Is hemispheric specialization important to scholastic achievement? *Cortex,* 1979, *15,* 97–107.

Tomlinson-Keasey, C., Kelly, R. R., & Burton, J. K. Hemispheric changes in information processing during development. *Developmental Psychology,* 1978, *14,* 214–223.

Trevarthen, C. B. Double visual learning in split-brain monkeys. *Science,* 1962, *136,* 258–259.

Trevarthen, C. B. Functional interactions between the cerebral hemispheres of the split-brain monkey. In G. Ettlinger (Ed.), *Functions of the corpus callosum.* London: Churchill, 1965.

Trevarthen, C. B. Brain bisymmetry and the role of the corpus callosum in behavior and conscious experience. In J. Cernacek & F. Podivinsky (Eds.), *Cerebral interhemispheric relations.* Bratislava, Czechoslovakia : Publishing House of the Slovak Academy of Sciences, 1972.

Trevarthen, C., & Sperry, R. W. Perceptual unity of the ambient visual field in human commissurotomy patients. *Brain,* 1973, *96,* 547–570.

Trevarthen, C. B. Analysis of cerebral activities that generate and regulate consciousness in commissurotomy patients. In S. J. Dimond & J. G. Beaumont (Eds.), *Hemisphere function in the human brain.* London: Elek Science, 1974. (a)

Trevarthen, C. B. Functional relations of disconnected hemispheres with the brain stem and with each other: Monkey and man. In M. Kinsbourne & W. L. Smith (Eds.), *Hemispheric deconnexion and cerebral function.* Springfield, Ill.: Charles C Thomas, 1974. (b)

Tsao, Y. C., Feustel, T., & Soseos, C. Stroop interference in the left and right visual fields. *Brain and Language,* 1979, *8,* 367–371.

Tsunoda, T. Tsunoda's method: A new objective testing method available for the orientation of the dominant cerebral hemisphere towards various sounds and its clinical use. *Indian Journal of Otology, Rhinology and Laryngology,* 1966, *18,* 78–88.

Tsunoda, T. Functional differences between right- and left-cerebral hemispheres detected by the key-tapping method. *Brain and Language,* 1975, *2,* 152–170.

Turkewitz, G. The development of lateral differences in the human infant. In S. Harnad, R. W. Doty, L. Goldstein, J. Jaynes, & G. Krauthamer (Eds.), *Lateralization in the nervous system.* New York: Academic Press, 1977. (a)

Turkewitz, G. The development of lateral differentiation in the human infant. *Annals of the New York Academy of Sciences,* 1977, *299,* 309–317. (b)

Turner, S., & Miller, L. K. Some boundary conditions for laterality effects in children. *Developmental Psychology,* 1975, *11,* 342–352.

Tweedy, J. R., Rinn, W. E., & Springer, S. P. Performance asymmetries in dichotic listening: The role of structural and attentional mechanisms. *Neuropsychologia,* 1980, *18,* 331–338.

Uhrbrock, R. S. Laterality in art. *Journal of Aesthetics and Art Criticism,* 1973, *32,* 27–35.

Umiltà, C., Bagnara, S., & Simion, F. Laterality effects for simple and complex geometrical figures and nonsense patterns. *Neuropsychologia,* 1978, *16,* 43–49.

Umiltà, C., Brizzolara, D., Tabossi, P., & Fairweather, H. Factors affecting face recognition in the cerebral hemispheres: Familiarity and naming. In J. Requin (Ed.), *Attention and performance VII.* Hillsdale, N.J.: Lawrence Erlbaum, 1978.

Umiltà, C., Frost, N., & Hyman, R. Interhemispheric effects on choice reaction times to one-, two- and three-letter displays. *Journal of Experimental Psychology,* 1972, *93,* 198–204.

Umiltà, C., Rizzolatti, G., Marzi, C. A., Zamboni, G., Franzini, C., Camarda, R., & Berlucchi, G. Hemispheric differences in the discrimination of line orientation. *Neuropsychologia,* 1974, *12,* 165–174.

Umiltà, C., Salmaso, D., Bagnara, S., & Simion, F. Evidence for a right hemisphere superiority and for a serial search strategy in a dot detection task. *Cortex,* 1979, *15,* 597–608.

Uyehara, J. M., & Cooper, W. A. Hemispheric differences for verbal and nonverbal stimuli in Japanese- and English-speaking subjects assessed by Tsunoda's Method. *Brain and Language,* 1980, *10,* 405–417.

Vaid, J., & Genesee, F. Neuropsychological approaches to bilingualism. *Canadian Journal of Psychology,* 1980, *34,* 417–445.

Vanden-Abeele, J. Comments on the functional asymmetries of the lower extremities. *Cortex,* 1980, *16,* 325–329.

Van Den Abell, T., & Heilman, K. M. Lateralized warning stimuli, phasic hemisphere arousal and reaction time. Presented before the International Neuropsychologic Association, Minneapolis, 1978.

Vandenberg, S. G. *Progress in human behavior genetics.* Baltimore, Md.: Johns Hopkins University Press, 1968.

Vandenberg, S. G., & Kuse, A. R. Spatial ability: A critical review of the sex-linked major gene hypothesis. In M. A. Wittig & A. C. Petersen (Eds.), *Sex-related differences in cognitive functioning.* New York: Academic Press, 1979.

Van Lancker, D. Heterogeneity in language and speech. *Working Papers in Phonetics, No. 29,* 1975.

Van Lancker, D., & Fromkin, V. A. Hemispheric specialization for pitch and "tone": Evidence from Thai. *Journal of Phonetics,* 1973, *1,* 101–109.

Van Lawick-Goodall, J. *In the shadow of man.* London: Collins Publishers, 1971.

Vargha-Khadem, F., & Corballis, M. C. Cerebral asymmetry in infants. *Brain and Language,* 1979, *8,* 1–9.

Varney, N. R., & Benton, A. L. Tactile perception of direction in relation to handedness and familial handedness. *Neuropsychologia,* 1975, *13,* 449–454.

Vellutino, F. R. Toward an understanding of dyslexia: Psychological factors in specific reading disability. In A. L. Benton & D. Pearl (Eds.), *Dyslexia: An appraisal of current knowledge.* Oxford: Oxford University Press, 1978.

Vellutino, F. R., Pruzek, R. M., Steger, J. A., & Meshoulam, U. Immediate visual recall in poor and normal readers as a function of orthographic-linguistic familiarity. *Cortex,* 1973, *9,* 370–386.

Vellutino, F. R., Steger, J. A., DeSetto, L., & Phillips, F. Immediate and delayed recognition of visual stimuli in poor and normal readers. *Journal of Experimental Child Psychology*, 1975, *19*, 223-232.

Vellutino, F. R., Steger, J. A., & Kandel, G. Reading disability: An investigation of the perceptual deficit hypothesis. *Cortex*, 1972, *8*, 106-118.

Vernon, M. D. *Backwardness in reading: A study of its nature and origin.* Cambridge: Cambridge University Press, 1957.

Vernon, M. D. *Reading and its difficulties: A psychological study.* Cambridge: Cambridge University Press, 1971.

Vernon, M. D. Variability in reading retardation. *British Journal of Psychology*, 1979, *70*, 7-16.

Vignolo, L. A. Evolution of aphasia and language rehabilitation: A retrospective exploratory study. *Cortex*, 1964, *1*, 344-367.

Virostek, S., & Cutting, J. E. Asymmetries for Ameslan handshapes and other forms in signers and nonsigners. *Perception and Psychophysics*, 1979, *26*, 505-508.

Von Bonin, G. & Bailey, P. Pattern of the cerebral isocortex. *Primatologia*, 1961, *2*, (10), 1-42.

Von Economo, C., & Horn, L. Uber windungsrelief, masse und rindenarchitektonik der supratemporalfläche, ihre individuellen und ihre seitenunterschiede. *Zeitschrift für die Gesamte Neurologie und Psychiatrie*, 1930, *130*, 678-757.

Vroon, P. A., Timmers, H., & Tempelaars, S. On the hemispheric representation of time. In S. Dornic (Ed.), *Attention and performance VI.* New York: John Wiley, 1977.

Waber, D. P. Sex differences in cognition: A function of maturation rate? *Science*, 1976, *192*, 572-574.

Waber, D. P. Cognitive abilities and sex-related variations in the maturation of cerebral cortical functions. In M. A. Wittig & A. C. Petersen (Eds.), *Sex-related differences in cognitive functioning.* New York: Academic Press, 1979.

Wada, J. A new method for the determination of the side of cerebral speech dominance. A preliminary report on the intracarotid injection of sodium amytal in man. *Medical Biology*, 1949, *14*, 221-222.

Wada, J., & Rasmussen, T. Intracarotid injection of sodium amytal for the lateralization of cerebral speech dominance. Experimental and clinical observations. *Journal of Neurosurgery*, 1960, *17*, 266-282.

Wada, J. A., Clarke, R., & Hamm, A. Cerebral hemispheric asymmetry in humans. *Archives of Neurology*, 1975, *32*, 239-246.

Walker, S. F. Lateralization of functions in the vertebrate brain: A review. *British Journal of Psychology*, 1980, *71*, 329-367.

Wallace, R. J. S-R compatibility and the idea of a response code. *Journal of Experimental Psychology*, 1971, *88*, 354-360.

Walsh, K. W. *Neuropsychology: A clinical approach.* Edinburgh: Churchill Livingstone, 1978.

Walters, J., & Zatorre, R. J. Laterality differences for word identification in bilinguals. *Brain and Language*, 1978, *6*, 158-167.

Wanner, E., Teyler, T. J., & Thompson, R. I. The psychobiology of speech and language: An overview. In J. E. Desmedt (Ed.), *Language and hemispheric specialization in man: Cerebral evoked response potentials.* Basel: Karger, 1977.

Ward, T. B., & Ross, L. E. Laterality differences and practice effects under central backward masking conditions. *Memory and Cognition*, 1977, *5*, 221-226.

Warm, J. S., Richter, D. O., Sprague, R. L., Porter, P. R., & Schumsky, D. A. Listening with a dual brain: Hemispheric asymmetry in sustained attention. *Bulletin of the Psychonomic Society*, 1980, *15*, 229-232.

Warren, J. M. Handedness and cerebral dominance in monkeys. In S. Harnad, R. W. Doty, L. Goldstein, J. Jaynes, & G. Krauthamer (Eds.), *Lateralization in the nervous system.* New York: Academic Press, 1977.

Warren, J. M. Handedness and laterality in humans and other animals. *Physiological Psychology*, 1980, *8*, 351-359.

Warren, L. R., & Marsh, G. R. Changes in event related potentials during processing of Stroop stimuli. *International Journal of Neuroscience*, 1979, *9*, 217-223.

Warrington, E. K. Constructional apraxia. In P. J. Vinken & G. W. Bruyn (Eds.), *Handbook of clinical neurology* (Vol. 4). Amsterdam: Elsevier/North-Holland Biomedical Press, 1969.

Warrington, E. K. Concrete word dyslexia. *British Journal of Psychology*, 1981, *72*, 175–196.

Warrington, E. K., & Pratt, R. T. C. Language laterality in left-handers assessed by unilateral E.C.T. *Neuropsychologia*, 1973, *11*, 423–428.

Warrington, E. K., & Taylor, A. M. Two categorical stages of object recognition. *Perception*, 1978, *7*, 695–705.

Weber, A. M., & Bradshaw, J. L. Levy and Reid's neurological model in relation to writing hand/posture: An evaluation. *Psychological Bulletin*, 1981, *90*, 74–88.

Webster, W. G., & Thurber, A. D. Problem-solving strategies and manifest brain asymmetry. *Cortex*, 1978, *14*, 474–484.

Weigl, E. On the problem of cortical syndromes. In M. L. Simmel (Ed.), *In the reach of mind: Essays in memory of Kurt Goldstein*. New York: Springer, 1968.

Weinstein, E. A. The brain and disorders of communication: Affections of speech with lesions of the non-dominant hemisphere. *Research Publications of the Association for Research in Nervous and Mental Disease*, 1964, *42*, 220–228.

Weinstein, E. A., & Keller, N. J. A. Linguistic patterns of misnaming in brain injury. *Neuropsychologia*, 1963, *1*, 79–90.

Weinstein, S. Functional cerebral hemisphere asymmetry. In M. Kinsbourne (Ed.), *Asymmetrical function of the brain*. Cambridge: Cambridge University Press, 1978.

Weiskrantz, L. Varieties of residual experience. *Quarterly Journal of Experimental Psychology*, 1980, *32*, 365–386.

Weiss, M., & House, A. S. Perception of dichotically presented vowels. *Journal of the Acoustical Society of America*, 1973, *53*, 51–58.

Wepman, J. M. *Recovery from aphasia*. New York: Ronald, 1951.

Werner, H. *Comparative psychology of mental development*. New York: International Universities Press, 1948.

Wernicke, C. *Der Aphasische SymptomenKomplex*. Breslau: Cohn & Weigert, 1874.

Westheimer, G., & Mitchell, D. E. The sensory stimulus for disjunctive eye movements. *Vision Research*, 1969, *9*, 749–755.

Wexler, B. E., & Heninger, G. R. Effects of concurrent administration of verbal and spatial visual tasks on a language-related dichotic listening measure of perceptual asymmetry. *Neuropsychologia*, 1980, *18*, 379–382.

Wheatley, G. H. The right hemisphere's role in problem solving. *Arithmetic Teacher*, 1977, *25*, 36–39.

Whitaker, H. A. Bilingualism: A neurolinguistics perspective. In W. C. Ritchie (Ed.), *Second language acquisition: Issues and implications*. New York: Academic Press, 1978.

Whitaker, H. A., & Ojemann, G. A. Lateralization of higher cortical functions: A critique. *Annals of the New York Academy of Sciences*, 1977, *299*, 459–473.

White, M. Laterality differences in perception: A review. *Psychological Bulletin*, 1969, *72*, 387–405.

White, M. J., & White, K. G. Parallel-serial processing and hemispheric function. *Neuropsychologia*, 1975, *13*, 377–381.

Wickelgren, W. A. Relations, operators, predicates, and the syntax of (verbal) propositional and (spatial) operational memory. *Bulletin of the Psychonomic Society*, 1975, *6*, 161–164.

Wigan, A. L. *A new view of insanity. The duality of the mind proved by the structure, functions and diseases of the brain, and by the phenomena of mental derangement and shewn to be essential to moral responsibility*. London: Longman, Brown, Green, & Longmans, 1844.

Wilkins, A., & Stewart, A. The time course of lateral asymmetries in visual perception of letters. *Journal of Experimental Psychology*, 1974, *102*, 905–908.

Wilson, D. Paleolithic dexterity. *Royal Society of Canada, Proceedings and Transactions*, 1885, *3*, 119–133.

Witelson, S. F. Hemisphere specialization for linguistic and nonlinguistic tactual perception using a dichotomous stimulation technique. *Cortex*, 1974, *10*, 3–17.

Witelson, S. F. Sex and the single hemisphere: Specialization of the right hemisphere for spatial processing. *Science*, 1976, *193*, 425–427. (a)

Witelson, S. F. Abnormal right hemisphere specialization in developmental dyslexia. In R. M. Knights & D. J. Bakker (Eds.), *The neuropsychology of learning disorders. Theoretical approaches*. Baltimore: University Park Press, 1976. (b)

Witelson, S. F. Anatomic asymmetry in the temporal lobes: Its documentation, phylogenesis, and relationship to functional asymmetry. *Annals of the New York Academy of Sciences,* 1977, *299,* 328–354. (a)

Witelson, S. F. Developmental dyslexia. Two right hemispheres and none left. *Science,* 1977, *195,* 309–311. (b)

Witelson, S. F. Early hemisphere specialization and interhemispheric plasticity: An empirical and theoretical review. In S. J. Segalowitz & F. A. Gruber (Eds.), *Language development and neurological theory.* New York: Academic Press, 1977. (c)

Witelson, S. F. Neuroanatomical asymmetry in left-handers: A review and implications for functional asymmetry. In J. Herron (Ed.), *Neuropsychology of left-handedness.* New York: Academic Press, 1980.

Witelson, S. F., & Pallie, W. Left hemisphere specialization for language in the newborn: Neuroanatomical evidence of asymmetry. *Brain,* 1973, *96,* 641–646.

Witelson, S. F., & Rabinovitch, M. S. Hemispheric speech lateralization in children with auditory-linguistic deficits. *Cortex,* 1972, *8,* 412–426.

Witkin, H. A. A cognitive-style approach to cross-cultural research. *International Journal of Psychology,* 1967, *2,* 233–250.

Wittig, M. A., & Petersen, A. C. (Eds.). *Sex-related differences in cognitive functioning.* New York: Academic Press, 1979.

Wold, R. M. Dominance—fact or phantasy: Its significance to learning disabilities. *Journal of the American Optometric Association,* 1968, *39,* 908–916.

Wolff, P. H. The development of manual asymmetries in motor sequencing skills. *Annals of the New York Academy of Sciences,* 1977, *299,* 319–328.

Wolff, P. H., & Hurwitz, I. Sex differences in finger tapping: A developmental study. *Neuropsychologia,* 1976, *14,* 35–41.

Wolff, P. H., Hurwitz, I., & Moss, H. Serial organization of motor skills in left and right handed adults. *Neuropsychologia,* 1977, *15,* 539–546.

Wood, F. Theoretical, methodological, and statistical implications of the inhalation rCBF technique for the study of brain-behavior relationships. *Brain and Language,* 1980, *9,* 1–8.

Wood, F., Stump, D., McKeehan, A., Sheldon, S., & Proctor, J. Patterns of regional cerebral blood flow during attempted reading aloud by stutterers both on and off haloperidol medication: Evidence for inadequate left frontal activation during stuttering. *Brain and Language,* 1980, *9,* 141–144.

Woods, B. T. Observations on the neurological basis for initial language acquisition. In D. Caplan (Ed.), *Biological studies of mental processes.* Cambridge, Mass.: MIT Press, 1980.

Wussler, M., & Barclay, A. Cerebral dominance, psycholinguistic skills and reading disability. *Perceptual and Motor Skills,* 1970, *31,* 419–425.

Wyke, M., & Ettlinger, G. Efficiency of recognition in left and right visual fields. *Archives of Neurology,* 1961, *5,* 659–665.

Wyke, M. A. Musical ability: A neuropsychological interpretation. In M. Critchley & R. A. Henson (Eds.), *Music and the brain.* London: Heinemann, 1977.

Yakovlev, P. I. Morphological criteria of growth and maturation of the nervous system in man. *Research Publications of the Association for Research into Nervous and Mental Diseases,* 1962, *39,* 3–46.

Yakovlev, P. I. A proposed definition of the limbic system. In C. H. Hockman (Ed.), *Limbic system mechanisms and autonomic function.* Springfield, Ill.: Charles C Thomas, 1972.

Yakovlev, P. I., & Lecours, A. R. The myelogenetic cycles of regional maturation of the brain. In A. Minkowski (Ed.), *Regional development of the brain in early life.* Oxford: Blackwell, 1967.

Yakovlev, P. I., & Rakic, P. Patterns of decussation of bulbar pyramids and distribution of pyramidal tracts on two sides of the spinal cord. *Transactions of the American Neurological Association,* 1966, *91,* 366–367.

Yamamoto, M. Developmental changes for hemispheric specialization of tactile recognition by normal children. *Perceptual and Motor Skills,* 1980, *51,* 325–326.

Yeni-Komshian, G. H., & Benson, D. A. Anatomical study of cerebral asymmetry in the temporal lobe of humans, chimpanzees, and rhesus monkeys. *Science,* 1976, *192,* 387–389.

Yeni-Komshian, G. H., & Gordon, J. F. The effect of memory load on the right ear advantage in dichotic listening. *Brain and Language,* 1974, *1,* 375–381.

Yin, R. K. Looking at upside-down faces. *Journal of Experimental Psychology,* 1969, *81,* 141–145.

Yin, R. K. Face recognition by brain-injured patients. A dissociable ability? *Neuropsychologia,* 1970, *8,* 395–402.

Young, A. W. Methodological and theoretical bases of visual hemifield studies. In J. G. Beaumont (Ed.), *Divided visual field studies of cerebral organization.* New York: Academic Press, 1981. (a)

Young, A. W. Asymmetry of cerebral hemispheric function during development. In J. W. T. Dickerson & H. McGurk (Eds.), *Brain and behavior: A developmental perspective.* Glasgow: Blackie, 1981. (b)

Young, A. W., & Bion, P. J. Identification and storage of line drawings presented to the left and right cerebral hemispheres of adults and children. *Cortex,* 1981, *17,* 97–106. (a)

Young, A. W., & Bion, P. J. Accuracy of naming laterally presented known faces by children and adults. *Cortex,* 1981, *17,* 97–106. (b)

Young, A. W., Bion, P. J., & Ellis, A. W. Studies toward a model of laterality effects for picture and word naming. *Brain and Language,* 1980, *11,* 54–65.

Young, A. W., & Ellis, A. W. Asymmetry of cerebral hemispheric function in normal and poor readers. *Psychological Bulletin,* 1981, *89,* 183–190.

Young, G. Manual specialization in infancy: Implications for lateralization of brain function. In S. J. Segalowitz & F. A. Gruber (Eds.), *Language development and neurological theory.* New York: Academic Press, 1977.

Young, J. Z. *A model of the brain.* Oxford: Oxford University Press, 1976.

Zaidel, D., & Sperry, R. W. Performance on the Raven's Coloured Progressive Matrices Test by subjects with cerebral commissurotomy. *Cortex,* 1973, *9,* 34–39.

Zaidel, D., & Sperry, R. W. Some long-term motor effects of cerebral commissurotomy in man. *Neuropsychologia,* 1977, *15,* 193–204.

Zaidel, E. Linguistic competence and related functions in the right cerebral hemisphere of man following commissurotomy and hemispherectomy. Unpublished doctoral dissertation, California Institute of Technology, 1973.

Zaidel, E. Auditory vocabulary of the right hemisphere following brain bisection or hemidecortication. *Cortex,* 1976, *12,* 191–211.

Zaidel, E. Concepts of cerebral dominance in the split brain. In P. A. Buser & A. Rougeul-Buser (Eds.), *Cerebral correlates of conscious experience.* Inserm Symposium No. 6. Amsterdam: Elsevier/North-Holland Biomedical Press, 1978. (a)

Zaidel, E. Auditory language comprehension in the right hemisphere following cerebral commissurotomy and hemispherectomy: A comparison with child language and aphasia. In A. Caramazza & E. B. Zurif (Eds.), *Language acquisition and language breakdown: Parallels and divergencies.* Baltimore: Johns Hopkins University Press, 1978. (b)

Zangwill, O. L. *Cerebral dominance and its relation to psychological function.* Edinburgh: Oliver & Boyd, 1960.

Zangwill, O. L. Dyslexia in relation to cerebral dominance. In J. Money (Ed.), *Reading disability: Progress and research needs in dyslexia.* Baltimore: Johns Hopkins University Press, 1962.

Zangwill, O. L. The brain and disorders of communication. The current status of cerebral dominance. *Research Publications of the Association for Research in Nervous and Mental Disease,* 1964, *42,* 103–118.

Zangwill, O. L. Speech and the minor hemisphere. *Acta Neurologica et Psychiatrica Belgica,* 1967, *67,* 1013–1020.

Zangwill, O. L. Thought and the brain. *British Journal of Psychology,* 1976, *67,* 301–314.

Zangwill, O. L. Aphasia and the concept of brain centers. In G. A. Miller & E. Lenneberg (Eds.), *Psychology and biology of language and thought: Essays in honor of Eric Lenneberg.* New York: Academic Press, 1978.

Zangwill, O. L., & Blakemore, C. Dyslexia: Reversal of eye-movements during reading. *Neuropsychologia,* 1972, *10,* 371–373.

Zenhausen, R. Imagery, cerebral dominance and style of thinking: A unified field model. *Bulletin of the Psychonomic Society,* 1978, *12,* 381–384.

Zigler, E., & Seitz, V. On "An experimental evaluation of sensorimotor patterning": A critique. *American Journal of Mental Deficiency,* 1975, *79,* 483–492.

Zoccolotti, P., & Oltman, J. Field dependence and lateralization of verbal and configurational processing. *Cortex,* 1978, *14,* 155–168.

Zurif, E. B. Auditory lateralization: Prosodic and syntactic factors. *Brain and Language,* 1974, *1,* 391–404.

Zurif, E. B. Language mechanisms: A neuropsychological perspective. *American Scientist,* 1980, *68,* 305–311.

Zurif, E. B., & Bryden, M. P. Familial handedness and left–right differences in auditory and visual perception. *Neuropsychologia,* 1969, *7,* 179–187.

Zurif, E. B., & Carson, G. Dyslexia in relation to cerebral dominance and temporal analysis. *Neuropsychologia,* 1970, *8,* 351–361.

Zurif, E. B., & Mendelsohn, M. Hemispheric specialization for the perception of speech sounds: The influence of intonation and structure. *Perception and Psychophysics,* 1972, *11,* 329–332.

Zurif, E. B., & Sait, P. E. The role of syntax in dichotic listening. *Neuropsychologia,* 1969, *8,* 239–244.

Author Index

Subject Index